the fast 800 GLP-1 recipe book

the fast 800 GLP-1 recipe book

ON, OFF & AFTER

Your *food first* solution for safe and speedy weight loss

DR CLARE BAILEY MOSLEY
& DR JACK MOSLEY
with NICOLA GRAIMES

First published in Great Britain in 2026
by Short Books, an imprint of
Octopus Publishing Group Ltd
Carmelite House
50 Victoria Embankment
London EC4Y 0DZ
www.octopusbooks.co.uk

An Hachette UK Company
www.hachette.co.uk

The authorized representative in the EEA is
Hachette Ireland, 8 Castlecourt Centre, Dublin 15,
D15 XTP3, Ireland (email: info@hbgi.ie)

Distributed in the US by Hachette Book Group,
1290 Avenue of the Americas, 4th and 5th Floors,
New York, NY 10104

Distributed in Canada by Canadian Manda Group,
664 Annette St, Toronto, Ontario, Canada M6S 2C8

ISBN 9781780726373
eISBN 9781780726380

A CIP catalogue record for this book is available
from the British Library.

Printed and bound in Europe.

10 9 8 7 6 5 4 3 2 1

Publisher: Jo Morrell
Commissioning Editor: Katie Forsythe
Recipe Contributors: Dr Clare Bailey Mosley,
Nicola Graimes and Caroline Barton
Project Editor: Jo Roberts-Miller
Editorial Assistant: Sarah Ramnath-Budhram
Nutritional Analysis: Fiona Hunter
Design, Photography and Art Direction: Smith & Gilmour
Food Stylist: Annie Rigg
Assistant Food Stylist: Lucy MacLeod
Props Stylist: Jenny Iggleden
Hand Models: Lily and Oscar Smith
Senior Production Manager: Katherine Hockley

MIX
Paper | Supporting responsible forestry
FSC® C011124
www.fsc.org

Contents

Foreword by Professor Susan Jebb

For nearly two decades now my research teams have been testing ways that we can support people to manage their weight. This work has emphasised what a difference it can make if we provide support to people to make changes to their diet.

Total diet replacements have transformed the way we treat people with type 2 diabetes and helped many more people wanting to lose weight to improve their health and cut their risk of heart disease. These diets, where people replace all their usual food with specially formulated, nutritionally complete products, before gradually returning to food, can help people to lose around 15 kg in six months. Alongside support from a trained coach, this programme is now offered by the NHS for people recently diagnosed with diabetes. Around a third of people who complete the programme are free of diabetes one year later.

But many people are reluctant to try this approach. If you love food, then the idea of a diet often based on soups and shakes for many weeks isn't much fun. Food matters, not just for health, but for our connections with family and friends and it can feel isolating to eat apart. Many people we spoke to asked how they could achieve the same results by preparing their own food.

So, we moved on to study lower carbohydrate diets – cutting out sugary foods and replacing staple carbohydrates with smaller portions of unrefined, fibre-rich carbs, while filling up on vegetables instead. We are excited to be finishing the DIAMOND trial, a project that Dr Clare Bailey Mosley was a part of at the very beginning, which shows that with the right diet and good support, diabetes can be put into remission for some people and many more can lose weight and gain better control of their blood sugar.

Now that new weight-loss medications are available some people are asking whether we need diets at all. This alarms me – all the evidence says that the two need to go hand-in-hand. The drugs are very good at reducing your appetite, but they don't ensure you get the nutrition you need. In clinical trials people typically cut their calorie intake by 15-25% because the drugs make you feel fuller for longer and reduce some of the automatic impulses to eat. That gives you more freedom to make informed choices about what to eat, and we are quickly learning how to optimise diets for people taking these new medications.

The key step is to ensure that the food you choose maximises the nutritional value. Making sure you keep up your protein intake by basing meals around poultry, pulses, fish or meat, with plenty of vegetables and carefully chosen sources of unrefined carbohydrate to boost fibre intake and nourish our gut microbiota, means you can maximise the health benefits. These diets build meals around fresh ingredients to provide essential micronutrients and important phytochemicals.

In our research studies trial we are able to provide lots of advice and support from practice nurses and trained coaches, but we know it can be hard to make changes on your own. Good, evidence-based advice on what to eat is important so that you don't waste time and money on things that don't move the dial. Reliable recipes can make all the difference to sticking with the programme and in the end it's adherence that matters most. What starts as a diet needs to transition to a new way of eating for life. I am thrilled that more and more people are discovering the power of food to improve their health.

Susan Jebb OBE, PhD, FRCP (Hon), FMedSci
Professor of Diet and Population Health,
University of Oxford

A word from Dr Clare Bailey Mosley

The world of weight loss and nutrition has changed dramatically over the last 15 years or so, and we have come a long way in our understanding of weight loss and nutrition. Most of us now know that our diet can have a huge impact on our wellbeing and that by eating well we can transform our health from the inside out. I have seen this in my own family. My husband, Michael Mosley, was able to lose 9kg and reverse his type 2 diabetes by following an intermittent fasting approach (the 5:2 diet). We used to think that type 2 diabetes was an irreversible disease with seemingly inevitable and devastating consequences. However, the pioneering work of Professor Roy Taylor and his team has shown that diabetes *can* be sent into remission.

For those living with obesity and poor metabolic health, losing 10 per cent of your bodyweight can dramatically improve your health, such as lowering blood pressure and cholesterol, improving cardiovascular health and achieving better blood sugars. But, more than this, it can cut your risk of a range of conditions, from non-alcoholic fatty liver disease, certain cancers and dementia, to depression and anxiety. You are also likely to see an improvement in sleep (even correcting symptoms of sleep apnoea), while energy levels improve, arthritis can reduce and so much more.

Losing weight fast

In the past, we were taught that rapid weight loss and 'crash' dieting were dangerous and led to 'yoyo' weight loss and gain. But now we realise that for many people losing weight quickly is the most effective and sustainable way to kick-start their health journey and see fast improvements in metabolic health.

Of course, rapid weight loss is not suitable for everyone, and we have a 3-step programme offering different options according to where you are in your weight-loss journey. This structured 12-week programme can be done fast, especially if you have a lot to lose, or do intermittent fasting at your own pace, or simply by following a way of life based on a nutrient-rich, Mediterranean-style diet.

The 800- to 900-calorie 12-week 'path to remission' programme, led by Professor Taylor, is currently being successfully rolled out on the NHS using soups and shakes. It is this research that forms the foundation of the Fast 800 programme.

The rise of weight-loss drugs

GLP-1 medications were initially used to treat type 2 diabetes. When it was shown that they could aid weight loss, they exploded in popularity and their rise has been meteoric. It's now seemingly easier than ever to lose weight fast. Many people see these drugs as a quick fix that will solve their weight-loss challenges. My son Jack is also a doctor and has written a bestselling book on this subject – *Food Noise* – that explains how they work and weighs up their pros and cons. Jack has joined with me to write this book and shares his insight, as he is an expert on GLP-1s.

For many people, the weight-loss medications will reduce cravings and give them relief from their relentless food noise – that constant chatter in your head that urges you to grab an extra tasty treat – which leads to weight loss. However, these drugs may not work for everyone. There are considerable possible side effects, as with any medication. For those people for whom the medication does work, when their appetite is suppressed, they might find they do not eat much at all. This can lead to them struggling to get all of the essential nutrients that their body needs, in particular, protein, fibre, vitamins and minerals. This lack of nutrition can have significant consequences for their health.

On the other hand, for those people who navigate the issues that come with taking the drugs and are successful in achieving their goal weight, they may be scared to stop taking them because of concerns that their food noise will return and their weight will creep back up. The answer is to make sustainable healthy lifestyle changes. Building healthy habits right from the start can make all the difference going forward.

Who is this book for?

The Fast 800 programme is the original rapid weight-loss plan, proven to work long-term, enabling you to embed healthy habits to sustain healthy weight loss. I'm always amazed by the countless people who have been helped by this approach – the more than 15,000 reviews on Amazon with 4.7 ratings are a testament to the fact that the Fast 800 changes lives. But it is not all about rapid weight loss, whether or not you are on the weight-loss medication. This is a flexible programme that you can follow at your own pace – either intensively, with intermittent fasting, including the 5-2 diet, or as a way of life. This final maintenance stage is the 'off ramp' to keep you on track, however your journey starts. Using the Fast 800 principles will encourage you to lose weight well and keep it off for good, one healthy meal at a time. It's for anyone who:

- Would like to lose weight fast. Maybe you're considering trying the GLP-1 medications or want to try and lose weight without them.
- Is on the weight-loss drugs and wants to eat healthily. You may have very little appetite but want each meal to be as nutrient rich as possible.
- Has reached their goal weight and wants to move into the maintenance phase. Whether you've been using weight-loss drugs or not, you're keen to keep the weight off for good, while also enjoying delicious, nourishing food.

Wherever you find yourself on this journey, we hope that this book is helpful and inspires you to eat well and embrace healthy and sustainable habits.

Thinking about food first

We like to call this a 'food first' approach. If you're considering trying the weight-loss drugs, we encourage you to give the Fast 800 programme a go initially, to see if it works for you. This has the added benefit of having far fewer side effects, being more affordable and sustainable. However, we understand that many people will need extra help. And if you are taking the GLP-1s, our aim is to help you stay nourished, so that your body has everything it needs to function well.

This will build good eating habits that you can rely on if you decide to come off the medication, leaving you feeling confident in maintaining your health and weight loss. For more support go to thefast800program.com.

All of the 135 brand-new recipes in this book are designed to be simple to prepare and delicious to eat, with maximum nutritional benefits. We've purposely tried to keep ingredients and cooking times to a minimum to help you fit these meals into your daily life (especially helpful if you have very little appetite on the GLP-1s and may not feel like cooking).

I've also included recipes that can be prepared using an air fryer and meals that can be batch cooked, so you can cut down on cooking if you are short of time. And we also have plenty of healthy treats, too. Once you reach the maintenance phase, it's possible to bulk up the recipes with extra fibre or protein, so that you get maximum nutrition and feel full for longer.

I hope you enjoy cooking and eating these recipes as much as I do.

Clare x
@drclarebaileymosley

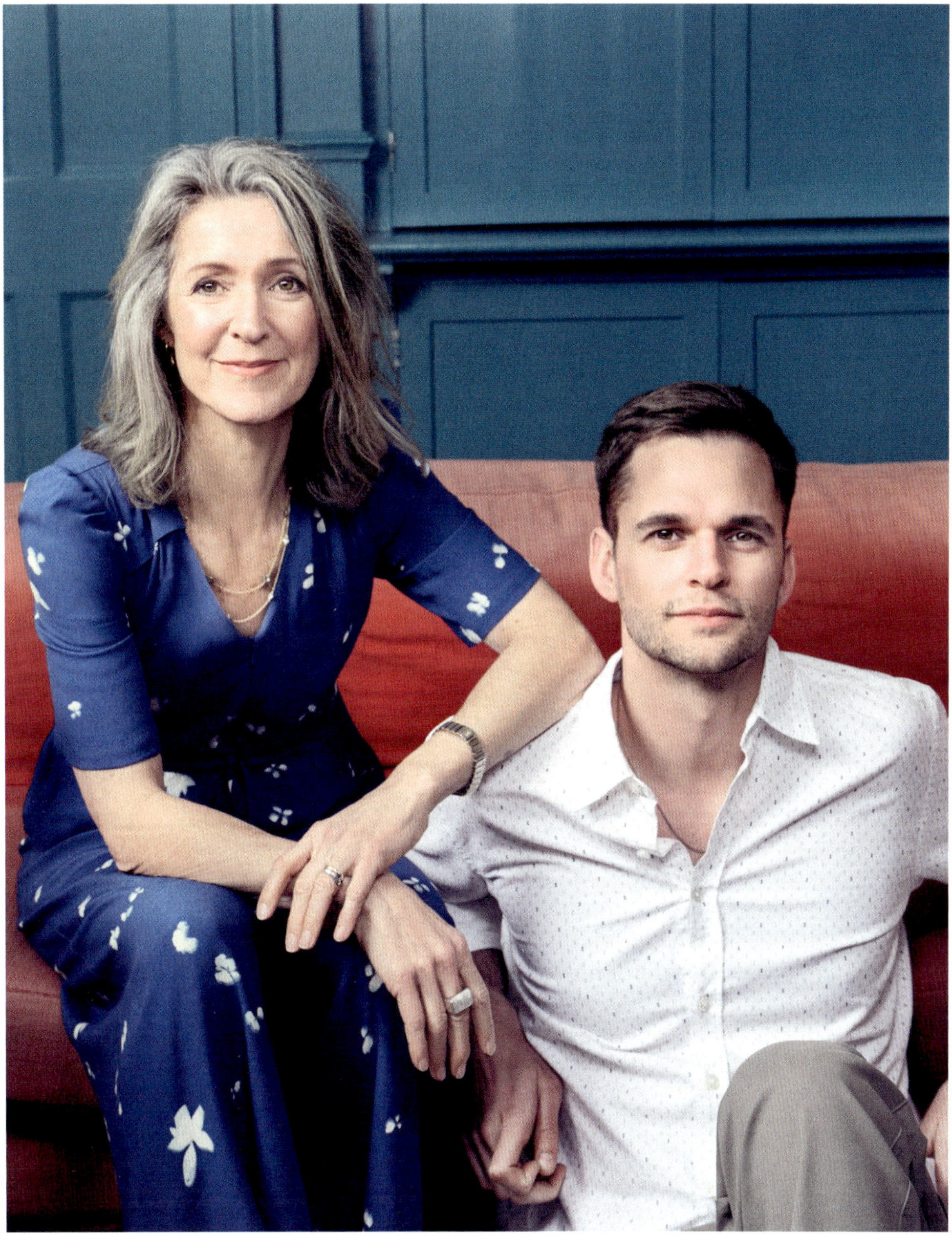

A word from Dr Jack Mosley

There are many valid and evidence-based dietary approaches to losing weight and improving your overall health, from fasting, rapid weight loss and the Mediterranean-style diet to GLP-1-assisted weight loss. As the saying goes, 'All roads lead to Rome', but some routes may be better for you than others!

Food noise and the GLP-1s

When I wrote my book, *Food Noise*, all about the GLP weight-loss drugs and how they work to silence our cravings, the term was still quite new. Food noise is that continuous mental chatter in your head about food. It is often different from physical hunger and the volume is often turned up when you are bored, tired, stressed or sad. With food noise, your brain wants reward or relief. Countless people now recognise that their experience of food noise is one of the things that makes it really hard for them to eat healthily and lose weight. Comfort eating is a science-backed phenomenon.

Losing weight with willpower alone can be really difficult. We are surrounded by tempting foods at every turn. Foods that are designed by scientists to trigger our food noise. These foods are often called UPFs (ultra-processed foods) and, while they are engineered to taste delicious, eating too much of them will inevitably be bad for our health, as they are usually high in sugar, poor-quality fats and excess salt, as well as containing very few nutrients. And it's extremely hard not to eat too much of them – these foods have been created to make us crave more. My dad, Michael Mosley, almost certainly had food noise when it came to his favourite chocolate treats – my mum used to have to hide them in the house because he couldn't stop himself from eating them all in one go!

We now know that certain people have their food noise turned up louder than others, as a result of genetic and environmental factors and through no fault of their own. Your brain is telling you that you need that sugary, salty snack, sometimes even when your body is full.

Our modern food environment is packed with foods that train our brains to seek quick reward. With the sight, sound and smell of these tempting components of the Western diet being ever-present in our lives, it was not surprising that the GLP-1 weight-loss drugs captured the headlines so dramatically.

The pros and cons of the diet drugs

GLP-1 medications represent a turning point: they achieve weight loss previously only seen with surgery, but with drugs alone and have a more favourable side-effect profile than past treatments. The drugs muffle your food noise and have been shown to lead to rapid weight loss, with some users with obesity losing between 15 to 20 per cent of their bodyweight within 1 year. New and stronger medications, known colloquially as 'reta' or retatrutide, may be even more effective and have been shown in trials to lead to as much weight loss as bariatric surgery (a major surgical procedure that restricts stomach size).

Although the risk to reward benefit of these medications outweighs anything we have seen in the past, there are potential side effects to watch out for. There are the immediate possible side effects, including nausea, constipation, vomiting and diarrhoea, as well as some much more serious side effects, although rare, including gallstones, pancreatitis and bowel blockages. Patients will react differently to the medications and some may find that the drugs are not an option for them, as the side effects are too severe.

There are other consequences that need to be considered, too. If you don't eat a nutrient-rich diet while on the drugs, because of your loss of appetite, you are at risk of nutrient deficiencies such as iron, B12, folate, calcium and fibre. This is why it is essential to eat a well-balanced diet. Studies show that 25 to 40 per cent of any weight lost is 'lean body mass', a key component of muscle, so eating enough protein and trying some resistance exercises, like lifting weights, is essential if you want to maintain muscle while losing weight.

Life after weight loss

What happens when you stop taking the medication? Unfortunately, the latest evidence suggests your weight could pile back on. It is true that weight regain can occur with any kind of diet or weight-loss plan, but the rate at which weight is regained after stopping the GLP-1 weight-loss drugs is much faster than after following a 'conventional' diet. This can mean your metabolic health markers, such as your cardiovascular health, blood pressure, glucose levels and inflammation, will likely *rise* as the weight comes back. As weight regain after stopping the drugs is a big concern for many people who are using them, we recommend following a healthy Mediterranean-style, lower-carb diet, along with some intermittent fasting in the form of the 5:2 diet, cutting your intake to 800–1000cals, two days a week, and eating normally the rest of the rest of the time.

Using nutrition to silence your cravings and feel full for longer

There is still much research to be done on the GLP-1 medications and whether they should be lifelong medications or only used in the short-term. But we do know that a focus on dietary habits and lifestyle changes is vital to get long-term, sustainable results.

It is vital to eat filling foods with plenty of protein, healthy fats and fibre. This can help support natural satiety signals in the gut, including GLP-1, and can make it easier to stay satisfied while following a reduced-calorie approach. This ties into the 'food first' mantra that my mum talks about above; whether you are on the medications or not, you need to consider the food you eat so that your body gets the vital fuel it needs to function well.

Before considering medication, weigh up the risks and rewards of taking it. Losing weight, eating well and feeling good is all about what suits *you*. If you choose to try the GLP-1 weight-loss medications, this book is packed with delicious and nutritious recipes that will nourish you while you are taking them. If not, don't worry, the fantastic recipes will suit a rapid weight-loss journey without medication, too, whether you are on a fasting journey or you just wish to follow a lower carb Mediterranean-style diet. The great thing about these recipes is they are both easy to make and delicious to eat. No more rooting around the far-flung corners of the supermarket for niche ingredients, and no more whiling away your entire evening cooking.

Whatever option you choose, I wish you all the very best and hope that you enjoy creating and eating the meals within these pages.

Jack
@dr.jack.mosley

Introduction

What is the Fast 800?

This diet is designed to be flexible, while incorporating the best science-based advice. All the meals are based on a lowish-carb Mediterranean-style way of eating, but how you manage the 800–1000cals days is down to you. There is also a less intensive option.

Most people choose to kickstart their diet with the fast-track plan of 800–1000cals a day, every day for 2 weeks, then review their progress. If you do have a lot to lose – and if the diet suits – you can continue this for up to 3 months at a time. If you don't have much weight to lose, or wish to do it more slowly, you can move on to the New 5:2 – consuming 800–1000cals a day for 2 days a week and on the other days continuing to eat a healthy, Med-style diet, keeping carb intake lowish and watching portion size.

You could also add in a relatively new form of intermittent fasting called Time Restricted Eating (TRE), whereby you eat all your calories within a narrow time window each day – usually within 10–12 hours. This extends the length of your normal overnight fast (when you are sleeping and not eating), giving your body an opportunity to burn fat and do essential repairs. (For more information see page 19.)

As with any diet, the Fast 800 may not suit everyone, so check with your health professional first (see page 20).

If you're using the GLP-1 weight-loss drugs, we urge you to follow the Fast 800 plan as far as possible; if you don't feel hungry, we have delicious nutrient-rich small bites that are simple to prepare and will help stimulate your taste buds. The recipes have been created to maximise your essential nutrients so you get what you need, in particular adequate protein and fibre.

A Mediterranean-style diet

While 'lowish' in carbohydrates, this is not a very restrictive diet as you will see in the delicious variety of healthy, flavourful recipes. However, it does mean reducing or avoiding sugary, starchy and ultra-processed foods (UPFs), such as white bread, white pasta, rice and potatoes, as well as many processed breakfast cereals, since these readily convert to sugars in your body.

As a general principle, the Med-style way of eating is about consuming whole foods, including those cooked from scratch. Mindful of our time-poor lives, I've tried to keep the recipes as simple as possible. We've also shared tips on how to create some of the recipes using an air fryer.

The great thing about eating a Med-style diet, rather than a low-fat one, is that you can enjoy plenty of healthy fats like olive oil, avocados, some full-fat dairy, nuts, seeds and oily fish – all the kinds of ingredients that make food tasty and filling. They also have anti-inflammatory properties, as well as helping us absorb important nutrients and vitamins, including the important fat-soluble vitamins A, D, E and K, essential for healthy vision, bones, immunity and more. The Med-style diet also includes fish and some dairy and meat, however there are lots of meat-free recipes too. The programme also includes recipes for luscious and colourful vegetables, fruit, wholegrains, beans and lentils, for much needed extra fibre. The intention is to combine protein and fibre in every meal, while delivering healthy weight loss.

So, what's out and what's in?

For the past 50 years we have been told to keep our consumption of fat to a minimum for fear that it will block our arteries and cause a heart attack. To compensate for this, we were encouraged to eat at least a third of our calories as starchy carbohydrates, in many cases putting up blood sugars and driving obesity. Likewise, the official line has commonly been to advise people to eat three meals a day, with snacks between meals and before bed if we got hungry. As a result, many of us are eating six times a day, leaving our metabolism constantly battling to keep sugar levels in the normal range. And given that most of us eat more than we burn, these extra calories usually end up getting stored as fat.

However, the good news is that in the past decade there has been a whole body of exciting new research that has turned standard dietary advice on its head. Studies have shown that, unlike the widely advocated 'slow and steady' approach, rapid weight loss helps people lose weight faster, get closer to their goal and help keep the weight off. By combining moderately low-carb, Mediterranean-style diet with a limit of 800–1000cals, you have a highly effective way to lose weight, restore blood sugars and re-set your metabolism.

Remission

Common chronic conditions caused by poor metabolic health that can improve or go into remission following a programme like this.

- Type 2 diabetes
- Heart disease (e.g. coronary artery disease and heart failure)
- Stroke
- Hypertension (high blood pressure)
- Non-alcoholic fatty liver disease (NAFLD)
- Polyendocrine Metabolic Ovarian Syndrome (PMOS)
- Chronic kidney disease (CKD)
- Obesity
- Sleep apnoea
- Cognitive decline / Alzheimer's (sometimes called 'Type 3 diabetes')
- Gout
- Depression and anxiety (linked via inflammation and insulin resistance)
- Osteoarthritis (via weight-related joint stress and inflammation)
- Retinopathy and vision loss (especially in diabetes)

What's out

1 Sugary, starchy and processed foods

It is increasingly clear that we should avoid sweet, starchy and highly processed foods where possible. These are foods packed with the perfect combination of sugar, fats, refined carbs, salt and flavourings in order to light up the reward centre in our brains. They are designed to be over-eaten. They will undo much of the benefit you get from eating healthily and are often toxic for the important microbes living in our guts that produce substances to keep us healthy and boost our mood. Be kind to these vital bugs and they will take care of you...

We describe the Fast 800 as a lowish carbohydrate diet. This is because not all carbs are equal. Refined and starchy carbs, such as white bread or white rice, are very rapidly broken down, causing a spike in blood sugars and encouraging fat storage and weight gain. What's more, they've had much of the nutrients stripped away from the original grain, including much of the fibre, B vitamins, minerals and phytonutrients. So, remember to cut down on the white stuff. Limit your white pasta, white bread and potatoes, too.

However, not all carbs are bad. More complex carbohydrates, like wholegrains, beans or lentils, are slower to break down as they contain more fibre. As a result, they release less sugar and do so more slowly, leaving you feeling full for longer, while the fibre in them makes its way down to the large intestine, where those helpful microbes convert it into important substances that help keep us well.

2 Hidden sugars

Sadly, we are surrounded by hidden sugars – they are found in all sorts of foods, including savoury snacks and takeaways, and can be very hard to spot. Check the ingredients in any ready-made convenience food, and the word 'sugar' may not appear at the top of the list, or indeed appear at all, despite it being included in significant quantities. Sugar often appears under alternative names, such as maltose, dextrose, fructose, glucose, lactose – of which there are 50–60 variations, many of which you won't even recognise. Add all these together and sugar can turn out to be the main ingredient.

Fruit contains lots of health-promoting phytonutrients and fibre, but it is best to eat fruit during or after a meal to reduce sugar spikes. It's far better to eat the whole fruit than to have it in the form of juice, as the juicing process removes much of the fibre and turns a healthy food into a sugary one. Try to make the fruit a low-sugar variety, such as berries, apples or pears, rather than sweet tropical fruits.

Alcohol is another challenge – it behaves like sugar, breaking down rapidly and causing a sugar spike. A single glass of wine can contain between 200–300cals and ends up stored in the liver as fat, causing inflammation. Spirits tend to contain slightly less sugar. But because alcohol disinhibits us, we are more likely to eat crisps or go for a takeaway when we've been drinking! So, for many reasons, we recommend moderation and to avoid alcohol on a fasting day.

And what's in

1 Protein

It has become increasingly clear that protein is key to regulating your appetite and your general health. Protein is required by every cell and organ in the body, including the immune system and brain. It maintains your muscle mass and metabolism, as well as helping you to feel full. However, unlike carbohydrates and fat, your body is unable to store protein.

Your body also isn't able to tell you what you are lacking, so if you aren't getting enough protein, you will continue to feel hungry, even if you have eaten enough, and you are likely to go on eating until you have satisfied your body's protein needs – and this drives weight gain. This is known as the 'protein leverage hypothesis'. So, it's important to get enough protein on a daily basis: you should aim for a minimum of 60g a day and perhaps 10–20g on top of that, if you are older, bigger, very active or are choosing the rapid weight-loss approach. Eating sufficient protein is particularly important if you are using the weight-loss medications, in order to protect your muscle mass. It is also especially important when on an 800–1000 calorie day to ensure you get the minimum requirement of protein.

To help you do this, we have included the protein content in our recipes, which are carefully calibrated to help give you adequate amounts and top-ups. We also offer suggestions for how to add protein top-ups (see page 272), so that you can adapt salads or veg dishes according to your own taste. Getting enough protein can be challenging for vegetarians, and even more so for vegans, who might be advised to take quality, low-sugar, protein supplements (such as those in the Fast 800 – see suggestions on the website) or use a meal replacement protein shake on 800–1000 calorie days. Using good-quality, protein-rich, meal replacement shakes with natural ingredients (see thefast800.com for options) will also help on days when you have to rush out of the door with an instant breakfast, or as an alternative to grabbing a sandwich and crisps for lunch.

2 Fibre

Most of us don't get enough fibre either – the average in the Western diet is about half the necessary 30g a day. To get what your body requires, you need to eat seven or more portions of fruit and veg a day, as well as some wholegrains, beans and lentils. On a fasting day, it can be a challenge to get enough fibre, but you'll find that you get to love your veg, and a suitable meal replacement shake can also provide a top-up. We've added a list of fibre top-ups at the end of the book to help you boost your intake (see page 273). Fibre is particularly important if you are using GLP-1 weight-loss medication, as these drugs can slow down your digestion.

3 Non-starchy veg

We know that there are numerous benefits to eating more vegetables. This includes an impressive 16 per cent reduction in the risk of having a stroke for every added portion. When you are trying to lose weight or control your blood sugars, it is best to stick to non-starchy vegetables, i.e. those that are lower in carbs and hidden sugars, such as spinach, cabbage and broccoli. And we encourage you to embrace variety and enjoy generous portions.

Ideally, pile your plate with steamed greens, salad, or any of the other vegetables on the list at the back of the book (see page 274). They are so low in calories that they can be eaten freely, without counting. It's fine to add a dressing or sauce to your veg, but do remember to include those added calories in your daily tally.

That said, adding a little olive oil to your non-starchy 'free' veg is actually beneficial, as it can improve the absorption of nutrients. This is particularly important when it comes to the absorption of the fat-soluble vitamins A, D, E and K. In the big scheme of things, a little drizzle of olive oil here and there is fine. The message is: don't worry about occasional extra calories, if it helps you eat more veg... And since we also know that variety is key to us getting the nutrients we need, you might take this opportunity to push the boat out and try new veg. By eating different phytonutrients (the health-promoting substances produced by plants), you will contribute to your metabolic health and to reducing inflammation. That's why we are encouraged to 'eat a rainbow'. Embrace as many different coloured vegetables as you can – red salad leaves, purple broccoli or beetroot, yellow peppers, dark aubergines, as well as plenty of greens...

4 Natural unprocessed fats, mainly plant-based

When it comes to choosing oils, the least processed the better. Try and go for cold-pressed or extra-virgin oils, as they are unrefined and retain their natural nutrients – although they are more expensive, so buy what you can afford.

For frying at high temperatures, you can use a good-quality rapeseed oil. Extra-virgin olive oil is good for gentle frying and ideal for salads. Coconut oil, a bit like butter, is fine in moderation. I like the flavour it can give to some stir-fries and curries, and it provides a slightly sweet and flavoured alternative for baking.

As part of a healthy, Mediterranean-style diet, there are plenty of other 'good' fats to be found in the likes of oily fish, such as mackerel and salmon, as well as nuts and seeds, all of which have been shown to lower your risk of stroke and heart disease.

5 Dairy

We include a fair amount of full-fat dairy in our recipes because the evidence suggests that in moderation this is beneficial – and does not, contrary to some reports, lead to diabetes. Fermented dairy is best, and full-fat products are less processed. Full-fat Greek-style yoghurt, for example, doesn't usually contain the starchy thickeners and sugars or sweeteners that are added to enhance low-fat products. We love the creamy richness of it. I try to eat a variety of yoghurts and kefir to improve diversity.

6 Meat in moderation

Many of us are trying to eat less meat in general these days, particularly red meat, for both health and environmental reasons. But meat is an excellent source of good-quality protein and, as we have seen above, getting adequate protein can be a challenge on fasting days. So, we have included a number of meat-based recipes in the main section of the book, as well as some veg-based ones that contain small quantities of processed meat, such as bacon or chorizo, both to boost protein and add extra flavour. Try to buy better-quality, grass-fed varieties, if you can.

Good hydration with minimal calories

Most of us fail to drink enough fluid every day (the NHS recommends 6–8 glasses of water a day). And yet, keeping well hydrated is especially important on a fasting day or on GLPs. This is because when you are burning fat your body releases water. So, it is really important to add extra fluid to your diet, otherwise you will find that you are feeling feeble and exhausted. Even mild dehydration (just 1–2 per cent of bodyweight) can impair memory, mood and concentration. Interestingly, the GLPs appear to suppress the body's natural thirst signals, as well as your appetite.

People often assume that exhaustion is due to a calorie deficit, but our bodies are designed to manage short periods without eating much food. However, we can get dehydrated more quickly when losing weight, leaving you feeling exhausted, feeble, light-headed or suffering headaches. What's more, getting dehydrated can also cause constipation, a common issue, particularly with the weight-loss medication.

On an 800–1000cals fasting day, or on GLPs, you should drink an extra 1–1.5 litres of calorie-free fluids, mainly as water (and more if you are very active or the weather is hot). Sipping fluids can also distract you from cravings and reduce hunger between meals. Try to avoid drinks with sweeteners if you can. Here are some lovely ways to add flavour without significant calories – drinks that can be enjoyed any time, and that will not interfere with fat burning.

Cold refreshing drinks

We like water and drink it straight from the tap or filtered, and keep a bottle in the fridge. If you are inclined to forget to increase your fluid intake, try having a jug or bottle in the house that needs to be finished by the end of the day. Or carry a bottle with you. If you are not a fan of plain water, drink carbonated water for a bit of fizz.

For added flavour, put in a few berries or some fresh herbs, like mint, rosemary or thyme. You might add a squeeze of fresh lemon or lime, and drop a twist into the bottle. A slice or two of cucumber or courgette looks and tastes refreshing. For a stronger brew, keep a bottle of cooled fruit or herbal tea in the fridge.

Hot comforting drinks

Try to avoid putting milk in your tea or coffee between meals, as this adds calories and interferes with fat-burning – although, straight after a meal, a dash of milk in your drink is OK. Between meals, try taking your tea with a squeeze of lemon, drink black coffee or try sipping fruit teas. Or make your own herbal infusions, adding a handful of fresh herbs, such as mint, thyme or sage, to boiled water. I'm a big fan of mint tea, with its smooth feel and sweet scent. Mint grows wild in the garden or you can keep it in a pot and harvest the larger leaves. Steep some leaves in hot water for 5 minutes. A generous handful of mint leaves contains a surprising amount of nutrients, including iron, vitamin and antioxidants, which may help protect your cells from damage. Peppermint is also thought to improve digestion.

Green tea, meanwhile, has been shown to be one of the healthiest drinks on the planet. Thanks mainly to its antioxidant properties, it is thought to reduce the risk of heart disease, improve brain function, protect against some cancers, as well as support weight loss. However, green tea is an acquired taste, as it can be slightly bitter (that is part of what makes it so beneficial). We like to drink green tea with some finely sliced fresh root ginger (1cm unpeeled) and ½ teaspoon ground cinnamon stirred in to add a delicate sweetness. Allow the tea leaves and ginger to steep for 3–5 minutes, then remove them before you drink.

The Fast 800 – a quick recap

STAGE 1

Rapid weight loss

By combining calorie restriction (800–1000cals) with a low-carbohydrate, Mediterranean-style diet you are more likely to get into fat burning – ketosis. Along with rapid weight loss, you will probably feel better, more energetic and have more mental clarity. We recommend you start with the intensive stage if possible. By sticking to 800–1000cals a day, every day, for at least two weeks, you will kickstart your weight loss and improve your metabolic health.

Why 800–1000cals? Because this is low enough to induce mild ketosis, which is associated with fat burning, but high enough to ensure you get the nutrients you need.

After two to three weeks, pause and reflect on how it is going. If you are losing weight and not struggling with the diet, then carry on. You can continue this approach until you reach your goal, or for up to 12 weeks.

If you are using the GLP-1 medications, you will likely find that your appetite has decreased and you are eating far fewer calories than usual. We recommend that you try to consume at least 800cals a day to keep your energy up and ensure you get all of the vital nutrients that your body needs.

For convenience, some people find it helpful during the rapid weight-loss stage to make up some of their meals as shakes, which also helps them get enough protein and fibre. Visit thefast800.com, where you will find a range of ready-made meal replacement shakes with a Med-style formation and decent protein content to help fill the gap. You can also find a variety of protein powders.

STAGE 2

Intermittent fasting with the New 5:2

When you get close to your target weight, or if you are struggling on the rapid weight-loss stage, you can swap to an intermittent fasting pattern – eating 800–1000cals on just a couple of days a week. Your weight-loss rate will be slower on this regime, but it has been shown to be highly sustainable, and one of the most effective ways to lose weight and keep it off. A 2025 study, which compiled 20 different studies, found that the 5:2 diet led to more fat loss, more loss of fat around the waist and improved BMIs, as well as a greater reduction in cholesterol and blood pressure, when compared to 'usual advice'. We recommend that, rather than reducing your calories to 500–600, as in the original 5:2 Fast Diet, you should stick to 800–1000cals on fasting days.

For those using weight-loss drugs, you may find that intermittent fasting for 1 or 2 days each week works well when you start to come off the medication. Later in the book we have included some tips to quieten your cravings if they start to return (see pages 22–4).

STAGE 3

The maintenance programme

Once you've hit your goal, you can continue with a healthy Mediterranean way of eating, not calorie counting but exercising portion control. For this 'maintenance phase', you can go on using most of the recipes in this book; just double up portions, add extra protein (see page 272) and a few tablespoons of high-fibre, unrefined carbs, such as beans, lentils or wholegrains (see page 273), here and there, and you are set for life. You can enjoy the occasional treat, but try to maintain a diet low in sugar and moderately low in starchy carbs to help prevent sugars creeping up or weight piling back on. The message is: relax a bit, but not too much!

If your weight increases or your new outfit starts to feel tight, you know what to do...

Adding in Time Restricted Eating

TRE is a form of fasting whereby you extend your overnight fast to restrict your eating window during the day. There is evidence that going 12 or even 14 hours without food gives your body and metabolism a chance to recover and focus on other functions, such as 'spring cleaning' old and damaged cells, and helping you switch from burning sugar to burning fat.

So how do you do this? Well, if you stop eating by 8pm and don't start again till 8am – that is a 12-hour overnight fast (i.e. 12:12). You can then build up to a 14-hour fast, which means eating all your day's food in a 10-hour window (14:10). Many people find that eating in a narrower window makes it easier to manage a fast day.

Either way, it is a good habit for all of us to get into, as calories eaten within a few hours of bedtime are more likely to be stored as fat.

	STAGE 1 **Rapid weight loss**	STAGE 2 **The New 5:2**	STAGE 3 **Maintenance**
how TO FAST	**800 – 1000 cals a day** (for up to 12 weeks)	**800 – 1000 cals 2 days a week** (intermittent fasting)	**No calorie counting, but portion control** (consider a weekly fast day – 6:1)
what TO EAT	**Lowish-carb Mediterranean-style diet** (or replace up to half your calories with meal-replacement shakes)		**Lowish-carb Med-style diet** (watching portion size)
when TO EAT	**Optional TRE 12:12 or 14:10** (Time Restricted Eating)		

Getting started

1 Write down what you want to achieve

Think about why you want to lose weight. What difference will it make? What changes do you want to see? And how important is it to you? What will success look and feel like? Your personal goal may be to lose the weight around your middle; or to bring about a general improvement in your overall health, energy and mood. Reminding yourself about what motivates you will help keep you on track. How will you know when you get there?

2 Make your kitchen 'hygienic'

This isn't about how clean and tidy your kitchen is; it means clearing away temptation, hiding (or even getting rid of) all convenience foods, snacks, biscuits, white bread or whatever your weaknesses are.

3 Tell people you are doing the diet

This helps you to hold yourself to account and increases commitment and success.

SAFETY: Exclusions and cautions

This diet is not suitable for teenagers, or if you're breastfeeding, pregnant or undergoing fertility treatment. Do not follow the diet if you are underweight or have an eating disorder. Discuss with your GP if you are on medication or if you have a medical condition, including diabetes, low or high blood pressure, retinopathy, gallstones or epilepsy. Nor should you do this if you are frail, unwell or while doing endurance exercise. (For more detailed information see thefast800.com/faqs/)

Extra support

It can make a real difference to have a partner, family member or diet buddy doing the diet with you in some way. Try to enlist friends, family, colleagues and anyone interested to help keep you motivated. For more information, see our website thefast800.com where you can access the Fast 800 Online Programme to help you stay on track and integrate the Fast 800 into your life.

As well as support from family, friends and the Fast 800 network, if you are struggling to reach protein and/or fibre targets, or would like some meal replacement solutions, go to our website or follow these links:

Clear Protein
https://thefast800.com/meal-replacements/clear-protein-apple-blackcurrant/

Fibre Blend
https://thefast800.com/meal-replacements/cloudy-apple-fibre-blend/

Sleep Blend
https://thefast800.com/meal-replacements/lemon-sleep-blend/

Protein Bars
https://thefast800.com/meal-replacements/dark-chocolate-raspberry-protein-bar-box-of-12/

Side effects of *The Fast 800*

Dehydration
The most commonly reported side effects when people begin the Fast 800 are headaches, constipation, feeling light-headed and fatigued. These are mainly due to not drinking enough added water. When you burn excess fat, you also lose fluid, which can leave you dehydrated. (For more on how to stay hydrated see page 17.) As for constipation, again, keeping well hydrated helps keep things soft – and make sure you are eating enough fibre-rich food.

Getting used to fibre
We try to include plenty of fibre in the recipes in the form of non-starchy vegetables, including beans, lentils and wholegrains. However, as most people have a low fibre intake, it can take time for your gut to get used to more fibre. Take it slowly, otherwise you may encounter wind or loose stools. See page 273 to find fibre top-ups that will help you adapt.

Low blood pressure
Within days of embarking on a low-calorie diet like the Fast 800, you may see a drop in your blood pressure, which is a common benefit, but if you are on medication, particularly for blood pressure, or have a medical condition, it is important that you speak to your health professional before starting as your medication may need reducing (see SAFETY: Exclusions and cautions, opposite). It can help to use a home blood pressure monitor, particularly at first.

Feeling rough at first
Flicking the metabolic switch so that your body goes from burning sugar to burning fat can leave you feeling a bit off-colour for a few days, while your body's metabolism adapts. This is known as 'keto flu' and will pass within a matter of days. In fact, patients often tell me that they then feel better than they had done prior to starting the diet, with more energy, a sharper mind and fewer food cravings. Despite being on 800–1000cals, they find they are no longer feeling hungry all the time.

If your symptoms are severe or last longer than a week or so, it would be wise to discuss this with your health professional before continuing the diet. See thefast800.com for more information.

15 WAYS TO HELP YOU REACH YOUR GOALS AND SILENCE YOUR CRAVINGS

1 Avoid snacking between meals or late-night grazing
The trouble with snacking is that it reduces fat burning. If you must snack on a fasting day, eat a small portion of non-starchy veg, such as some broccoli or celery. Alternatively, try a few nuts (one portion is the amount that will sit on the palm of your hand) or a sliver of cheese.

2 Make your kitchen 'hygienic'
Control the food environment – that's your own house. Think of your weight-loss journey as an expedition and prepare accordingly – clear out the junk from your kitchen cupboards. Empty them of processed junk foods – willpower is overrated! It will be far harder to succumb to temptation and reach for your favourite sugary and salty snacks if they are not there.

3 Plan ahead
Willpower is fickle. Sometimes you have it, sometimes you don't. So best to assume it doesn't exist. Instead, plan to make things easier by ensuring that you have healthy, delicious alternatives to help you resist temptation. Don't go shopping when you're hungry!

4 Enlist your friends and family to support you
Explain what you are doing and why; perhaps you are wanting to reduce your blood sugars, or just to lose the extra weight that has been creeping on for years. Whatever your motivation, the more they understand what you are trying to achieve, the more they can support you. Be specific: 'Please don't offer me cake/another helping/ice cream...'

5 Add in TRE
This can enhance the effect of fasting on your weight loss and metabolic health (see page 19 for details).

6 Be more active
This is really important for your general health – switch the TV off, get up and go outside, walk more and try some strength-building exercises, as this increases your metabolic rate. A word of caution, though: while exercise is great for cardiovascular health, mood, strength and sleep, it is unfortunately a lousy way to lose weight. You need to run 36 miles to burn off a single pound of fat. So, go easy on the hard stuff at first, especially on fasting days – save that marathon training for a non-fast day, or when you are closer to your target weight or have finished the programme. Remember that taking a 10–15 minute walk after a meal can reduce blood sugars and aid weight loss.

7 Get enough sleep

We are increasingly aware of the impact that poor and disrupted sleep has on our brain and mood, leaving us irritable, with even less willpower than usual, and far more inclined to crave sweet and starchy foods. On average, people tend to consume around 350 extra calories after a poor night's sleep. Sleep deprivation creates a vicious cycle of weight gain, snoring and exhaustion. (See Michael's book, *4 Weeks to Better Sleep*, for the full lowdown on why we sleep and how to get more of it.)

8 De-stress

When we are stressed, we don't reach for the broccoli, we go for the biscuit tin. We want that sugar high. Many people self-soothe with sugary, salty and sweet foods to help manage their emotions, stress included! Meditation can be a great option for managing stress. (The Fast 800 book has some great advice on this; or go to thefast800.com.)

9 Keep a food mood diary

Many of us seek food for distraction, comfort or reward. Having a sugary, salty, fatty or carby treat gives us instant gratification, but can leave us feeling regret or guilt. Keep a food mood diary to help you understand when you are eating for hunger and when you are eating for emotional reasons (e.g. stress, boredom or loneliness). Write down what you eat and when, and how you feel before and after; you can then take steps to address the emotions without the need for snacking.

10 Practise 'urge surfing'

Urge surfing (developed by psychologists Alan Marlatt and Judith Gordon) is a mindfulness technique that can help address cravings. Like a wave, urges and cravings often pass over time. Ride that wave instead of succumbing to it. Instead of ruminating on your urges, 'ride them out' using an adapted version of urge surfing, the 3 Ns:

- Notice the craving;
- Name what you feel (e.g. this is an urge, not hunger);
- Nurture yourself – take a few deep breaths and consider an alternative way to soothe yourself, other than that sweet treat (e.g. a walk around the block).

Some people find it helpful to write down their craving intensity (out of 10) before and after they try the 3 Ns. Any improvement in your craving score is a bonus. Writing it down also helps you increase your understanding of your own cravings, quite often 'this too shall pass'.

11 Eat filling foods

Some foods naturally keep us full for longer and keep our cravings at bay. Fill up on protein, healthy fats and fibre, and swap unhealthy ultra-processed snacks for delicious, satisfying healthy alternatives.

12 Think positively
Celebrate how much fitter and healthier you feel than you did before. A Mediterranean-style diet can lift your mood and, paired with exercise, can help create a virtuous cycle of feeling good, which makes it easier to stick to eating well.

13 Challenge your inner critic and cultivate your inner coach
We can all fall into that trap of criticising ourselves; 'I have no willpower' or 'I'm useless'. But remember, the widespread availability of sweet, salty and fatty delights is designed to overcome your good intentions of healthy eating. They are designed to be addictive. Instead, turn your inner critic into a supportive health coach or a friend, and remind yourself how much progress you have made so far.

14 Eat mindfully
Take time to savour your food to enjoy the taste of it, to appreciate the smell and the texture. Eating mindfully is much easier if you are sitting at a dinner table rather than in front of the TV. It has been associated with less impulsive eating of junk, smaller portion sizes and healthier meals. It allows you to enjoy your food and appreciate it, instead of wolfing it down at speed.

15 And if you fall off the wagon...
Please be assured that all is not lost. We all have bad days when we return to unhealthy food choices! Just start again the next day. The sooner you get back on track, the better. Be kind to yourself, it's just a blip.

What is food noise?

The meteoric rise in popularity of weight-loss jabs has brought a new phrase into the modern vocabulary – 'food noise'. This refers to the internal chatter many people experience when it comes to food and hunger. Some lucky souls rarely 'hear' it, but plenty of other people live with a near-constant, rolling, food-related dialogue in their heads: they can't stop themselves thinking about planning their next meal, imagining the taste of it, wanting to eat it, or just looking at images of food online.

On a basic level, we need food noise in order to survive – it is all part of the message signalling that goes from our gut to our brain, telling us we are hungry and must take in some fuel. But for many people, food noise is so incessant and intrusive that it drives over-eating and a very unhealthy obsession with food.

For many users, the GLP-1 medications either hugely reduce food noise or they silence it altogether. Then, when you do eat, some users report being more inclined to crave healthy and wholesome food – the thought of booze or anything fatty or sugary makes them feel queasy. This factor alone makes the food restriction required for rapid weight loss so much easier to tolerate.

For those thinking of starting weight-loss medication

If you are thinking of starting GLP-1s, before you do, stop and think – are weight-loss drugs right for you? It is a big undertaking, costly and not without possible side effects. It might be wise to give the Fast 800 method a try first, as many thousands have done successfully before.

And just because your friend, neighbour, work colleague or partner is using weight-loss drugs, it doesn't mean this route is appropriate for you. If you have any doubts about whether it is the right course, I urge you to arrange a face-to-face consultation with a qualified health professional for an assessment. Don't rush into trying to get hold of these drugs without properly thinking through what you're doing.

Ask yourself, am I prepared for the ongoing cost? (The drugs are not a quick fix, and unless you change your diet and lifestyle, you might have to consider taking them for a prolonged period.) Am I prepared for possible side effects? Am I prepared to risk losing some enjoyment in food? How will I set myself up for success when I come off the weight-loss medications? Could I achieve the same results without medication?

Side effects of the GLP-1 medications

There can be significant side effects when using the GLP-1 weight-loss medications, and we have included details of the most common ones here. GLP-1s slow down the digestive tract. This is why problems can occur at both ends – nausea, vomiting, constipation and diarrhoea can ensue, but there are ways to try and mitigate this.

Nausea and vomiting

Nausea is extremely common among people using weight-loss medications. For many people this does dissipate over time, as you acclimatise to the dose, so be careful not to escalate the dose too quickly.

Vomiting can also occur, especially if you don't change the quality and quantity of what you eat. If you over-eat while on the medications, which is much easier to do with processed junk foods, you are more likely to vomit. Additionally, if you eat lots of fried foods and starchy carbs, like chips, this can also exacerbate vomiting. Every mouthful matters – food is competing for space in your now limited stomach space.

Constipation and diarrhoea

Constipation is often due to a number of factors. To start with, it can be caused by the slowing down of the bowel. However, it can also be exacerbated by a lack of fibre, fruit and veggies in the diet – essential roughage to keep those bowels plodding along nicely!

Paradoxically, diarrhoea can also be a side effect because GLP-1s can upset the coordination of the passage of food through your digestive tract.

Other uncomfortable gastro side effects can include bloating, reflux and eggy burps.

More serious side effects to be aware of, though relatively rare, include gallstones, pancreatitis and bowel blockages. This is a non-exhaustive list, so consult your doctor if you have any concerns or you think something isn't quite right.

GLP-1 weight-loss drugs Q&A

What are these drugs and how do they work? GLP-1 stands for Glucagon-like Peptide 1, which is a naturally occurring gut hormone. However, when we create our own version, it is broken down rapidly, in minutes. Some clever scientists figured out how to create a synthetic version that is broken down in not minutes, but days. The most important therapeutic effects of GLP-1 drugs, like Ozempic and Mounjaro, are three-fold: they help reduce blood sugar levels, by acting on the pancreas and liver. Slowing the emptying of stomach contents into the small intestines, further flattens blood sugar levels, while also increasing feelings of fullness. Thirdly, and most importantly, they act centrally on areas of the brain to reduce physical hunger and reward-driven hunger too (your food noise).

How do our bodies produce GLP-1 naturally? GLP-1 hormones are produced by the body in response to a meal. They are known as 'incretins' because they stimulate insulin in response to food consumption. They also help tell our bodies that we are full. GLP-1 is released shortly after we start eating and food enters our stomach and the early part of our small intestine. Protein, fibre and healthy fats are particularly potent at causing the release of our own natural GLP-1s. However, GLP-1 released by the body is broken down in minutes, whereas the synthetic GLP-1, found in medications like Ozempic, are chemically modified to take days to break down.

What are the benefits and drawbacks of the drugs? If you are overweight or living with obesity, it may be affecting your health, and the signs that this may be the case include high blood sugars, high cholesterol and high blood pressure, as well as a large number of obesity-related diseases. If you are living with obesity, obesity-related diseases or poor metabolic health, then losing weight can significantly improve your health. In trials, the weight-loss drugs were shown to lead to more than 15 per cent bodyweight loss over the course of a year. They have been associated with a reduction of heart disease, kidney disease, type 2 diabetes, fatty liver disease, sleep apnoea and perhaps even dementia. They are safer and more effective than any weight-loss medications that have previously been discovered. However, they are not without their risks, some of which I have discussed on page 25. Some of the downstream consequences are also worth understanding, including muscle loss. Malnutrition is another concern. Half of the people living with obesity have a micronutrient deficiency. If you are eating less – even of a poor-quality diet – you may be missing out on vital nutrients. Every bite counts when your food intake is inevitably restricted by the power of the medications.

Another thing to be aware of is the possible rapid return of your lost weight, which is something that can happen when you stop the medications, if your 'food noise' returns with a vengeance and your appetite races back. Studies show that after stopping the weight-loss medications, the average person has regained all the weight they initially lost by 20 months after stopping and those cardiometabolic markers have also returned to baseline. The weight regain is typically between 4 and 8 times faster after stopping the new generation of GLP-1s, compared to dieting without weight loss medications. This is why it is so vital to build healthy eating habits and lifestyle changes when you take the medications, so you can sustain weight loss once you stop them.

Why is it so important to maintain muscle while using losing weight? If you don't eat enough protein (at least 60g per day) when you are on weight-loss medications, your body will scavenge protein from your muscles, resulting in loss of lean muscle mass. So, it is important to include protein, such as fish, chicken, cheese, eggs, nuts or tofu, as a significant part of each meal. In the recipes we try to make sure that you get the nutrients you need, despite the calorie reduction.

Aerobic and strength-training exercises have been shown to be good for your heart, brain and mental health, as well as improving your overall mobility. But when you lose weight quickly, whether using weight-loss drugs or not, it's essential to maintain your lean muscle mass because when you lose weight rapidly, much of what you lose will be muscle.

Muscle really matters: it is metabolically active and requires more energy to maintain than fatty tissue. People with greater muscle mass burn more calories even when they are not exercising. Muscle keeps us young and fit, and it reduces the risk of type 2 diabetes and future frailty.

Eating plenty of protein will help protect your muscles, but exercise is an essential part of the muscle-preserving mix – in particular, resistance training. This is a type of exercise designed to increase the strength of our muscles, and it means repeatedly contracting the muscles against a heavy 'resistance' (such as a band or a weight). Many may think that these sorts of exercises are just for the young but they can benefit you at any age. Resistance training can take many forms. It could range from 'free weight' training, using dumbbells, barbells or kettlebells, to using machines in the gym. Bodyweight exercises, such as press-ups, squats or planks, are another option and can be easily carried out in the comfort of your home. Others may opt to use resistance bands, or train outdoors or in a group setting. Just pick what suits you best. Some people find group exercise a great option. We are social animals and it is a good way to meet others and improve our stamina and strength together. It may also provide you with more accountability and force you out of the door to attend a weekly or twice-weekly class. You are less likely to come up with an excuse not to go, if it has become embedded in your routine.

Why does fibre matter? Most of us eat about half the recommended fibre (which is around 30g of dietary fibre every day). It can be hard to achieve the recommended amount, particularly when you are reducing your calories. Aim to include good sources of fibre in every meal. Of course, once you are nearing your goal it will be easier to achieve a higher daily fibre count.

Most of the recipes here are paired with a combination of protein sources, as well as fibre. This means, including a wide variety of fibre-rich foods, such as beans, lentils, wholegrains, nuts and seeds, as well as vegetables –ideally unpeeled as that is where the best nutrients are stored. Fibre is important for maintaining a functioning digestive tract, something that will mitigate unwanted side effects, such as constipation or diarrhoea, both of which can be an issue with rapid weight loss, particularly on the GLPs. So, the better you feed your gut microbes with fibre, the more they look after you in return! With that in mind, we have found ways to slip extra fibre into meals that still taste delicious, as well as adding it to satisfying treats (for example, see page 260). Eating in this way, and with the support of a happy and healthy gut microbiome, your health and even your mood are bound to benefit.

FAQs

Does it matter if I eat 2 or 3 meals a day on a fast day? On the whole, it is probably easier to do 3 meals a day, but it's a matter of what works for you. We would advise, however, that you don't go down to one meal a day, particularly if it's soon before retiring to bed, as your body is more likely to treat it as a feast and store more fat. See the meal plans on pages 277–81 for more information.

Can I do it with shakes or protein powder, too? Yes, absolutely. We take a pragmatic view of meal replacement shakes. Eating real food is best, but if you are dashing out in a hurry and grabbing toast and jam for breakfast, or snatching a processed starchy lunch on the hoof, good-quality shakes are definitely preferable. They can help you top up the protein and nutrients you need, and leave you feeling full. Do choose carefully as many of those available are full of sugars and contain inadequate amounts of protein (see thefast800.com for suitable low-carb, Mediterranean-formula options).

Should I take multivitamins?
Our recipes are carefully balanced to include all the nutrients you need, but on a low-calorie diet it is not always easy to combine your meals for maximum nutritional variety, so we recommend taking a good-quality multivitamin on your 800–1000cals days as a back up.

What can I snack on? We encourage you to avoid snacking between meals as this stops fat burning and may put sugars up. But if you must, have a small handful of nuts (unsweetened as they become very moreish otherwise!), a few berries, or a handful of non-starchy veg, such as carrots, cauliflower or celery. Alternatively, try a hot or cold drink to help keep hunger at bay (see page 17).

Can I exercise on a fasting day? Doing more exercise helps us in lots of ways, including improving health and mood, but it's not a good way to lose weight. If you are already doing exercise and feel comfortable sticking with it on a fasting day, carry on with your current regime. But don't start a new, heavy programme or do endurance exercise on a fasting day. For those of you who have not been regular exercisers, you will find that as you lose weight you will feel better and have more energy and can get more active. Remember, it's not all about the gym. A lot of people surprise themselves and find they enjoy simple outdoor activities like walking or cycling. Walking with brief brisk bursts of 30–60 seconds can be a great way to start. And adding in some strengthening exercises will increase your muscle mass and improve your metabolism.

Can I exercise while I'm taking weight-loss drugs? In the big weight-loss drug studies, 25–40 per cent of the bodyweight lost was shown to be lean body mass, and the main component of that is muscle. Muscle and strength are associated with longevity, reducing frailty, a reduced risk of type 2 diabetes, and muscles burn more calories than fat. If you want to lose fat, while retaining muscle, the solution is fairly simple: increase your activity (consider basic strength training) while increasing your protein intake. To keep things very simple, you can start with 3 exercises from the comfort of your own home – press ups (starting from your knees, if necessary), lunges and squats. These require no weights, no gym and no equipment. Give it a go when you wake up in the morning and it will give you a nice endorphin buzz to start the day.

Aerobic and strength-training exercises have been shown to be good for your heart, brain and mental health, as well as improving your overall mobility. While it's certainly true 'you can't outrun a bad diet', exercising is a great way to achieve weight-loss maintenance aka keeping that weight off for the long term. Ingraining those habits early in the process is vital if you want to keep them up, if and when you stop the weight-loss medications.

I have lost weight but recently hit a plateau. What can I do? It is common for weight loss to happen in bursts. Initial weight loss can be deceptive, as early on it also includes fluid loss. But if you stick to 800–1000cals you are likely to go on losing weight. When the weight loss seems to stall, some people find adding in shakes as part of their daily quota on a fasting day can help. It's also worth checking that you are still in the 800–1000cals zone. However, we are all different and some people will find that their weight loss is slower.

Can I eat bread? When it comes to bread, it's about choosing carefully, as white bread and a slice of seeded wholemeal sourdough are like chalk and cheese. You can occasionally have a thin slice of wholegrain, seeded or sourdough bread on a non-fast day, but try to avoid it on a fasting day. When you are buying bread, try to make sure the fibre content is higher than 7g in 100g.

Will I feel hungry all the time on a fasting day? For the first few days you are likely to feel hungry, but most people find that this settles as their metabolism re-sets. People often tell me how surprised they are that, despite such a dramatic drop in their daily calorie intake, within a week or two, they are no longer hungry all the time.

What if I am using weight-loss drugs and don't feel hungry at all? It is still important to ensure you are nourishing your body with nutritious foods. Go through the motions, make simple meals that are packed with nutrients (such as the ones in this book). Don't waste your time grazing on junk. We want to make sure we are still getting enough protein, healthy fats, fibre, vitamins, minerals and polyphenols, too. If you really, really aren't eating, it may be that you are on too high a dose and perhaps it would be a better move to a lower dose. Consult your clinician if you are concerned.

Should I tell my doctor/health professional that I am doing a low-calorie diet? It is always a good idea to keep your health professional informed about a major change to your diet, particularly if you have a medical condition and/or are on medication (see SAFETY: Exclusions and cautions on page 20). It may help to print out a letter advising them about the diet, so they can monitor and support you in the process. This can be found at thefast800.com/healthcareprofessionals. Most health professionals will be aware of the 800-calorie approach and will be supportive.

Should I contact my doctor/health professional to inform them that I am using weight-loss medication, if they have not prescribed it? Yes. Jack is a doctor working in general practice and Clare is a retired GP. From their joint perspective, it is always important to have that sort of information available about a patient, because it can change their practice. What's more, if you are planning to have surgery any time soon, then it is absolutely vital to inform your doctor. GLP-1 medications dramatically slow down stomach emptying, which can increase risks during surgery if not managed appropriately.

I'm taking weight-loss medication and want to come off it. How do I do this? As of yet, there is no hard-and-fast rule here. It is not dangerous to stop suddenly; however, your food noise may come racing back more quickly. An alternative would be to slowly reduce the dose over time, so you can become used to your returning appetite. Whatever decision you choose, speak to whoever has prescribed it to you first.

Should I microdose my weight-loss medication? Microdosing is a fascinating area. However, I cannot in good faith recommend microdosing, when there hasn't been research to establish its safety or efficacy. Could the weight-loss drugs have extra benefits beyond weight loss and lower blood sugar? Possibly. However, as far as we know, the majority of the benefits are as a result of the weight loss.

Some useful tools and tricks

How to measure your waist accurately with a tape measure. Locate the top of your hip bone and the bottom of your ribs and measure halfway between them, typically this is just above the belly button. Wrap a measuring tape around the mid-section, and breathe out naturally.

A set of scales is useful, and you might also consider investing in a blood pressure monitor.

Keto stix (a urine dipstick to measure if you are in nutritional ketosis – i.e. burning ketones from fat instead of burning sugar); these can be helpful at first or if you hit a plateau. Please note that ketosis reduces after a few weeks, but weight loss continues, although at a slower rate.

Studies have shown that keeping a **diet journal** can be hugely helpful when you are trying to lose weight. Try our book *The Fast 800 Health Journal* to help monitor your progress and to keep yourself motivated.

Only minimal cooking equipment required! Useful kit includes: a stick blender, some digital kitchen scales, a set of measuring spoons, a small and medium saucepan, a flameproof casserole with well-fitting lid, a wide frying pan or wok, a metal baking tray, baking dish (optional), medium bowl, vegetable peeler, spiraliser (optional) and a good sharp knife.

Tips for using this book

- **Calorie counts** These refer to one individual serving, unless stated otherwise. Please be aware that we include calories as a rough guide only. There are significant variations between different nutritionists, counters and apps, so don't be too concerned by a few extra calories here or there.

- **Increase non-starchy veg and reduce calorie counting** We encourage you to enjoy green and non-starchy veg without counting calories. Pile half your plate with 'free' vegetables, such as leafy greens, salad leaves or celery, which have minimal calories but huge nutritional benefits (see page 274 for non-starchy greens and veg). It's fine to add a dash of olive oil or a little butter without counting, as it enhances the flavour and nutrients. And, of course, you might want to add a dressing or a teaspoonful of extra-virgin olive oil – in which case, see page 274 for calories.

- **Suggestions for non-fast days** We offer tips if you are on the New 5:2 or have moved on to a maintenance stage to adapt the recipes to make them more substantial. These might involve simply increasing or doubling the portion size, or adding a few tablespoons of brown rice or lentils, an extra glug of olive oil, a slice of seeded bread or extra vegetables.

- **Make the recipes suit you** These recipes are based on a Med-style way of eating, but can be adapted to fit different cuisines and tastes. Feel free to use alternative flavours, or add different herbs and spices – all of which have minimal impact on calories. The tastier and more satisfying you find your food, the more likely you are to stick to this way of eating.

SYMBOLS

We have added the following symbols to the bottom of each page, so you can quickly spot which recipes might suit you best.

VEGAN Vegan

VEGGIE Vegetarian

GLUTEN FREE Gluten free

NUT FREE Nut free

DAIRY FREE Dairy free

Freezer friendly

Super speedy

You will also find nutritional information above each recipe, including calories (cals), for each individual serving.

Although some of the recipes included here are vegan, the Fast 800 is not designed for vegans.

We have included adaptations for air fryers where appropriate.

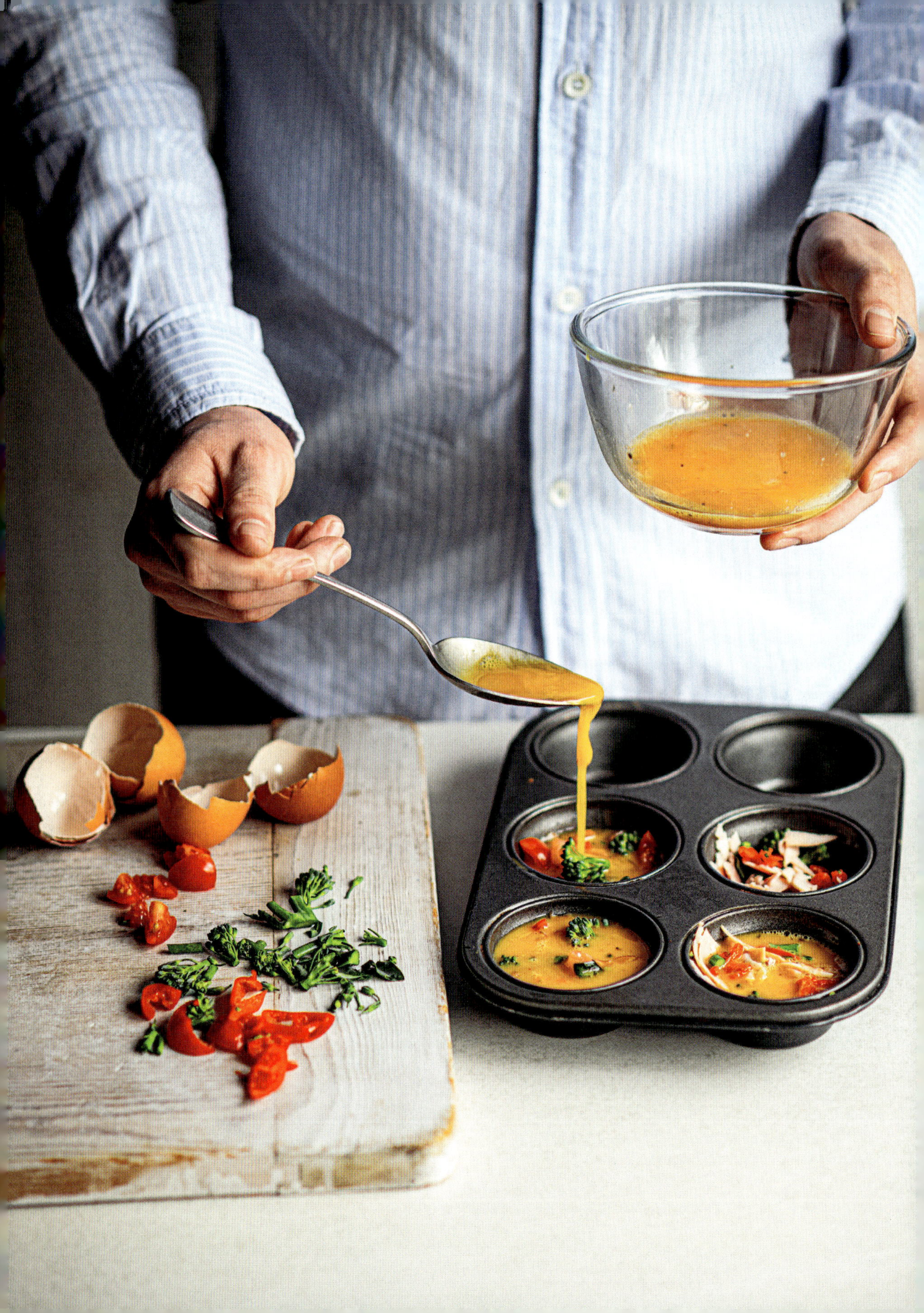

Breakfast and Brunch

UNDER 400 CALORIES

PER SERVING | **356cals** | PROTEIN **24.5g** | CARBS **19g** | FIBRE **1.5g**

Scrambled Eggs with Parmesan and Greens

SERVES **1** | PREP **5** mins | COOK **5** mins

Knob of butter
2 eggs
1 slice of sourdough, wholegrain, seeded or rye bread, toasted
Handful of baby spinach, rocket leaves or cooked greens
1 tbsp grated Parmesan

This is one of my go-to breakfasts – creamy scrambled egg, grated Parmesan and ground black pepper served on seeded sourdough toast, this delivers plenty of umami flavour and lots of protein.

1. Melt the butter in a small frying pan over a medium heat.

2. Break the eggs into a bowl and whisk with a fork. Add a pinch of salt and black pepper, then tip the eggs into the pan. Stir over the heat for a few minutes, until soft and creamy. Be careful not to overcook.

3. Place the toast on a plate and top with the spinach, rocket or greens. Spoon the eggs on to the veg, then sprinkle with the grated Parmesan. Finally, add some extra black pepper to serve.

NUT FREE

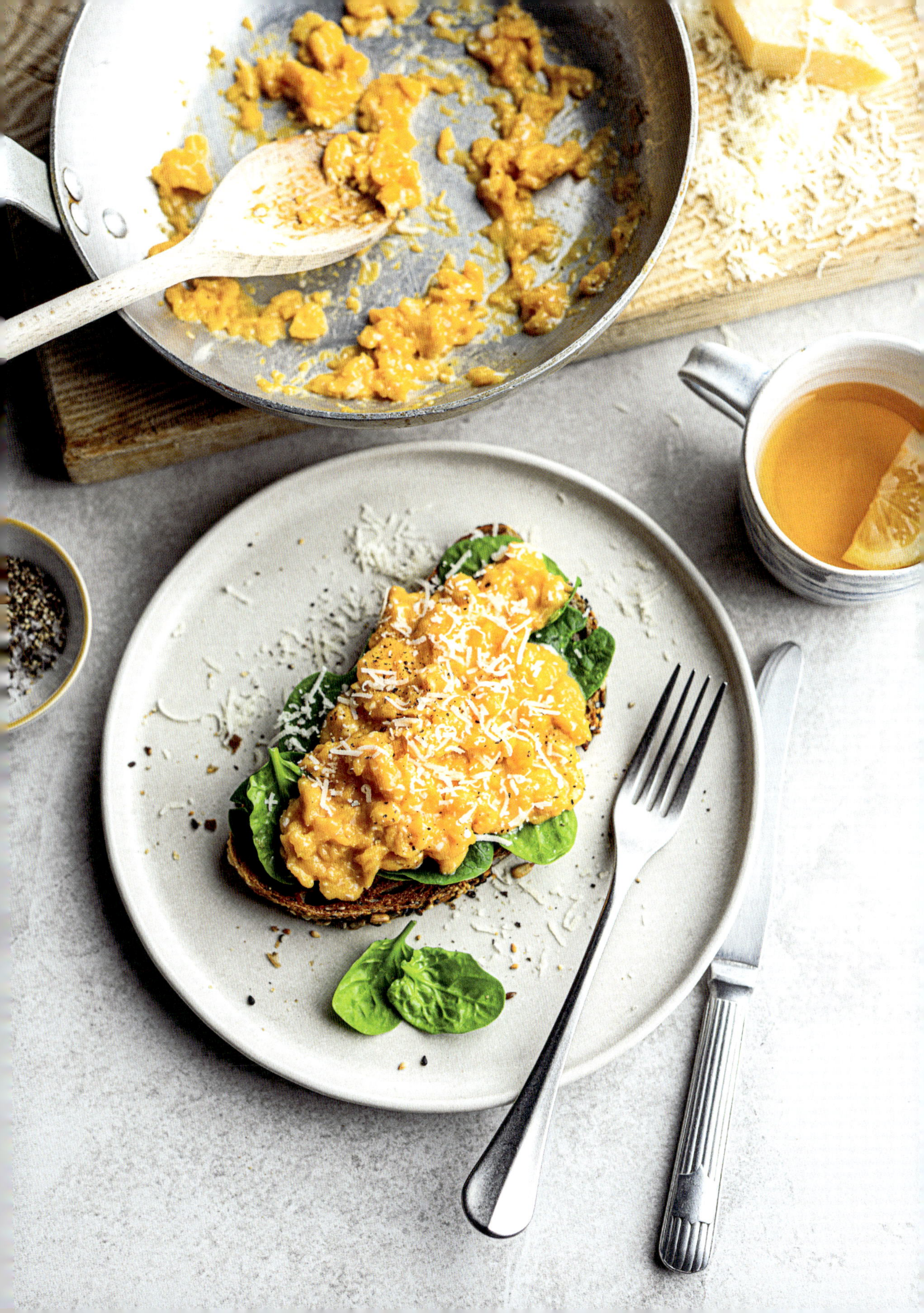

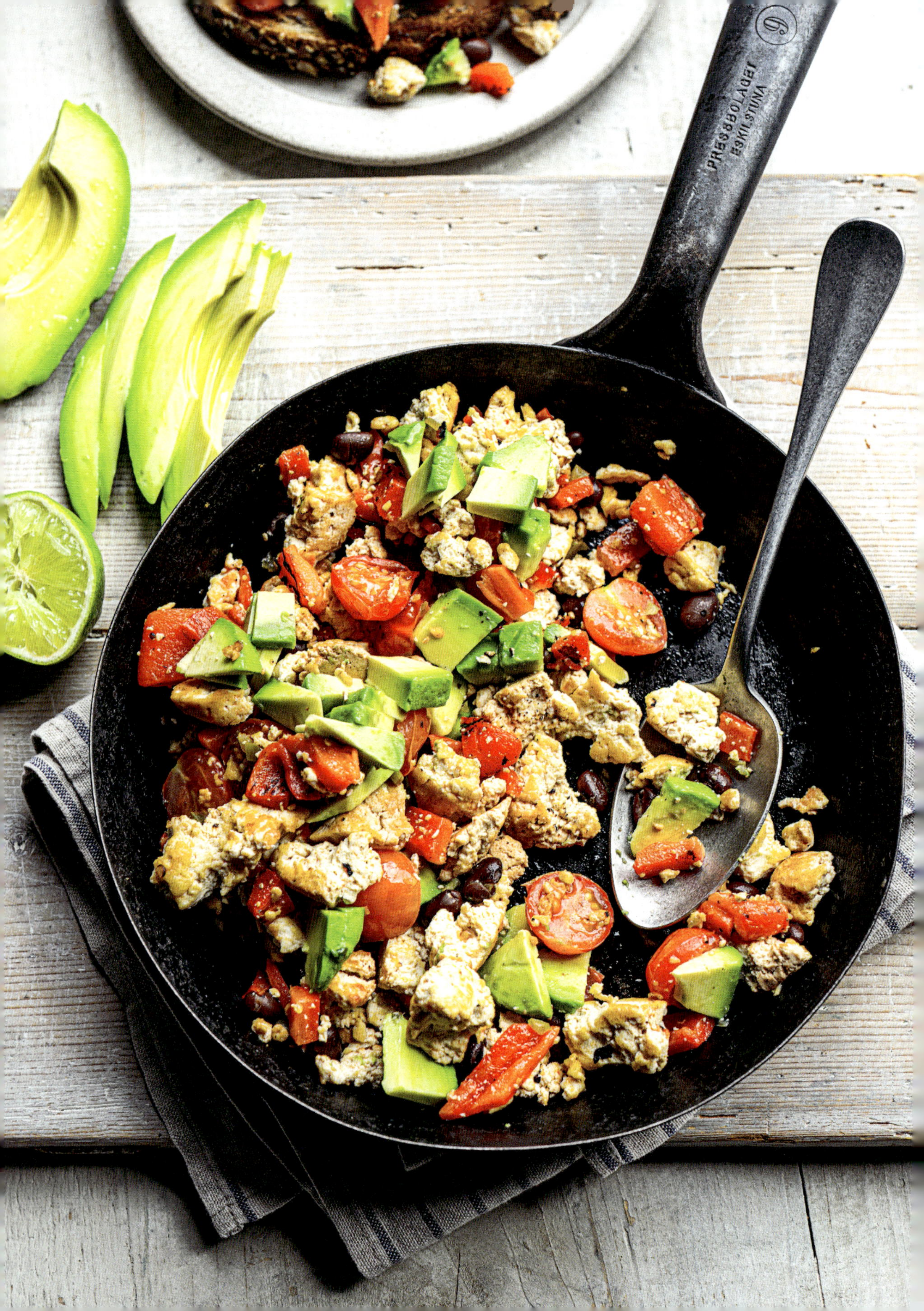
PRESSBOLAGET
ESKILSTUNA

PER SERVING | **432cals** | PROTEIN **24g** | CARBS **18g** | FIBRE **8g**

UNDER 500 CALORIES

Mexican-style Scrambled Tofu

SERVES 2 | PREP 10 mins | COOK 8 mins

1 tbsp olive oil
1 × 225g or 300g pack of smoked tofu, crumbled
8 cherry tomatoes, halved
2 tbsp cooked black beans
10g jalapeño peppers, diced (or to taste)
1 roasted pepper from a jar, roughly chopped
1 avocado, peeled, destoned and cubed
Juice of ½ lime
2 thin slices of wholegrain, seeded or sourdough bread, toasted

Spice up your scrambled tofu with a Mexican theme – mildly smoky, with sweet jalapeño peppers and soft black beans, this is made all in one pan. The black beans and avocado top up the fibre nicely. For extra protein and fibre, add 1–2 tablespoons of toasted seeds, or the Seedy Sprinkles from page 39.

1. Heat the oil in a small frying pan over a medium heat.

2. Add the tofu, cherry tomatoes, black beans, jalapeños and roasted pepper, and cook for 5 minutes, stirring occasionally.

3. Stir in the avocado, add a generous pinch of salt and black pepper, then squeeze in the lime juice.

4. Divide the toast between two plates then share the scrambled tofu between them to serve.

VEGAN | NUT FREE | DAIRY FREE

UNDER 300 CALORIES

PER SERVING | **290cals** | PROTEIN **17.5g** | CARBS **3g** | FIBRE **2.5g**

Harissa Scrambled Eggs

SERVES 2 | PREP 10 mins | COOK 8 mins

½ tbsp olive oil
8 cherry tomatoes
4 eggs
1 tsp harissa paste
½ avocado, peeled, destoned and sliced
1 tbsp Seedy Sprinkles (see opposite), to serve

Michael and I liked to jazz up our scrambled eggs, and it doesn't take much to change the flavour and make it more exotic. Perfect for a relaxed brunch.

1. Heat the oil in a frying pan over a medium heat. Add the tomatoes and cook for a couple of minutes.

2. Meanwhile, break the eggs into a bowl and whisk with a fork. Add the eggs to the pan, then drizzle in the harissa paste. Let the eggs cook for a few seconds undisturbed, then stir gently. Continue to cook until the eggs are mostly set.

3. Divide between two plates and serve with the sliced avocado and a scattering of seeds.

VEGGIE | GLUTEN FREE | NUT FREE | DAIRY FREE

SOY SEEDS PER TBSP	SEEDS WITH ZA'ATAR PER TBSP	SMOKY SEEDS PER TBSP
37cals	**43cals**	**39cals**
PROTEIN **1.5g**	PROTEIN **1.5g**	PROTEIN **1.5g**
CARBS **2g**	CARBS **2g**	CARBS **2g**
FIBRE **0.5g**	FIBRE **1g**	FIBRE **0.5g**

UNDER 100 CALORIES

Seedy Sprinkles

SERVES **4** | PREP **5** mins | COOK **5** mins

A choice of differently flavoured seedy sprinkles to scatter over the top of your boiled egg (see page 41), a salad or soup.

SOY SEEDS
4 tbsp mixed seeds
1 tsp reduced-salt light soy sauce

SEEDS WITH ZA'ATAR
4 tbsp mixed seeds
2 tsp za'atar

SMOKY SEEDS
4 tbsp mixed seeds
1 tsp hot or sweet smoked paprika
½ tsp garlic granules (optional)

1. Whichever your flavour, tip the seeds into a frying pan and spread out evenly. Toast over a low heat for 4–5 minutes, turning the seeds frequently until they start to colour and pop. Keep an eye on them as you don't want them to darken too much or burn.

2. Take the pan off the heat and tip them into a bowl, then stir in either the soy sauce, za'atar or smoked paprika and garlic granules, depending on your choice of flavouring. The seed mix can be stored in an airtight jar for up to 5 days.

VEGGIE · NUT FREE · DAIRY FREE

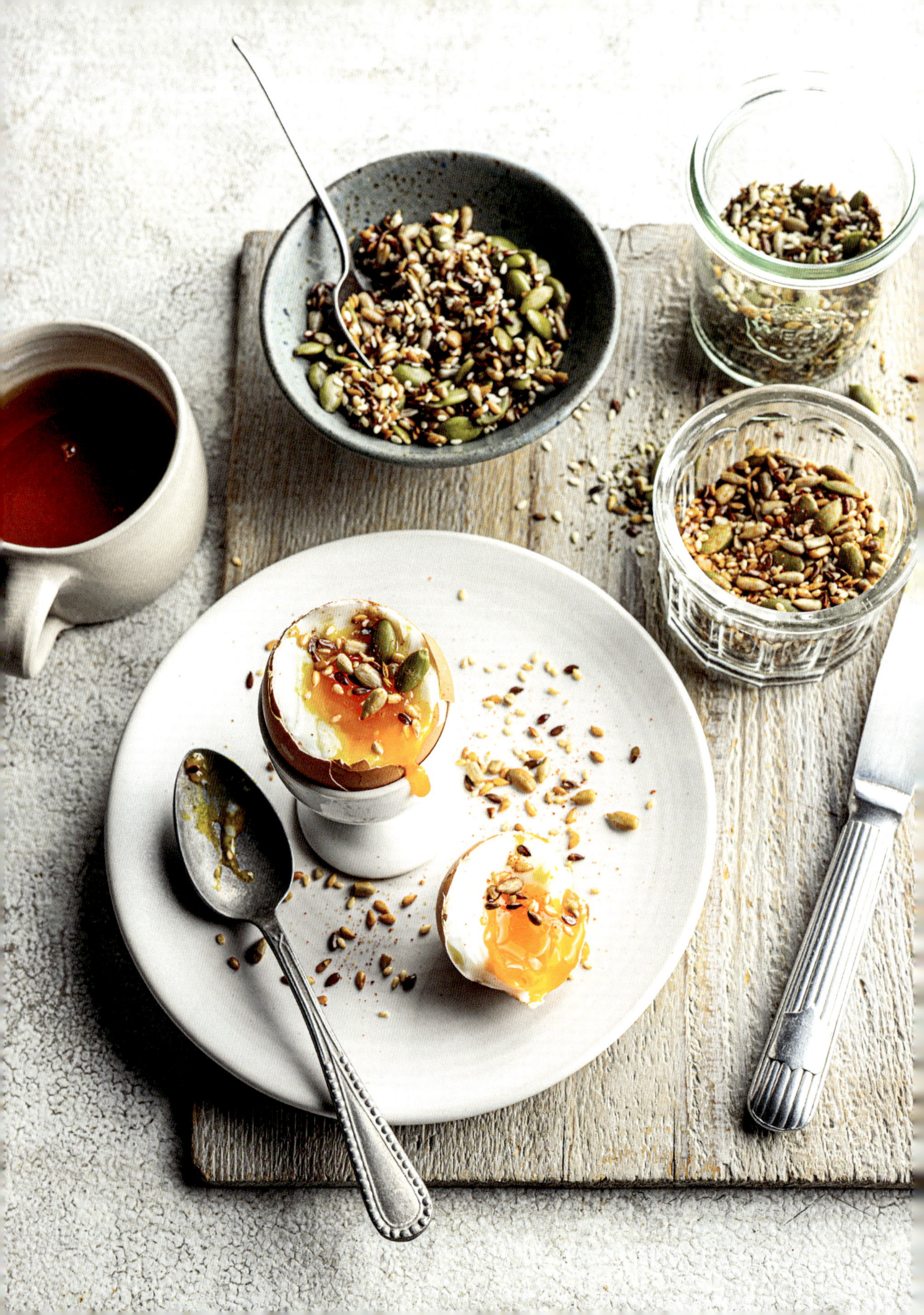

PER SERVING | 117cals | PROTEIN 9g | CARBS 2g | FIBRE 0.5g

UNDER 200 CALORIES

Boiled Egg with Seedy Sprinkles

SERVES 1 | PREP 2 mins | COOK 6 mins

1 medium egg, at room temperature
½ tbsp your choice of Seedy Sprinkles (see page 39)

A boiled egg makes a simple, high-protein start to the day. Here, it is served with your choice of flavoured seedy sprinkles to scatter over the top. Serve the egg with a slice of rye bread, cut into soldiers, if you like.

1. Bring a small saucepan of water to the boil. Reduce the heat to a simmer and carefully lower the egg into the pan. Cook for 6 minutes for a set white and runny yolk.

2. Transfer the egg to an egg cup, slice the top, and serve sprinkled with your choice of seeds.

VEGGIE | GLUTEN FREE | NUT FREE | DAIRY FREE

UNDER 400 CALORIES

PER SWEET SERVING	PER SAVOURY SERVING
318cals	**355cals**
PROTEIN **14.5g**	PROTEIN **15g**
CARBS **19g**	CARBS **18g**
FIBRE **3.5g**	FIBRE **4.5g**

High-protein Pancakes

SERVES **2** | PREP **18** mins | COOK **6** mins

40g rolled oats
100g cottage cheese
1 egg
1½ tbsp full-fat milk
1 tsp chia seeds
½ tsp baking powder
½ tsp ground cinnamon (if making the sweet version)
10g butter, for cooking

For the sweet topping
3 tbsp full-fat Greek yoghurt
Handful of berries (such as strawberries, blueberries or raspberries), or sliced banana
15g toasted hazelnuts or pecans, roughly chopped (optional)

For the savoury topping
50g cottage cheese
1 small avocado, peeled, destoned and sliced
2 tsp diced jalapeños (or 1–2 tsp sriracha)
1 tbsp Seedy Sprinkles (see page 39, optional)

With a few easy tweaks, these versatile and delicious pancakes provide a good amount of protein along with fibre, making them an excellent way to start the day, so you won't reach for a pastry mid-morning. The savoury version could also be served as a light meal or lunch, topped with a runny-yolked egg and rocket leaves.

1. Put all the pancake ingredients in a high-speed blender with a pinch of salt and blend for 1 minute until smooth and creamy. Set the batter aside for 15 minutes to let it rest.

2. Melt half the butter in a large, non-stick frying pan over a medium–low heat and swirl the pan to lightly coat the base. Add 3 tablespoons of batter per pancake to the pan and cook for about 2–3 minutes on each side until golden. Keep the pancakes warm in a low oven while you make the rest, if you have cooked them in batches. The quantity makes 4 in total.

3. Serve the pancakes with your choice of topping.

VEGGIE

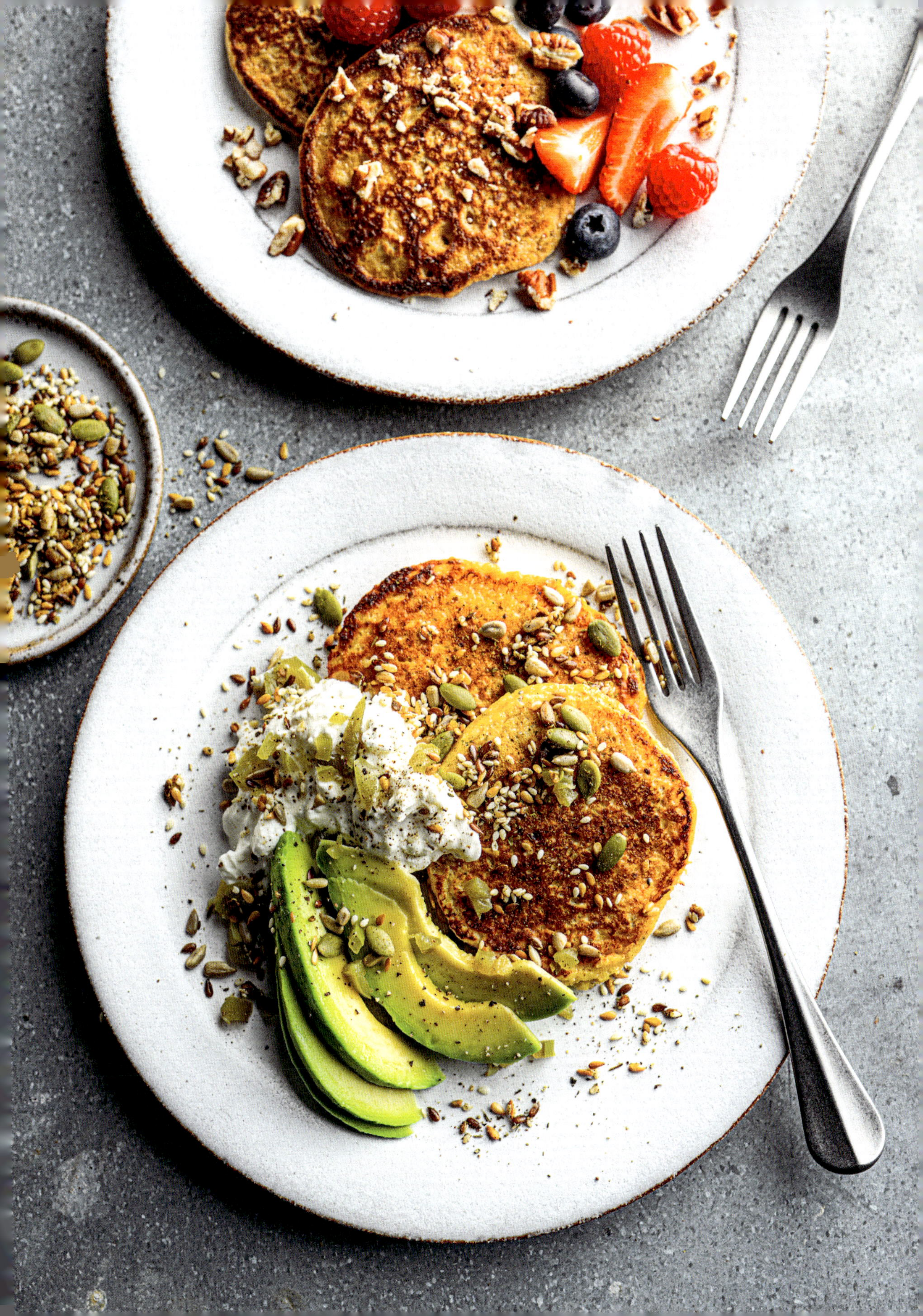

UNDER 500 CALORIES

PER SERVING | **434cals** | PROTEIN **14g** | CARBS **27g** | FIBRE **5g**

Creamy Quinoa Porridge

SERVES **2** | PREP **2** mins | COOK **15** mins

300ml full-fat milk
65g quinoa
2 tsp ground cinnamon
2 tbsp full-fat Greek yoghurt
60g pecans, chopped
1 small handful of berries

Quinoa is soft and slightly chewy. It delivers more fibre, and 2–3 times more protein than oat porridge. Unlike porridge, quinoa is a complete protein and contains all 9 essential amino acids, so that should set you up for the day!

1. Add the milk, quinoa and cinnamon to a small pan and place over a gentle heat. Bring to a simmer and cook for 15 minutes, stirring frequently, until cooked and creamy.

2. Remove from the heat and stir in the Greek yoghurt. Add a splash of water to loosen, if needed.

3. Divide between two bowls and top with the chopped pecans and a handful of berries to serve.

VEGGIE GLUTEN FREE

PER SERVING | **222cals** | PROTEIN **9g** | CARBS **15g** | FIBRE **4g**

UNDER 300 CALORIES

Make Your Own Muesli

MAKES 6 portions | PREP 10 mins

12 tbsp roughly chopped mixed nuts
12 tbsp rolled oats
6 tsp chia seeds
12 tbsp toasted spelt (I use Rude Health toasted spelt flakes)
6 tsp ground flaxseed
3 apricots, diced

Instead of rummaging through the cupboards to find the components of your favourite muesli, make it in large quantities, so that it is always ready to go. That way, you are less likely to go for the sweet processed version. You can use whichever nuts you like – they all provide a variation of nutrients depending on the nut. The toasted spelt adds crunch as well as fibre.

1. Combine all the ingredients in a large Kilner jar or airtight container.

2. For each serving, place 6 tablespoons of the muesli in a bowl and top with 115ml milk of choice. For extra protein add 2 tablespoons of Greek yoghurt, and if you still have a bit of a sweet tooth, add a dash of maple syrup, too.

VEGAN · GLUTEN FREE · DAIRY FREE

UNDER 200 CALORIES

PER MUFFIN | **118cals** | PROTEIN **9g** | CARBS **0.5g** | FIBRE **0.5g**

Easy Breakfast Eggy Muffins

MAKES **4** | PREP **15** mins | COOK **20** mins

1 tbsp olive oil or butter, for greasing
1–2 broccoli spears, chopped
4 eggs
1 slice of ham, torn (about 25g)
1 sweet piquanté pepper from a jar, sliced
1 slice of smoked salmon, torn (about 25g)
1 cherry tomato, sliced

These colourful and tasty muffins are perfect for a quick breakfast, but also ideal for a lunch box eaten cold. They'll make an ideal healthy snack if you have just one.

1. Preheat the oven to 190°C/Fan 170°C/Gas 5. Lightly grease 4 muffin holes with oil or butter.

2. Divide the broccoli between the 4 muffin holes.

3. Crack the eggs into a jug and whisk lightly with a fork. Season with salt and black pepper, then pour into the muffin holes.

4. Divide the ham and piquanté pepper between 2 holes, and the smoked salmon and cherry tomato between the 2 remaining holes. Cook in the preheated oven for 20 minutes or until firm.

5. Serve 1–2 muffins per person.

GLUTEN FREE NUT FREE

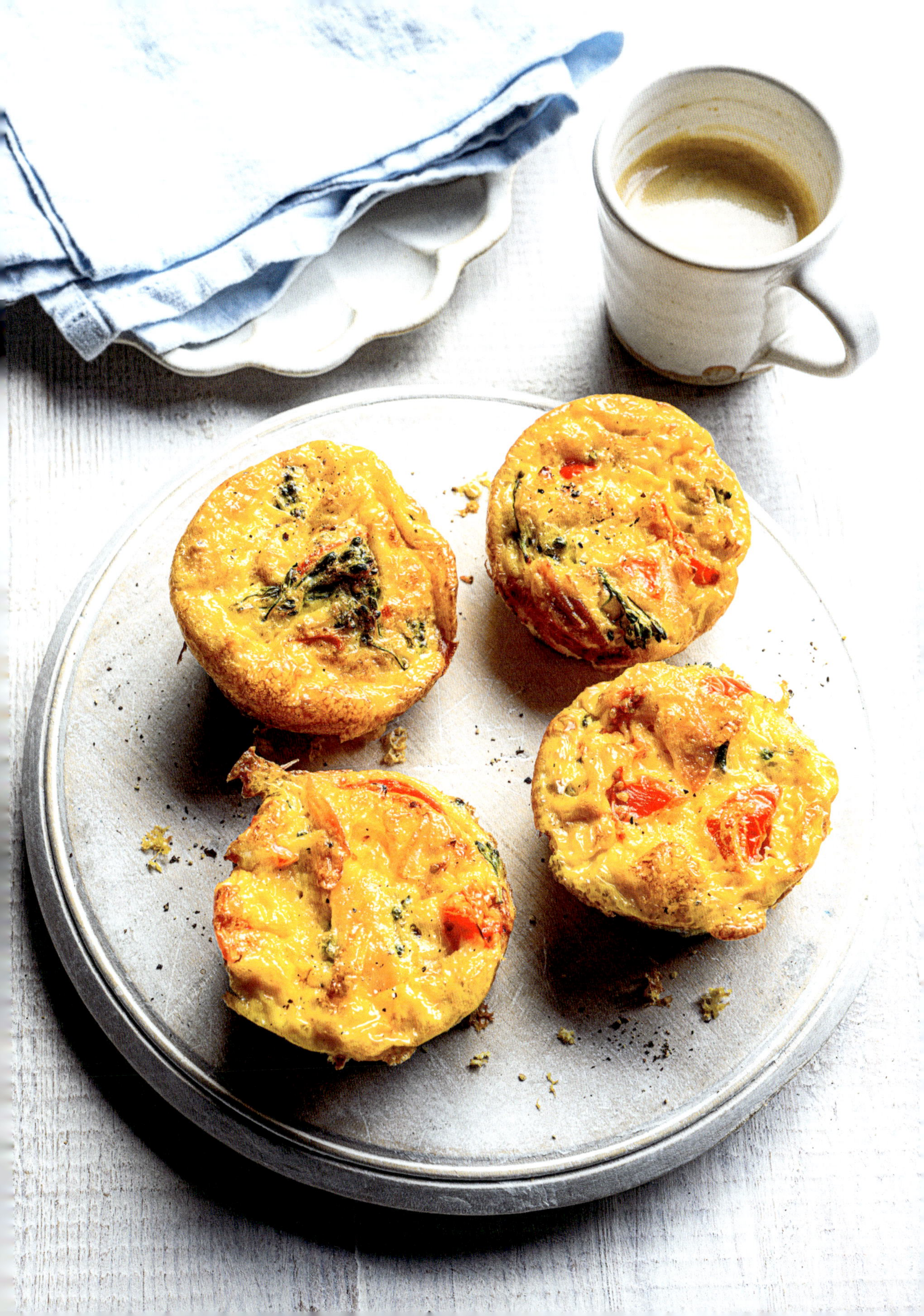

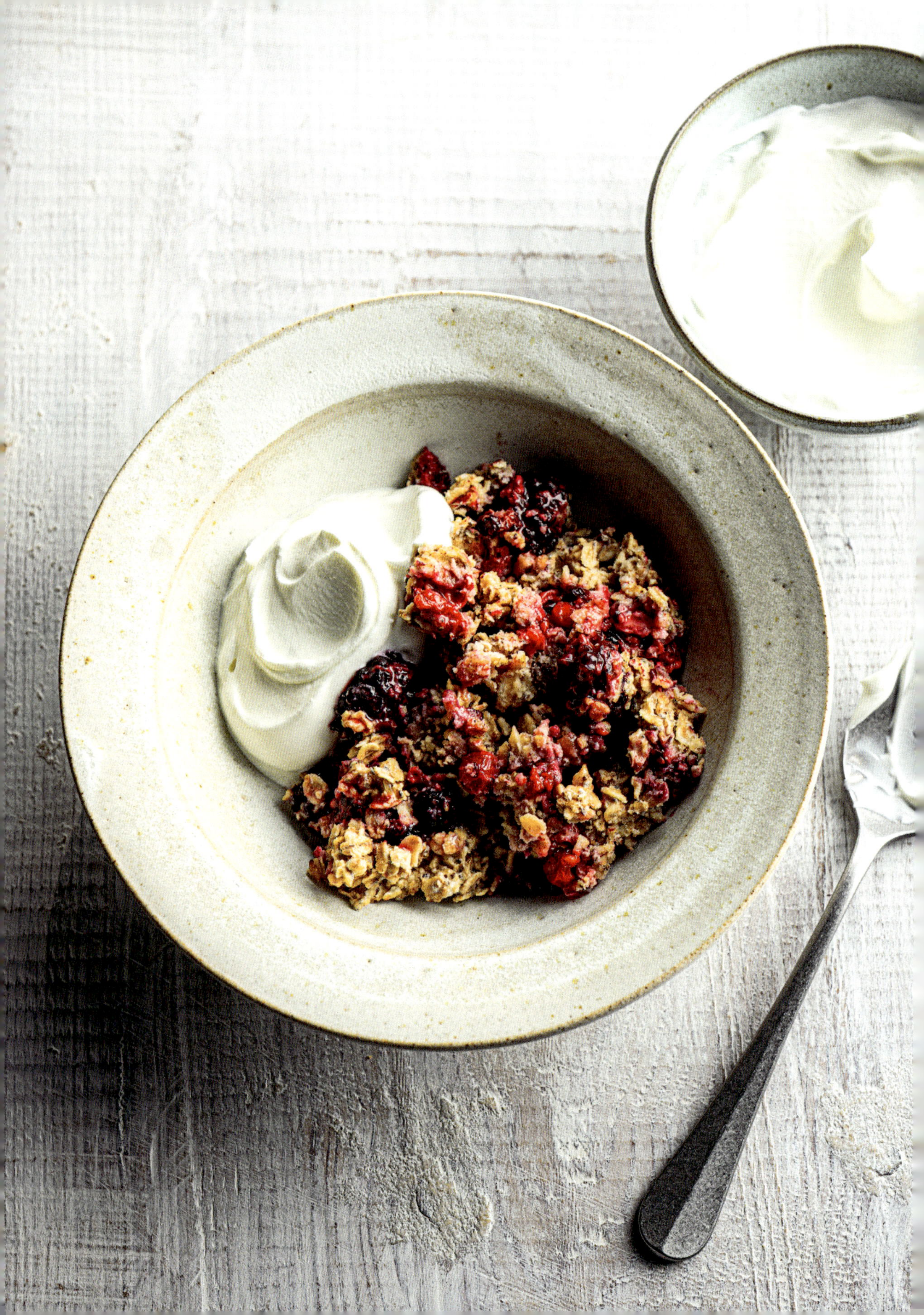

PER SERVING | **338cals** | PROTEIN **12g** | CARBS **28g** | FIBRE **7g**

UNDER 400 CALORIES

Baked Berry Oats

SERVES **1** | PREP **5** mins | COOK **20** mins

30g rolled oats
5g chia seeds
60ml unsweetened almond milk
50g assorted berries, fresh or frozen
¼ tsp vanilla extract
20g crunchy or smooth peanut butter
¼ tsp baking powder
30g full-fat Greek yoghurt

Luxurious comfort food, high in fibre and in protein, which will keep you feeling full for longer, thanks particularly to the chia seeds, oats and Greek yoghurt. It's a favourite from the Fast 800 programme. You could make this in larger batches, although you will need to extend the baking time – an extra 5–10 minutes per serve should work. Store leftovers in an airtight container in the fridge for up to 3 days or in the freezer for up to 2 months.

1. Preheat the oven to 200°C/Fan 180°C/Gas mark 6.

2. Mix all the ingredients except the yoghurt thoroughly in a small baking dish or oven-safe bowl.

3. Bake in the preheated oven for 15–20 minutes.

4. Set aside to cool for 5 minutes, then serve with the yoghurt on top.

VEGGIE GLUTEN FREE

UNDER 400 CALORIES

PER SERVING | **319cals** | PROTEIN **12.5g** | CARBS **26g** | FIBRE **4g**

Satisfying Raspberry Overnight Oats

SERVES 2 | PREP 5 mins

45g jumbo oats
1 tbsp chia seeds
½ tsp ground cinnamon
125ml full-fat Greek yoghurt
Squeeze of lemon
125ml milk, plus extra to serve
20g mixed nuts, chopped
Drizzle of maple syrup
30g raspberries

Perfect if you have to dash out in a hurry in the morning, as these oats are easy to take with you. Rich in protein and fibre, the second portion will keep an extra day in the fridge. Experiment with different fruit, including apples or other types of berries, and different spices, such as nutmeg, cardamom, or try chopped fresh mint.

1. Combine all the ingredients, except the raspberries, in a bowl, and mix well.

2. Divide the mixture between two bowls or jars, and top with the raspberries.

3. Cover with a lid or some cling film and place in the fridge overnight.

4. The next morning, the overnight oats will be ready for breakfast. Loosen with some extra milk, if necessary.

VEGGIE GLUTEN FREE

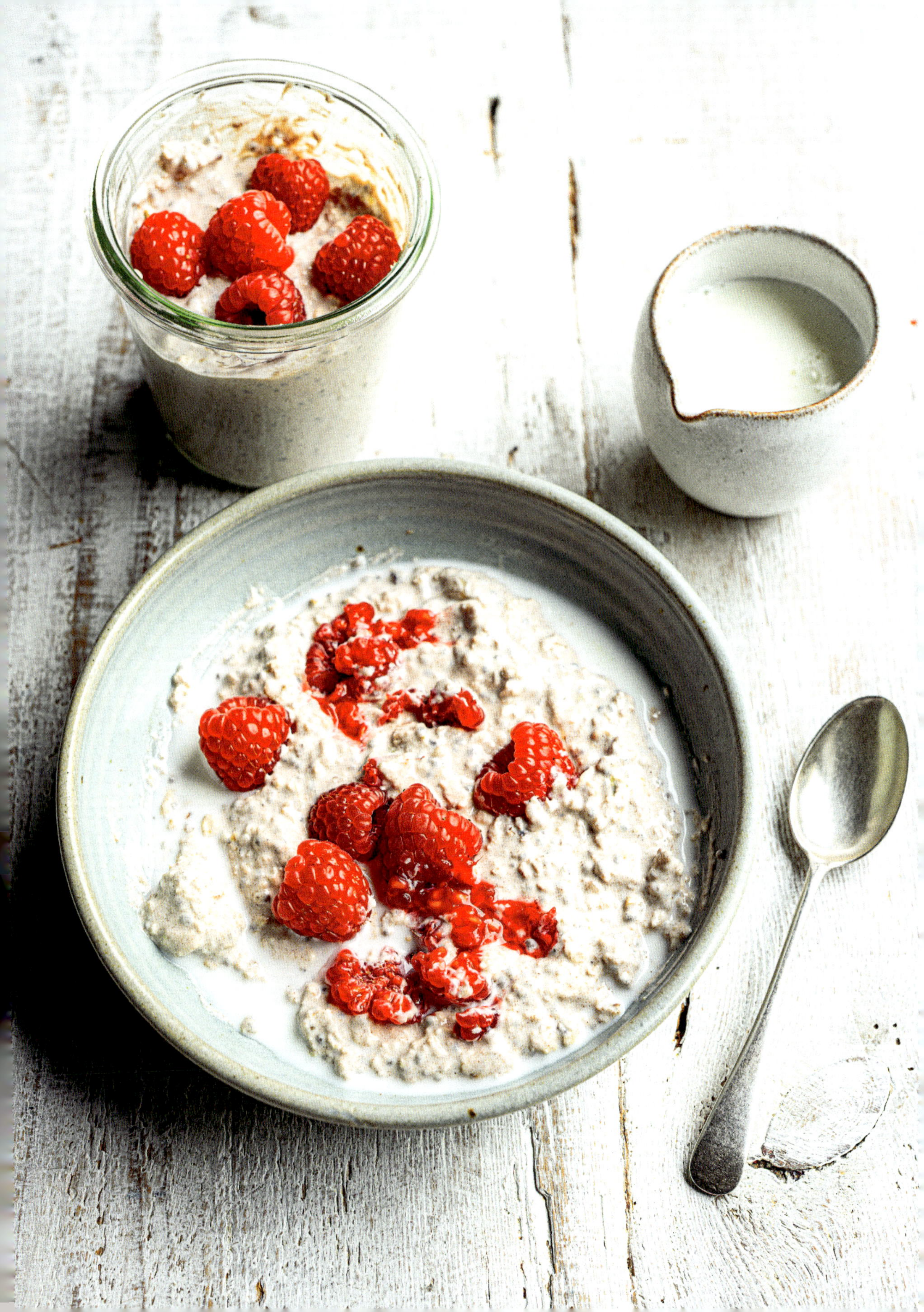

TOFU PROTEIN POTS 3 WAYS

Rich in protein, soft silken tofu is ideal for a creamy breakfast or a small dessert. If you aren't familiar with tofu, it is worth getting to know it as another easy source of quality protein. The base is the same with all three versions here. Apricot, blueberry or chocolate – take your pick!

UNDER 300 CALORIES

PER SERVING | **200cals** | PROTEIN **10g** | CARBS **21.5g** | FIBRE **6g**

Apricot Protein Pot

SERVES 1 | PREP 5 mins

⅓ × 300g pack of silken tofu
½ tsp vanilla extract
1 tsp chia seeds
½ tsp ground cardamom or ground cinnamon
4 apricots, snipped with scissors

For the hazelnut topping
5g hazelnuts, chopped
1 tsp maple syrup

1. Place the silken tofu, vanilla, chia seeds, cardamom and apricots in a small bowl and use a stick blender, or place in a food processor, and blitz for about 30–60 seconds until a smooth consistency.

2. Spoon into a serving bowl and sprinkle the chopped hazelnuts over the top. Drizzle with the maple syrup to serve. It can be eaten immediately but is also nice cold from the fridge. The protein pot will keep in the fridge for up to 3 days.

VEGAN GLUTEN FREE DAIRY FREE

PER SERVING | **118cals** | PROTEIN **8g** | CARBS **10.5g** | FIBRE **3.5g**

UNDER 200 CALORIES

Blueberry Protein Pot

SERVES **1** | PREP **5** mins

⅓ × 300g pack of silken tofu
½ tsp vanilla extract or ground cinnamon
1 tsp chia seeds
80g blueberries, plus a few extra to finish

1. Place all the ingredients in a small bowl and use a stick blender, or place in a food processor, and blitz for about 30–60 seconds until a smooth consistency.

2. Spoon into a serving bowl and scatter over the extra blueberries to serve. It can be eaten immediately but is also nice cold from the fridge. The protein pot will keep in the fridge for up to 3 days.

PER SERVING | **185cals** | PROTEIN **10g** | CARBS **19g** | FIBRE **5g**

UNDER 200 CALORIES

Chocolate Protein Pot

SERVES **1** | PREP **5** mins

⅓ × 300g pack of silken tofu
1 tsp vanilla extract or ground cinnamon
1 tsp chia seeds
1 level tsp unsweetened cocoa powder
1 Medjool date, pitted
Handful of fresh or frozen raspberries, to serve
A few walnuts, chopped, to serve (optional)

1. Place all the ingredients, except the raspberries and walnuts, in a small bowl and use a stick blender, or place in a food processor, and blitz for about 30–60 seconds until a smooth consistency.

2. Spoon into a serving bowl and scatter over the raspberries and walnuts, if using, to serve. It can be eaten immediately but is also nice cold from the fridge. The protein pot will keep in the fridge for up to 3 days.

VEGAN | GLUTEN FREE | NUT FREE | DAIRY FREE

UNDER 300 CALORIES

PER SERVING | **215cals** | PROTEIN **15g** | CARBS **16g** | FIBRE **2.5g**

Kipper on Toast with Roasted Peppers

SERVES 2 | PREP 2 mins | COOK 3 mins

1 kipper in a bag
1 red pepper from a jar, drained and sliced
2 slices of wholemeal, seeded or sourdough bread, toasted
Pinch of chilli flakes (optional)
1 tbsp roughly chopped parsley leaves
2 lemon wedges, to serve

Another family favourite; this is one of the quickest breakfasts and the kipper is almost ready by the time the toast pops up! Kippers are one of the best sources of fish oil, giving us omega 3, which most of us are not getting enough of – and the sweet peppers cut through the oil.

1. Remove the kipper from the packet. Separate the fillets and place them on a microwave-safe plate.

2. Scatter the slices of red pepper on top of the kipper fillets, then microwave on high for 2½–3 minutes.

3. Divide the toast between two plates. Place a kipper on each slice of toast, then season generously with freshly ground black pepper and chilli flakes, if using. Garnish with parsley and serve with a wedge of lemon.

NUT FREE DAIRY FREE

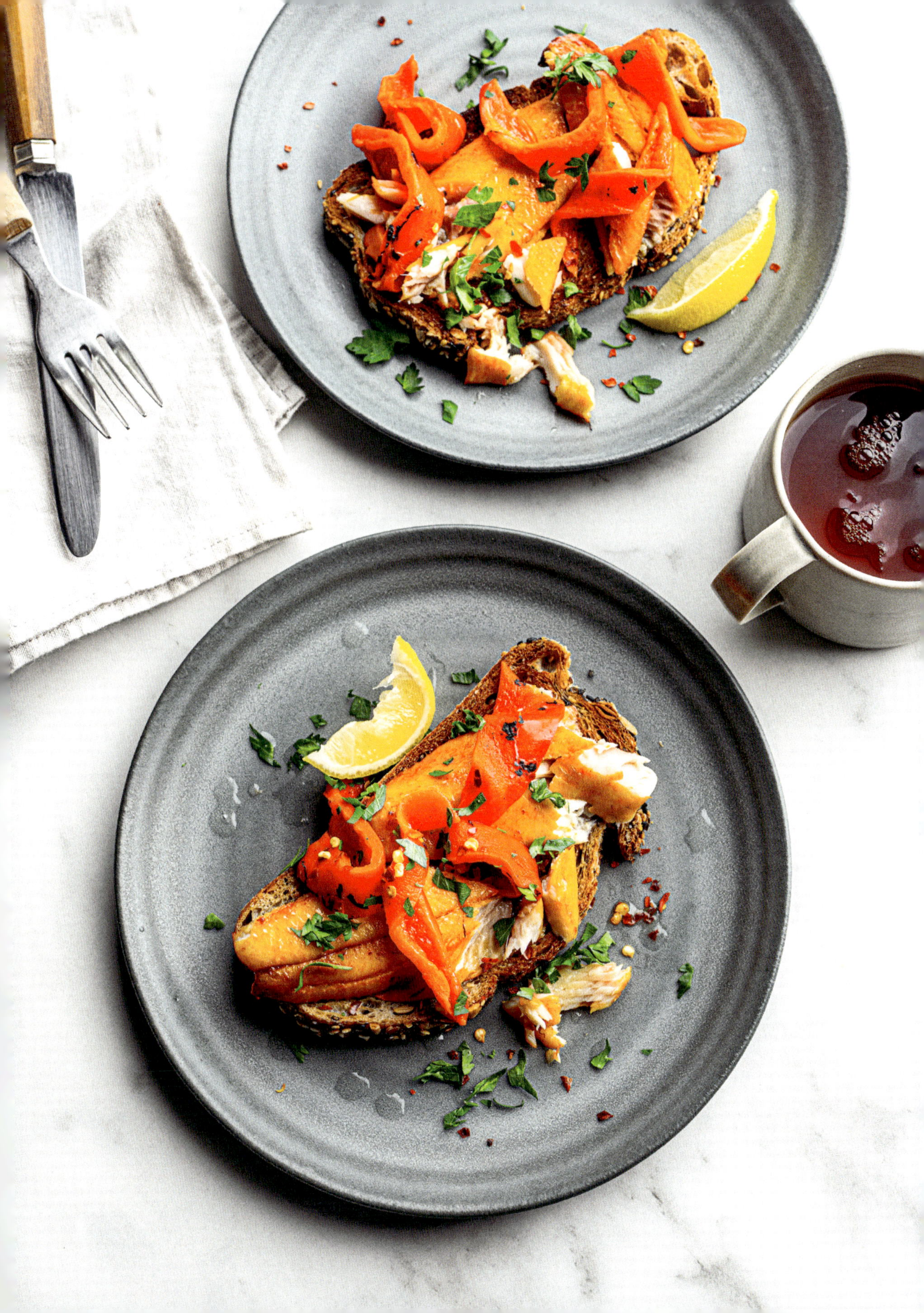

UNDER 300 CALORIES

PER 50G SERVING | **200cals** | PROTEIN **4g** | CARBS **15g** | FIBRE **2g**

Nutty Granola

SERVES **12** | PREP **15** mins | COOK **30** mins

200g coconut oil
100g Medjool dates, pitted
Generous pinch of flaked sea salt
4 tsp vanilla extract
4 egg whites
400g rolled oats
200g mixed nuts (or nuts of your choice)
100g ground flaxseed
2 tbsp maple syrup

Fill a jar with this delicious homemade nutty granola. Lightly sweetened with dates, I use it to scatter on my porridge, on desserts, on top of a pudding or eat it simply as a small snack. The nuts are natural powerhouses, packed with healthy nutrients.

1. Preheat the oven to 140°C/Fan 120°C/Gas 1. Line a baking tray with non-stick baking paper.

2. Place the coconut oil in a saucepan over a low heat to melt, or place in a microwave-safe bowl and melt in the microwave.

3. Meanwhile, place the dates, salt, vanilla extract and egg whites in a food processor and blitz, or tip into a jug and blitz with a stick blender, to form a paste.

4. Place the coconut oil, date paste, oats, nuts, flaxseed and maple syrup in a large bowl and stir well to combine.

5. Scatter the oat mixture into the prepared baking tray and press the mixture down so it clusters closely. Bake in the preheated oven for 25–30 minutes, or until lightly brown.

6. Turn the oven off and leave the oats to cool and crisp up before removing them from the oven.

7. Serve straight away or store in a sealed container.

VEGGIE GLUTEN FREE DAIRY FREE

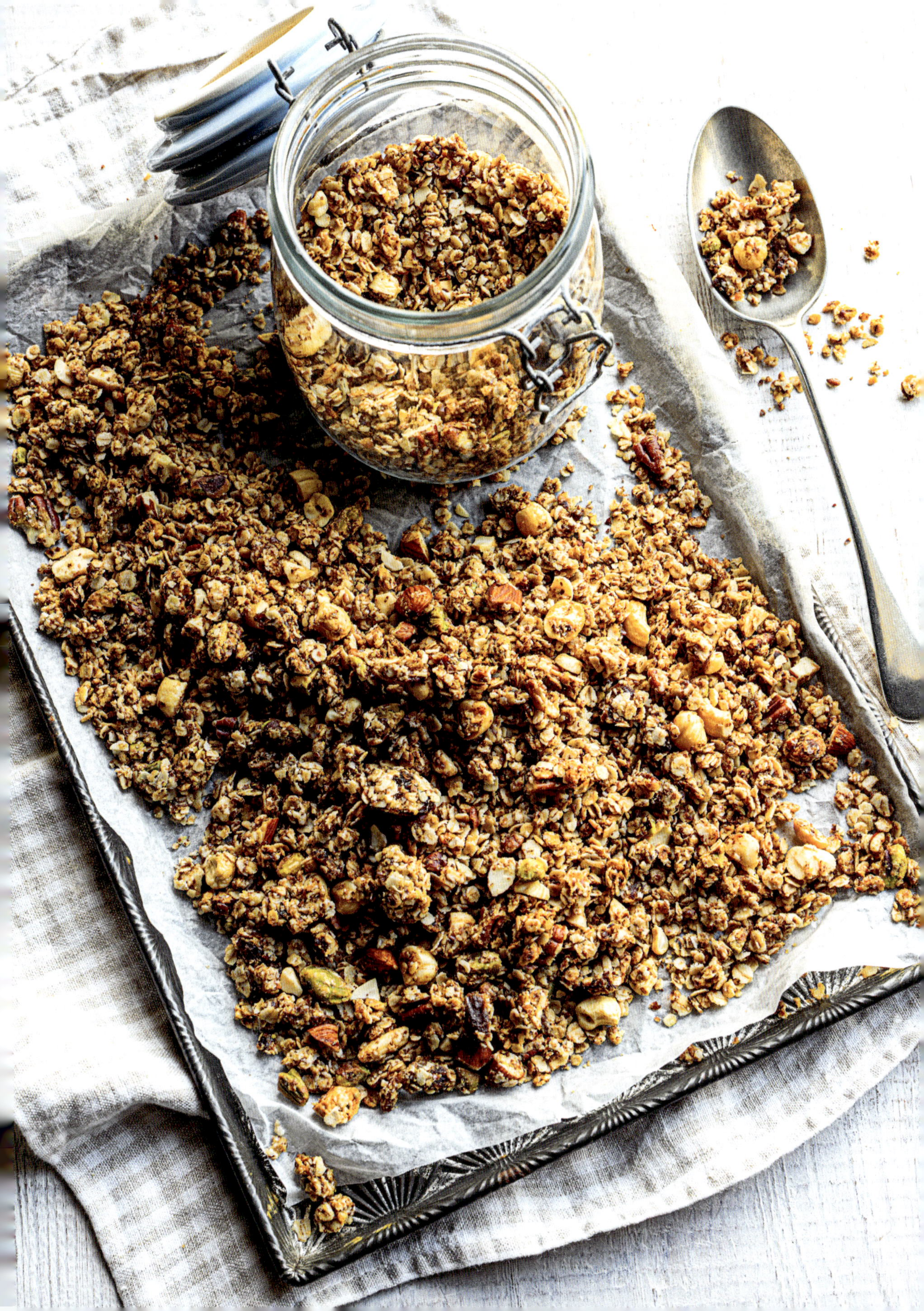

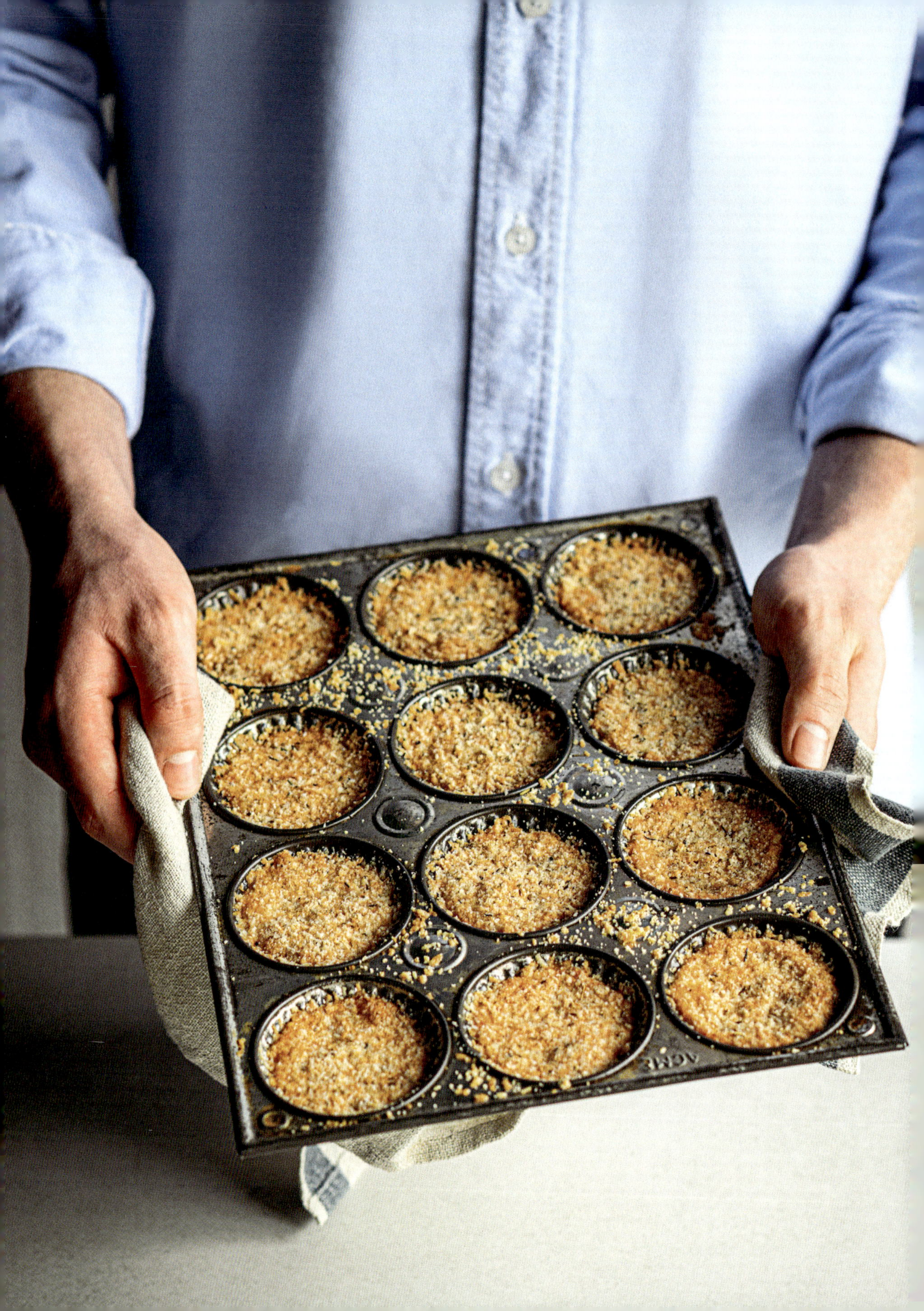

Light Bites and Drinks

UNDER 200 CALORIES

PER SERVING | **194cals** | PROTEIN **9.5g** | CARBS **17g** | FIBRE **3g**

Bruschetta with Prosciutto and Tomato

SERVES **2** | PREP **10** mins | COOK **2** mins

6 cherry tomatoes, quartered
A few sprigs of basil (about 10 leaves), torn
1 tbsp balsamic vinegar
1 tbsp olive oil
1 garlic clove, peeled and halved
2 thin slices of wholegrain, seeded or sourdough bread, toasted
4 slices of prosciutto

Such a timeless Mediterranean classic, and so easy. These bruschetta are fresh, herby and garlicky, topped with sweet tomatoes and thin slices of umami prosciutto and drizzled with sweet balsamic vinegar on a crunchy sourdough base.

1. Place the tomatoes, basil, vinegar and oil in a bowl and mix well. Season with ground black pepper.

2. Rub the garlic halves on the toast, then top with the tomatoes.

3. Share the bruschetta between two plates, then top with the prosciutto, sprinkle with some more black pepper and serve.

NUT FREE

DAIRY FREE

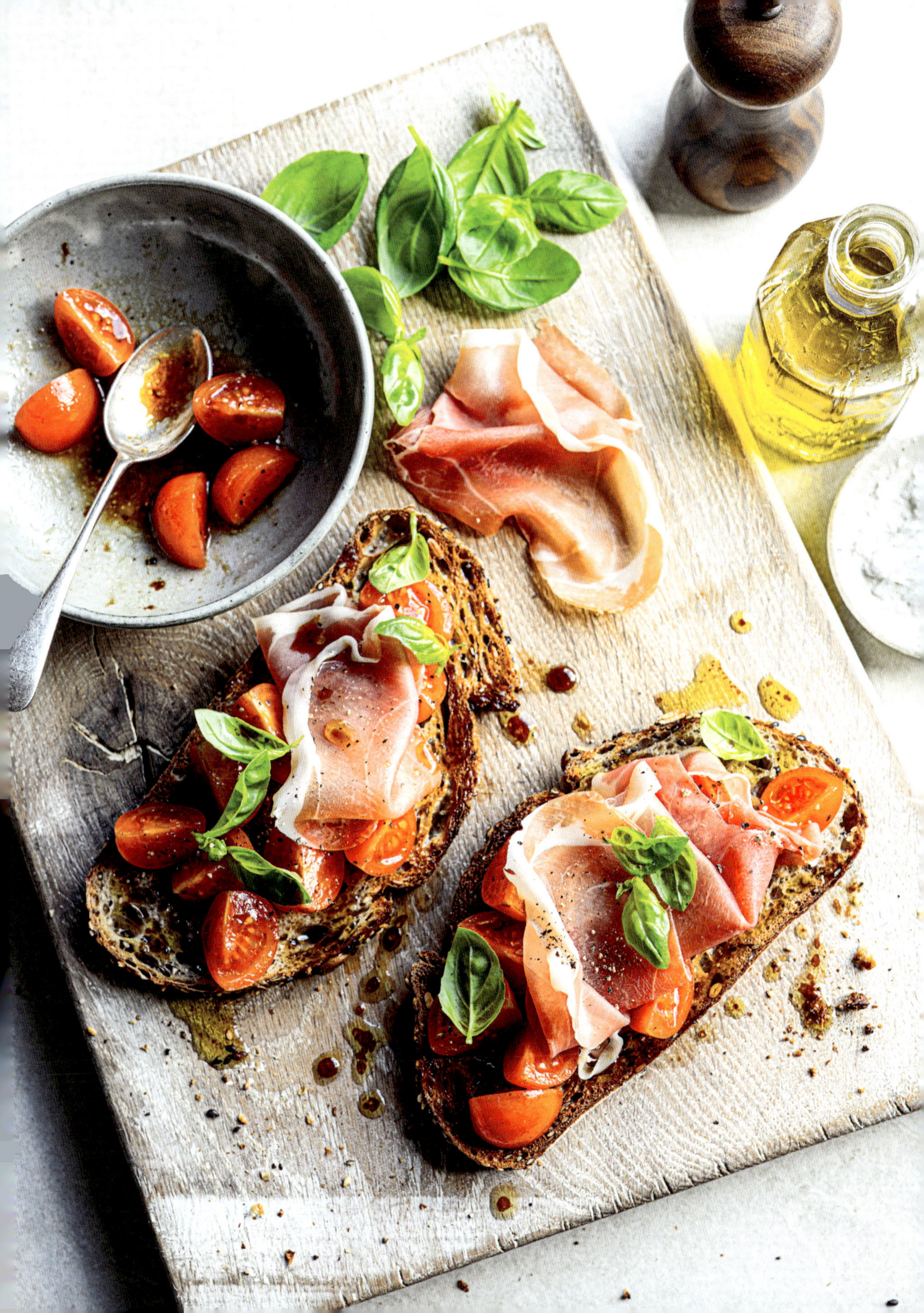

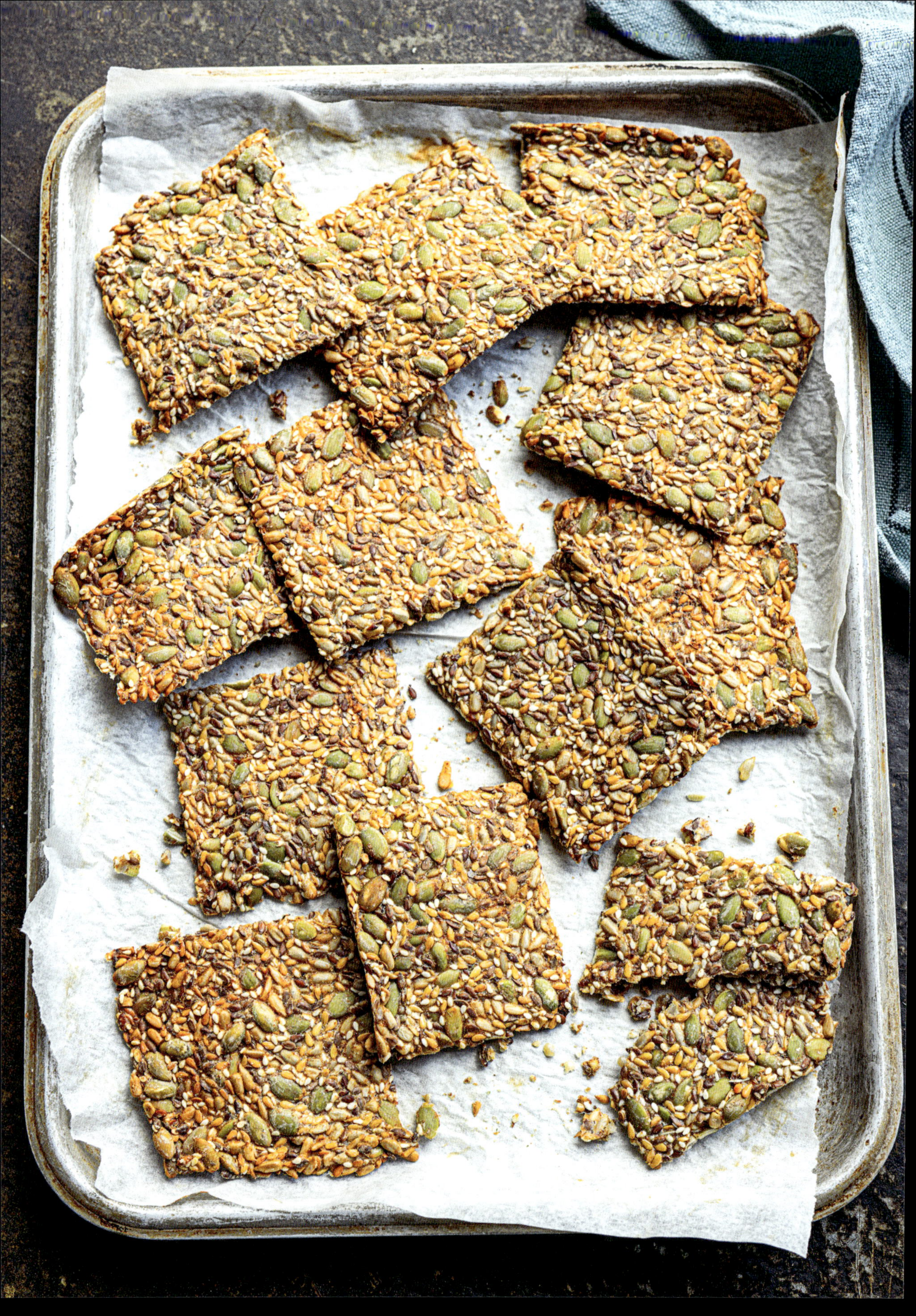

PER SERVING | **82cals** | PROTEIN **3g** | CARBS **7g** | FIBRE **1.5g**

UNDER 100 CALORIES

Miso Fibre Crackers

MAKES **12** | PREP **20** mins | COOK **20** mins

200g mixed seeds
60g wholemeal flour
1 tbsp miso paste

Once you've tasted these crunchy crackers, you won't bother with shop-bought again! You could add other flavours, such as garlic granules, chilli flakes, or dried herbs. If the crackers go soft before you've finished eating them, just crisp them in a hot oven for 5 minutes.

1. Preheat the oven to 190°C/Fan 170°C/Gas 5 and line a large baking tray with non-stick baking paper.

2. Combine all the ingredients in a bowl and season with a generous amount of ground black pepper. Pour in 200ml cold water and mix well. Set aside for about 15 minutes, until it thickens and feels tacky.

3. Using a spatula, spread the mixture onto the prepared baking tray in a thin layer. Score lines in the surface with the spatula to make around 12 crackers.

4. Bake in the preheated oven for about 15–20 minutes, until it is starting to turn golden in places. Avoid over-cooking, as the crackers may turn bitter.

5. Turn off the oven and leave the crackers to cool in the oven, with the door slightly ajar, so they crisp up. Store in an airtight container.

VEGAN | NUT FREE | DAIRY FREE

UNDER 300 CALORIES

PER SERVING | **251cals** | PROTEIN **15.5g** | CARBS **7g** | FIBRE **1g**

Mackerel with Horseradish and Beetroot Dip

SERVES **4** as a starter | PREP **10** mins

1 × 250g pack of peppered hot-smoked mackerel fillets
5 tbsp full-fat Greek yoghurt
2 tbsp creamed horseradish
160g cooked beetroot, diced

Full of colour and flavour, this dip includes two of Michael's favourite ingredients – mackerel and beetroot – with an extra punch from the horseradish. Beetroot is packed with heathly nitrates and fibre, as well as being known to lower blood pressure, and it supports digestion and athletic performance and more. Mackerel is one of the most nutrient-rich foods available, with omega-3 fish oil, which is important for the brain, bone health and immune function too.

1. Remove the skin from the mackerel fillets and discard. Shred the fillets and place in a bowl with all the other ingredients. Mix everything together well.

2. Add a little extra yoghurt to loosen, if needed. Serve as a colourful zingy dip with crudités.

GLUTEN FREE · NUT FREE

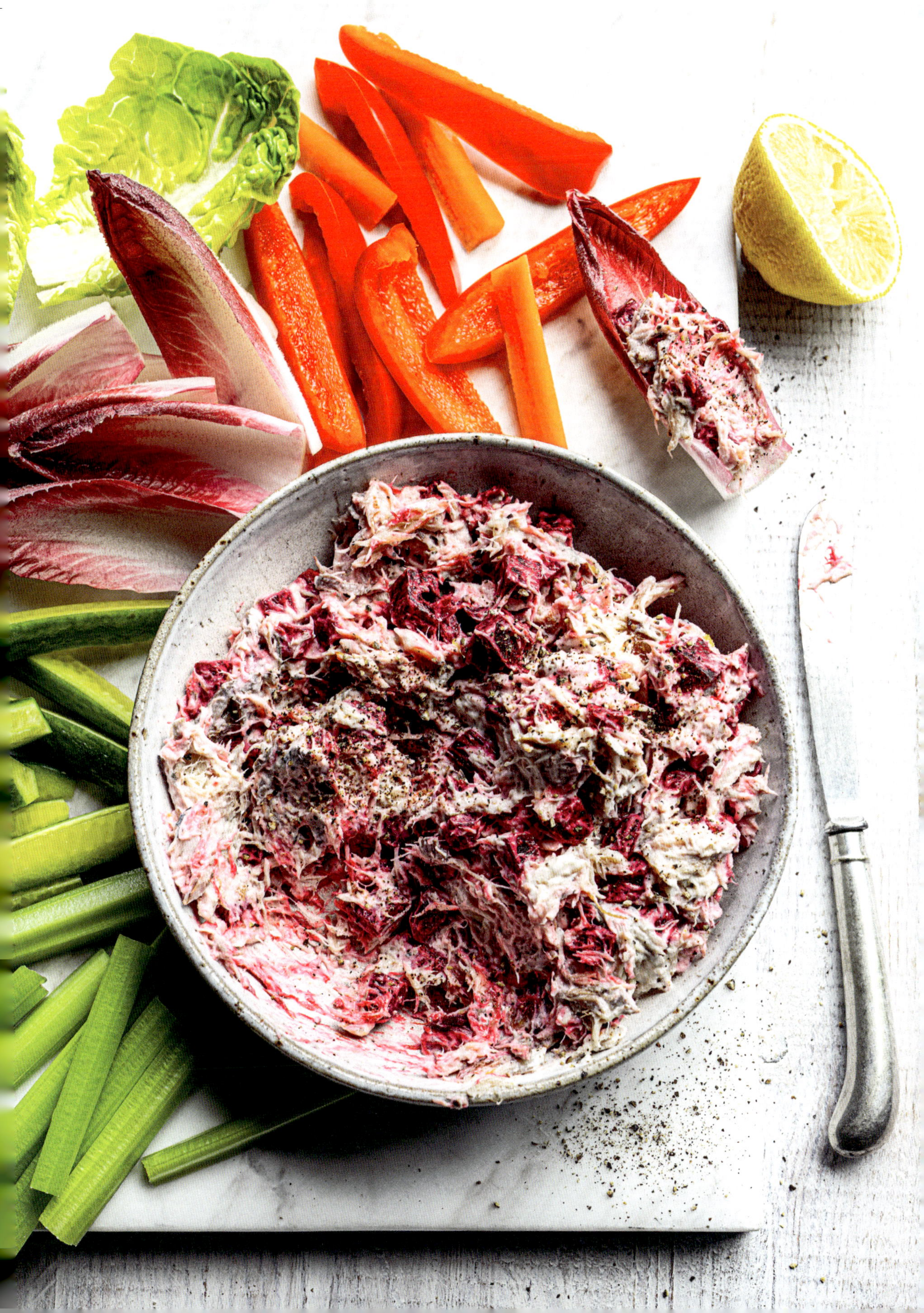

UNDER 200 CALORIES

PER SERVING | **124cals** | PROTEIN **4g** | CARBS **9g** | FIBRE **3g**

Crispy Miso Chickpeas

SERVES **4** | PREP **2** mins | COOK **30** mins

2 tbsp olive oil
1 tbsp miso paste
½ tsp sweet smoked paprika
Pinch of dried chilli flakes (optional)
210g cooked chickpeas (tinned or jarred, drained weight)

Sweet and savoury, perfect to nibble on, or scatter on a salad, soup or stew.

1. Preheat the oven to 190°C/Fan 170°C/Gas 5.

2. Combine all the ingredients, except the chickpeas, in a small bowl. Season generously with ground black pepper, and mix well.

3. Add the chickpeas, then turn to coat in the paste. Tip them into a small roasting tin and cook in the oven for about 30 minutes, stirring occasionally, until slightly brown but still soft.

VEGAN | GLUTEN FREE | NUT FREE | DAIRY FREE

PER SERVING | **113cals** | PROTEIN **3.8g** | CARBS **1.3g** | FIBRE **0.5g**

UNDER 200 CALORIES

Caprese Sticks

SERVES **5** | PREP **10** mins

100g fresh mozzarella, cut into bite-sized pieces, or baby bocconcini
Handful of fresh basil, leaves picked
100g cherry tomatoes
2 tbsp balsamic vinegar
2 tbsp extra-virgin olive oil

This easy, tasty delicacy is a favourite from the Fast 800 programme. It can be scaled up for the family or for a party! If bringing to a celebration, keep the vinegar and oil separate until ready to serve. Store any leftovers in an airtight container in the fridge for up to 3 days.

1. You will need 10 toothpicks, or small skewers.

2. Skewer a piece of mozzarella, then a basil leaf, then a tomato onto each toothpick/skewer. Repeat until all the ingredients have been skewered.

3. Arrange on a platter, drizzle with the balsamic vinegar and olive oil, and season with salt and pepper to serve.

GLUTEN FREE · NUT FREE

UNDER 500 CALORIES

PER SERVING | **406cals** | PROTEIN **18.5g** | CARBS **25.5g** | FIBRE **13g**

Crushed Pea and Edamame Toast with Avocado

SERVES 2 | PREP 15 mins | COOK 2 mins

125g frozen edamame beans
125g frozen peas
1 small avocado, peeled and destoned
1 tbsp green pesto
1 tbsp ground flaxseed
2 slices of wholegrain or seeded sourdough bread, toasted
Pinch of dried chilli flakes (optional)
2 lemon wedges, to serve

This green and luscious topping, rich in protein and fibre, makes a fab open sandwich when spread on wholemeal, seeded or sourdough toast. The edamame is a powerhouse of plant protein. Any leftovers will keep in the fridge for later.

1. Place the edamame and peas together in a bowl and pour over boiling water to defrost. Leave them for a couple of minutes, then drain.

2. Using a food processor or a stick blender, briefly blitz the edamame and peas. Season with salt and black pepper, then add the avocado and blitz again, leaving some texture.

3. Stir in the pesto and ground flaxseed, mixing it well.

4. Divide the toast between two plates, then spread with the pea mixture.

5. Serve sprinkled with a pinch of chilli flakes, if you like, and a wedge of lemon.

VEGGIE NUT FREE

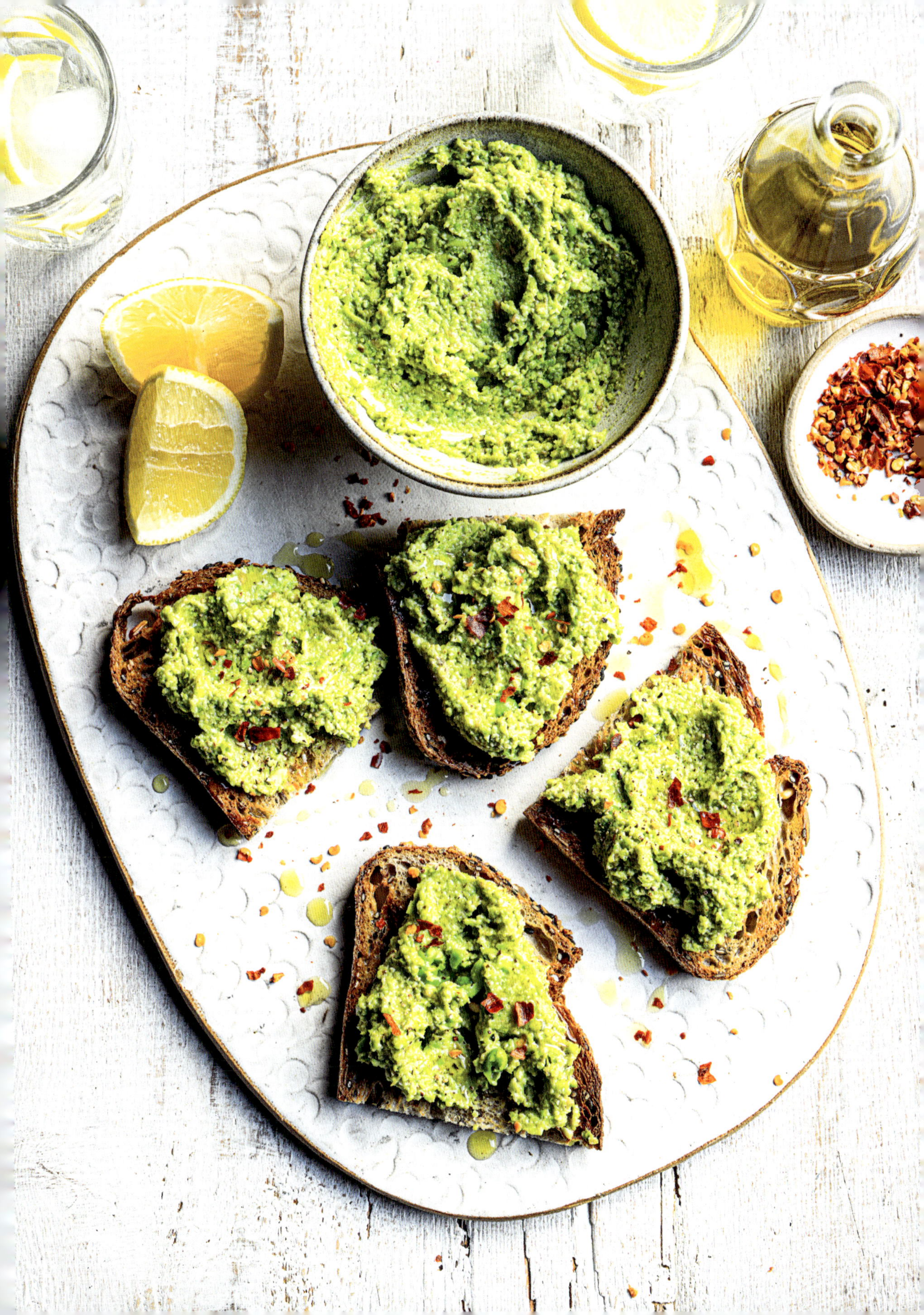

UNDER 200 CALORIES

PER SERVING | **193cals** | PROTEIN **8g** | CARBS **3.5g** | FIBRE **0.5g**

Savoury Nuts

SERVES 4 | PREP 5 mins | COOK 10 mins

120g mixed nuts, larger nuts roughly chopped
2 tsp coconut oil, melted
1 tsp medium curry powder
½ tsp flaked sea salt
½ tsp dried chilli flakes (optional)

Michael was a fan of flavoured nuts to fill a little gap when hungry – they are well known for their health benefits and steady release of energy, keeping you full for longer. They also have anti-inflammatory properties, bolstering your immune system, as well as providing important nutrients such as selenium and vitamin E. They can even provide some protection from heart disease and type 2 diabetes.

1. Preheat the oven to 180°C/Fan 160°C/Gas 4.

2. Place the nuts in a medium bowl. Add all the remaining ingredients and lots of ground black pepper. Toss everything together until the nuts are lightly coated.

3. Scatter over a baking tray and roast in the oven for 5 minutes.

4. Remove from the oven and turn the nuts. Return to the oven for a further 5 minutes, or until the nuts are lightly browned. Take care they don't burn.

5. Cool for a few minutes on the tray to allow to crisp a little, then transfer to a bowl. Serve slightly warm or leave to cool completely.

VEGAN GLUTEN FREE DAIRY FREE

PER SERVING | **92cals** | PROTEIN **4.5g** | CARBS **2g** | FIBRE **1g**

UNDER 100 CALORIES

Protein Crackers

MAKES 12 | PREP 10 mins | COOK 40 mins

120g ground almonds
225g cottage cheese
2 tbsp mixed seeds

Another example of marrying quality protein (cottage cheese) with fibre (seeds).

1. Preheat the oven to 170°C/Fan 150°C/Gas 3½ and line a large baking tray with non-stick baking paper.

2. Place all the ingredients in a bowl and mix well. Season with a good pinch of salt and freshly ground black pepper.

3. Spread the mixture onto the prepared baking tray. Place another sheet of baking paper over the top, then use a heavy pan to flatten the mixture down until it is 0.5cm thick.

4. Remove the top layer of baking paper, then transfer to the oven and bake for about 35–40 minutes, or until the surface is golden brown.

5. Take the tray out of the oven and cut into 12 squares. Slide the knife underneath and between the crackers to separate them. Return the tray to the oven, then turn the oven off. Leave the crackers to cool and crisp in the oven.

VEGGIE GLUTEN FREE

UNDER 100 CALORIES

PER SERVING | **64cals** | PROTEIN **3.5g** | CARBS **0.5g** | FIBRE **0.5g**

Easy Cheesy Crispy Biscuits

MAKES **12** | PREP **10** mins | COOK **25** mins

A simple crispy savoury snack, which also adds flavour and crunch to crumble on soup and scatter on salads.

1 tsp olive oil, plus extra for greasing
50g Parmesan, grated
50g Cheddar, grated
50g ground almonds
1 heaped tsp dried mixed herbs

1. Preheat the oven to 170°C/Fan 150°C/Gas 3½, and grease a 12-hole bun tin lightly with olive oil.

2. Combine all the ingredients in a bowl and mix well.

3. Add 1 tablespoon of the mixture to each of the bun holes, pressing down well.

4. Bake in the preheated oven for about 20–25 minutes, until golden and crisping.

5. Leave to cool in the tin for a few minutes, then transfer to a wire rack.

VEGGIE GLUTEN FREE

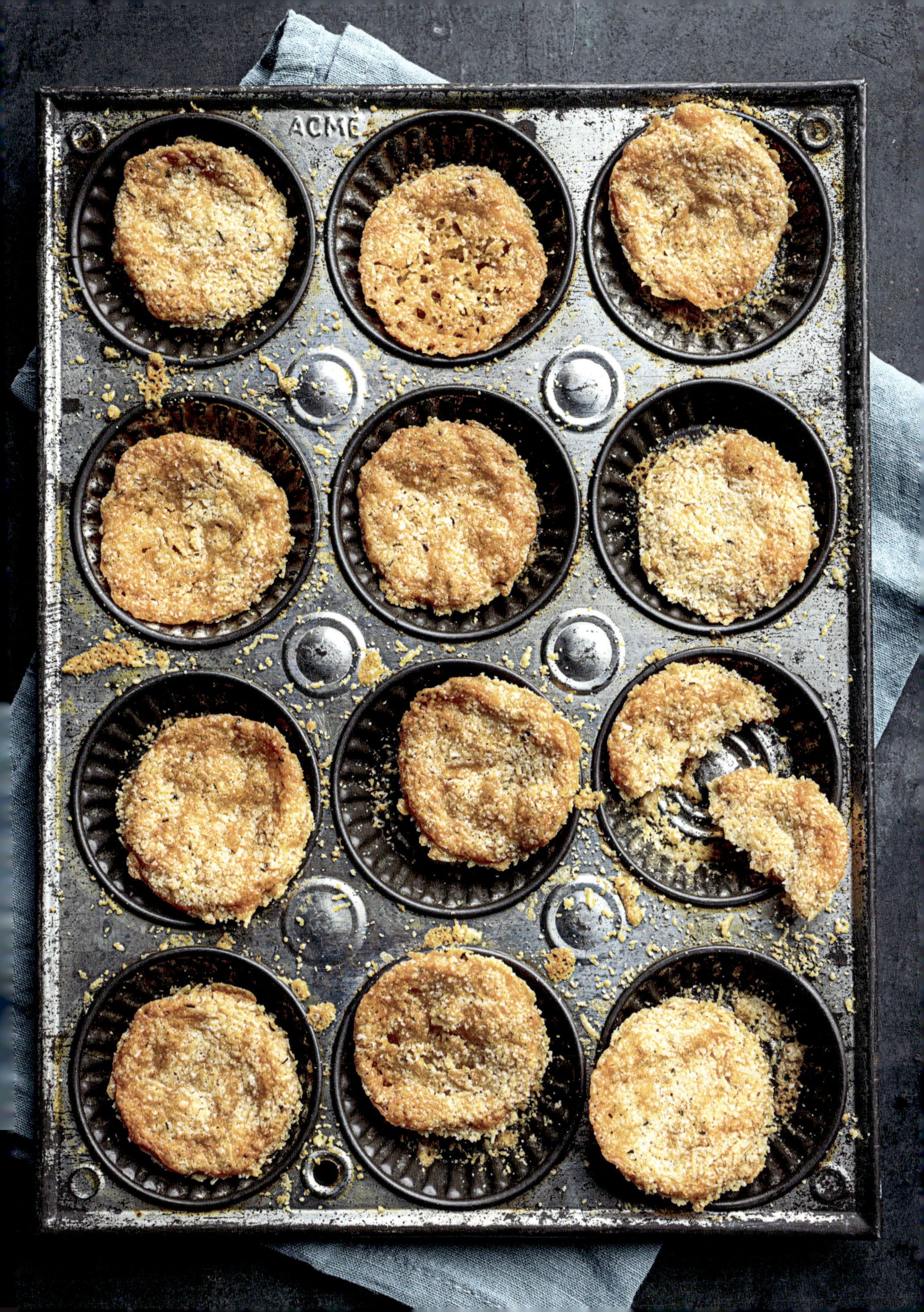
ACME

Fruit and Veg Blinis

Switching from starchy blinis and crackers can make all the difference when it comes to reducing sugar spikes. Here we make the base from sliced courgette and pear or apple. Whipped together in less than 5 minutes, they work for one, but can be expanded for more people, or even for a party.

UNDER 100 CALORIES PER SERVING | 57cals

Courgette and Prawn Cocktail Blinis

1 small–medium courgette (roughly 160g prepared weight), trimmed and cut into 12 slices about 0.5cm thick
12 tsp mayonnaise
24–36 small cooked prawns
Pinch of sumac or sweet paprika
Squeeze of lemon (optional)

1. Dollop 1 teaspoon of mayo on each slice of courgette and top with 2–3 prawns.

2. Season with a pinch of sumac or paprika, a pinch of salt and ground black pepper and a squeeze of lemon juice, if using.

GLUTEN FREE · NUT FREE

PROTEIN **4g** | CARBS **0g** | FIBRE **0.2g**

UNDER 100 CALORIES PER SERVING | 25cals

Courgette and Smoked Salmon Blinis

1 small–medium courgette (roughly 160g prepared weight), trimmed and cut into 12 slices about 0.5cm thick
12 tsp cream cheese
60g smoked salmon slices, roughly chopped
Squeeze of lemon (optional)

1. Dollop 1 teaspoon of cream cheese on each slice of courgette, then top with some smoked salmon.

2. Season with a pinch of ground black pepper and a squeeze of lemon juice, if using.

GLUTEN FREE · NUT FREE

PROTEIN **1.5g** | CARBS **0.5g** | FIBRE **0.2g**

UNDER 100 CALORIES PER SERVING | **15cals**

Courgette and Sweet Piquanté Pepper Blinis

1 small-medium courgette (roughly 160g prepared weight), trimmed and cut into 12 slices about 0.5cm thick
12 tsp cream cheese
6 sweet piquanté peppers from a jar, halved

1. Dollop 1 teaspoon of cream cheese on each slice of courgette, then top with half a pepper.

2. Season with a pinch of ground black pepper.

VEGGIE · GLUTEN FREE · NUT FREE

PROTEIN **0.5g** | CARBS **0.5g** | FIBRE **0.2g**

UNDER 100 CALORIES PER SERVING | **59cals**

Pear, Blue Cheese and Walnut Blinis

1 small pear or apple, cored and sliced into 4 discs (each about 0.5cm)
4 tsp blue cheese (such as St Agur)
4 walnut halves

1. Dollop 1 teaspoon of blue cheese on each slice of pear, then top with a walnut half.

2. Season with a pinch of ground black pepper.

VEGGIE · GLUTEN FREE

PROTEIN **2g** | CARBS **3g** | FIBRE **1g**

UNDER 100 CALORIES

PER SERVING | **0cals** | PROTEIN **0g** | CARBS **0g** | FIBRE **0g**

Aromatic Infusions

MAKES	PREP	COOK
1 litre	**2** mins	**5** mins

GINGER AND LEMON
2 thick slices of lemon
1cm piece of fresh root ginger, sliced

ROSEMARY AND MINT
1 sprig of rosemary
1 generous sprig of mint

LEMON AND THYME
2 thick slices of lemon
1 sprig of thyme

One of the side effects of losing weight is that, as you burn fat, you also lose water in your system. So, if you don't drink extra fluids, you are more likely to get dehydrated, leaving you feeling listless, headachy and suffering with constipation. This is often mistakenly blamed on lack of calories. Easily remedied – just add 1½ extra litres of water a day (and more if it is hot). These simple, flavoured infusions may be enough to help stave off dehydration. Be creative and add your own flavourings. My favourite is the zingy ginger and lemon.

1. Add your choice of flavourings to a pan and pour in 1 litre of water. Bring to the boil.

2. Turn off the heat and leave the aromatics to infuse for 4–5 minutes.

3. Pour the liquid through a sieve into a jug or bottle. Discard the aromatics and drink the infusion hot or cold. It will keep in the fridge for up to 5 days.

VEGAN | GLUTEN FREE | NUT FREE | DAIRY FREE

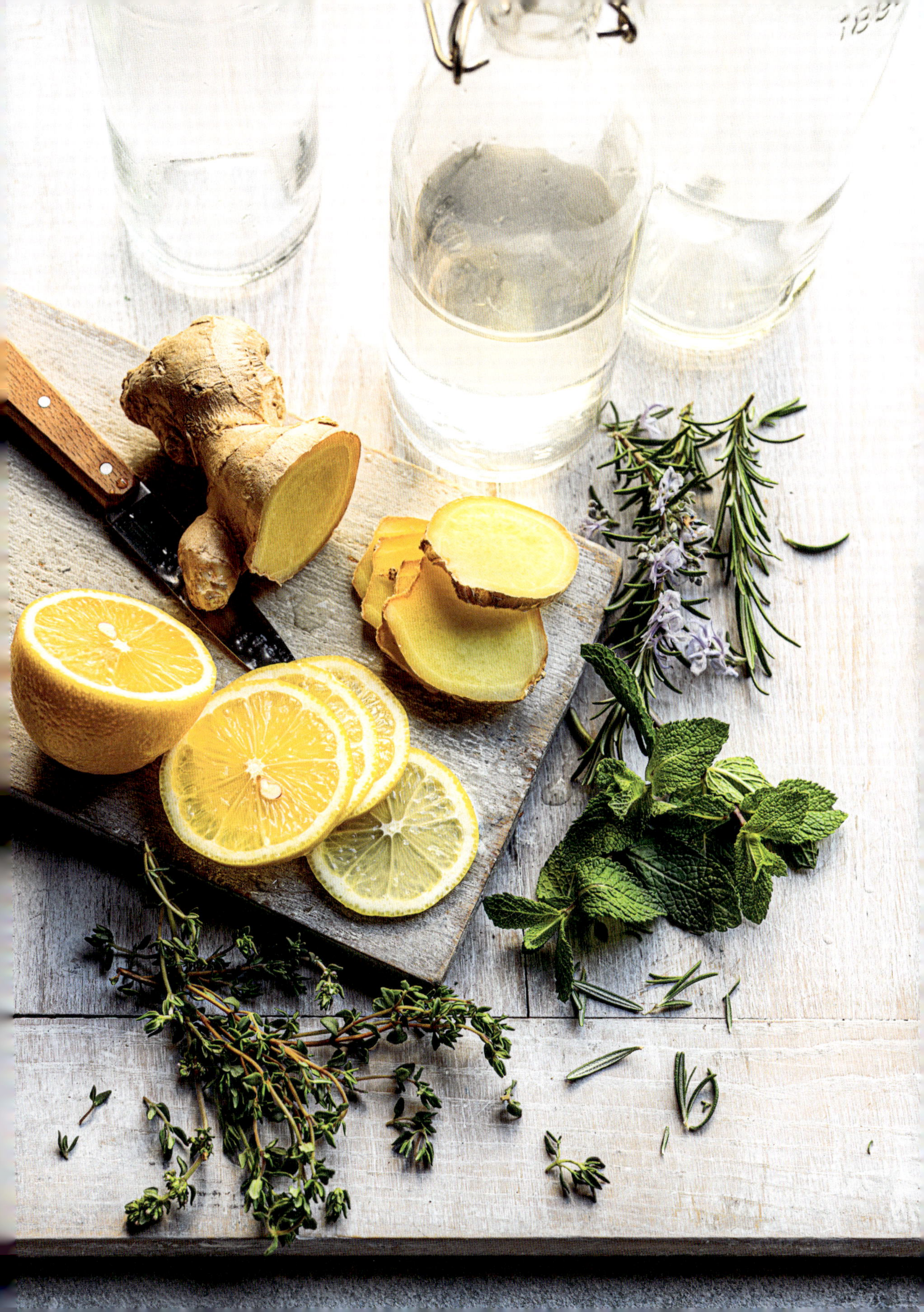

LUSCIOUS SMOOTHIES 4 WAYS

UNDER 300 CALORIES | PER SERVING | **271cals**

Mango and Vanilla

You can use Greek yoghurt or kefir – both give the smoothie a creamy texture and are good for the gut.

SERVES 2

250g fresh mango, cut into chunks (prepared weight)
2 tbsp milled mixed seeds (including sunflower, chia and flax)
4 tbsp full-fat Greek yoghurt or kefir
1 tsp vanilla extract
300ml full-fat milk

1. Put all the ingredients in a blender (or use a jug and a stick blender) and blitz until smooth and creamy.

PROTEIN **10g** | CARBS **27.5g** | FIBRE **5g**

UNDER 300 CALORIES | PER SERVING | **200cals**

Galia Melon and Almond

My nephew made this on a scorching hot day when he was little and I adopted it. So simple and filling.

SERVES 2

1 Galia melon, peeled, deseeded and roughly chopped
1 large tbsp almond butter (or peanut butter)
4 tbsp full-fat Greek yoghurt

1. Put all the ingredients in a blender (or use a jug and a stick blender) and blitz until smooth and creamy.

PROTEIN **6g** | CARBS **22g** | FIBRE **3g**

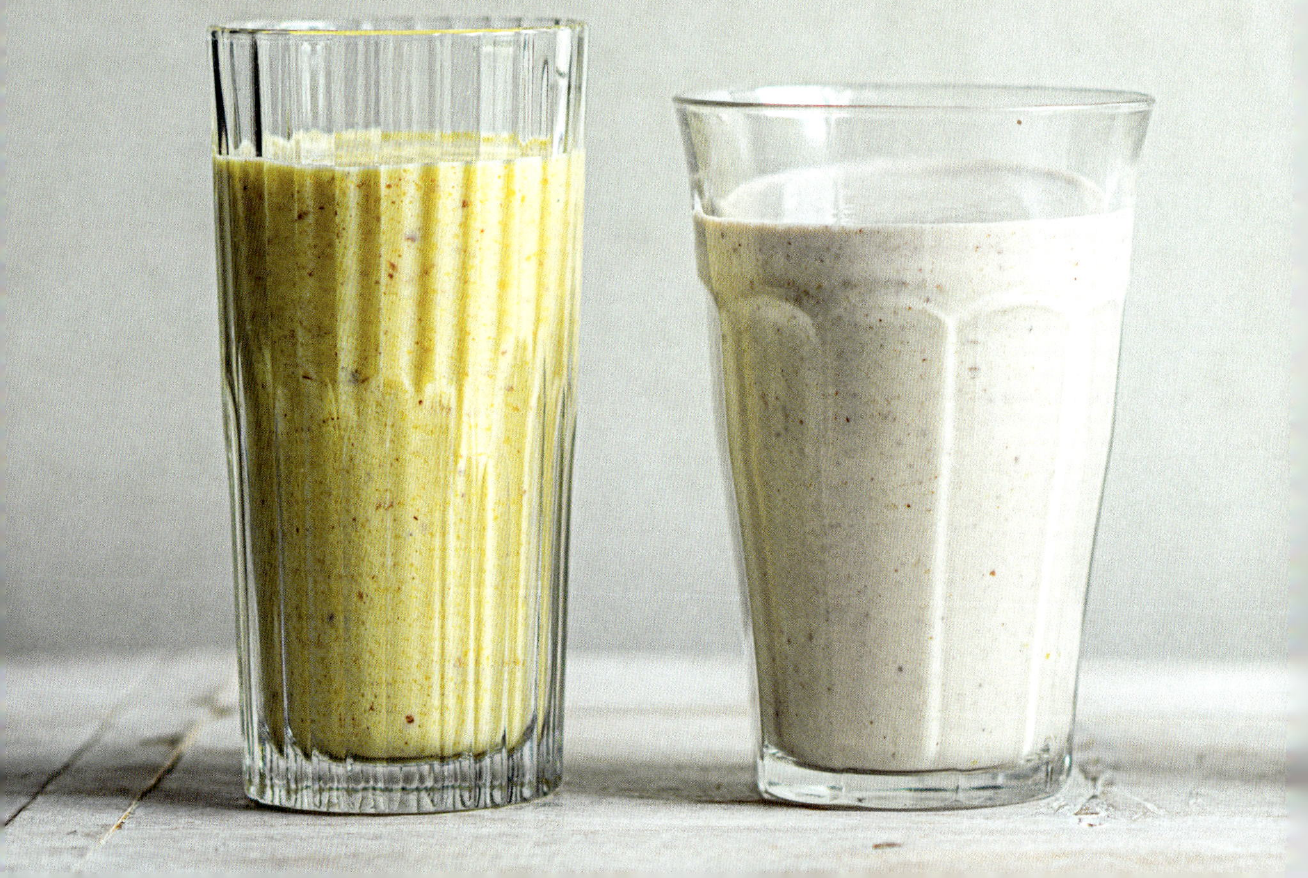

UNDER 400 CALORIES PER SERVING | **306cals**

Banana and Tahini

Tahini is high in protein and provides good monounsaturated fats, as well as containing essential minerals, including calcium and magnesium.

SERVES 2

2 small ripe bananas, peeled
2 tbsp milled mixed seeds (including sunflower, chia and flax)
4 tbsp full-fat Greek yoghurt
1 tbsp tahini
½ tsp ground cinnamon
300ml full-fat milk

1. Put all the ingredients in a blender (or use a jug and a stick blender) and blitz until smooth and creamy.

PROTEIN **11g** | CARBS **26g** | FIBRE **3g**

UNDER 300 CALORIES PER SERVING | **221cals**

Berry and Cinnamon

Ground cinnamon is a great way to add sweetness to a smoothie without reaching for sugar.

SERVES 2

200g frozen mixed berries, defrosted
1 ripe banana, peeled
2 tbsp milled mixed seeds (including sunflower, chia and flax)
1 tsp ground cinnamon
300ml kefir

1. Put all the ingredients in a blender (or use a jug and a stick blender) and blitz until smooth and creamy.

PROTEIN **9g** | CARBS **24.5g** | FIBRE **5g**

VEGGIE | GLUTEN FREE

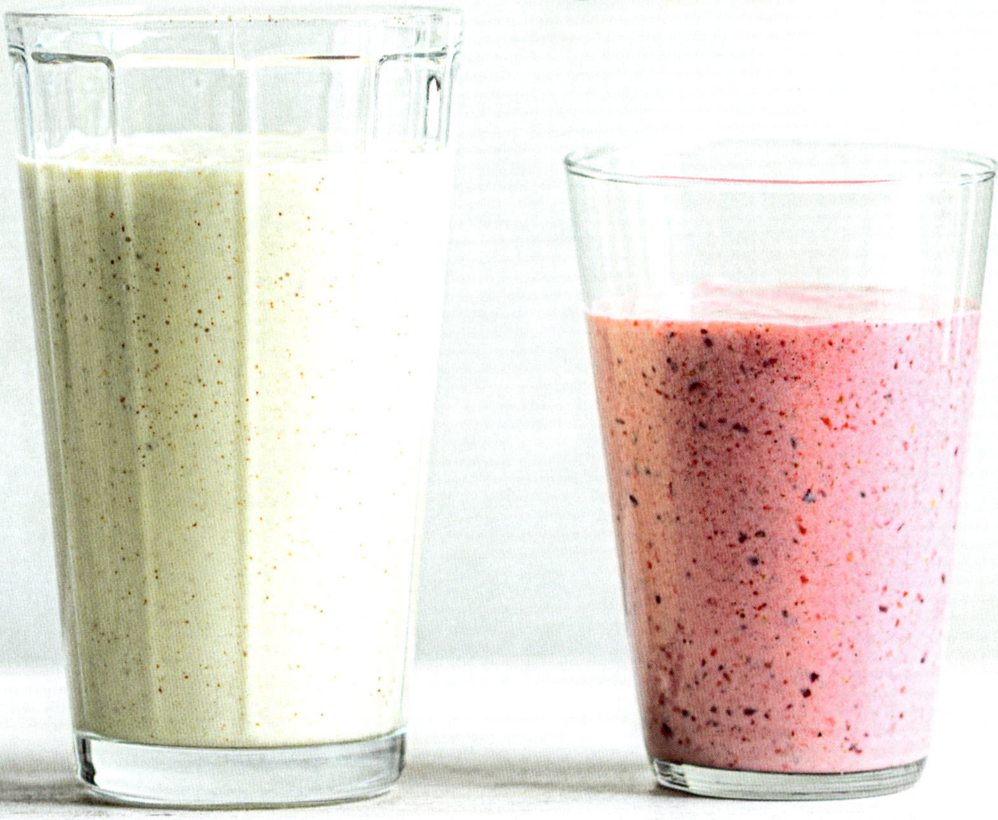

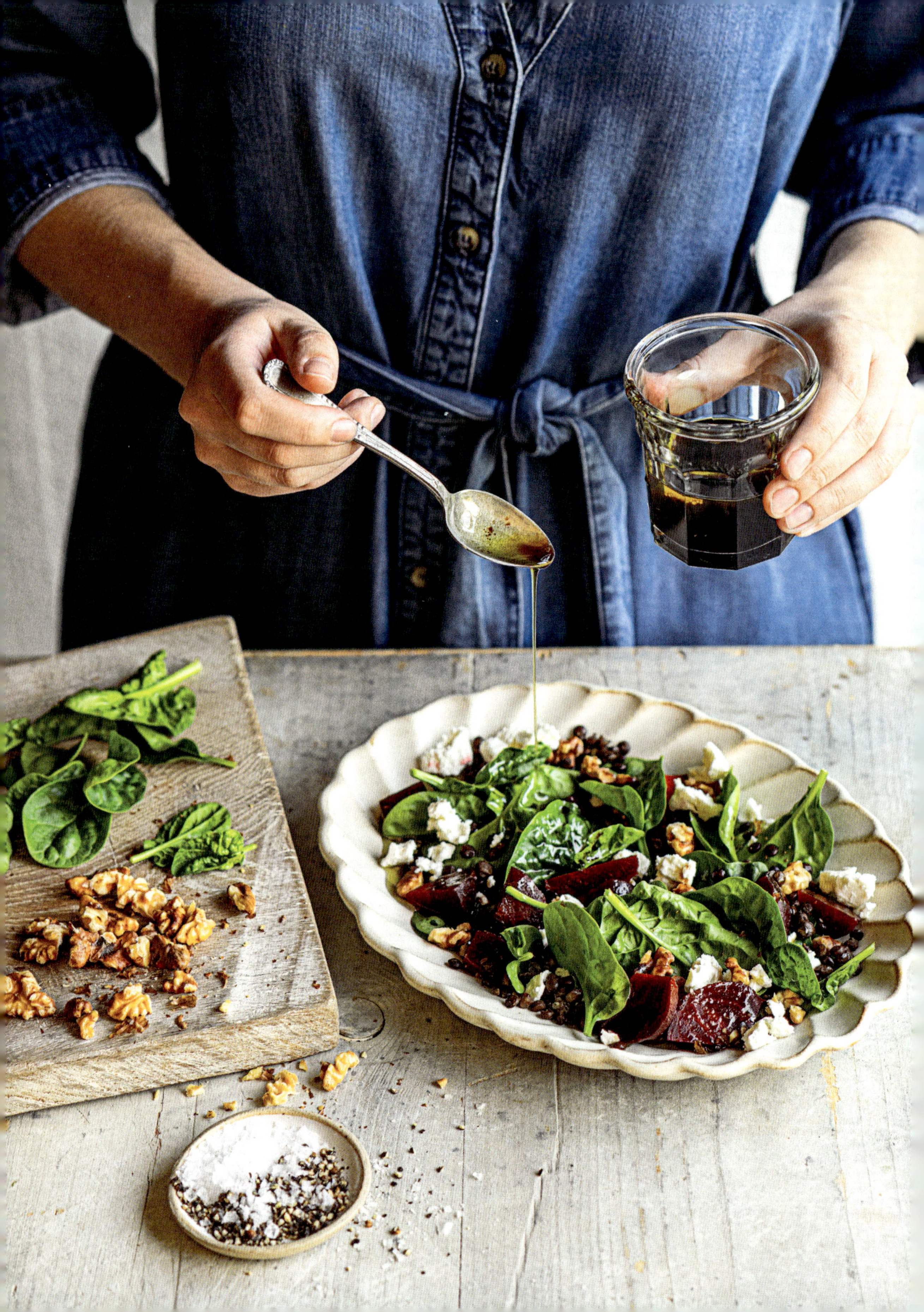

Lunch and Soups

UNDER 300 CALORIES

PER SERVING | 262cals | PROTEIN 16g | CARBS 27g | FIBRE 9g

Simple Minestrone

SERVES 3 | PREP 5 mins | COOK 35 mins

1 tsp olive oil
1 small onion, diced
1 tsp dried thyme
1 celery stick, diced
1 garlic clove, finely chopped
25g dried wholemeal pasta
50g cooked edamame beans (podded weight)
1 × 400g tin white beans (such as cannellini)
1 × 400g tin chopped tomatoes
Generous handful of finely sliced cabbage or cavolo nero
½ vegetable stock cube
3 tbsp grated Parmesan

This twist on the classic Italian vegetable, bean and pasta soup contains edamame, which bolsters the protein and fibre, while the Parmesan adds even more protein.

1. Place the oil in a saucepan over a medium heat. Add the onion, thyme and celery and cook for 4–5 minutes, stirring occasionally. Add the garlic and cook for another minute.

2. Pour in 100ml water and add the pasta, edamame, the beans with their liquid, the chopped tomatoes, shredded cabbage and the stock cube. Bring up to the boil, then reduce the heat, cover with a lid and simmer for 30 minutes, adding a splash more water, if needed.

3. Serve topped with a tablespoon of Parmesan per person.

NUT FREE

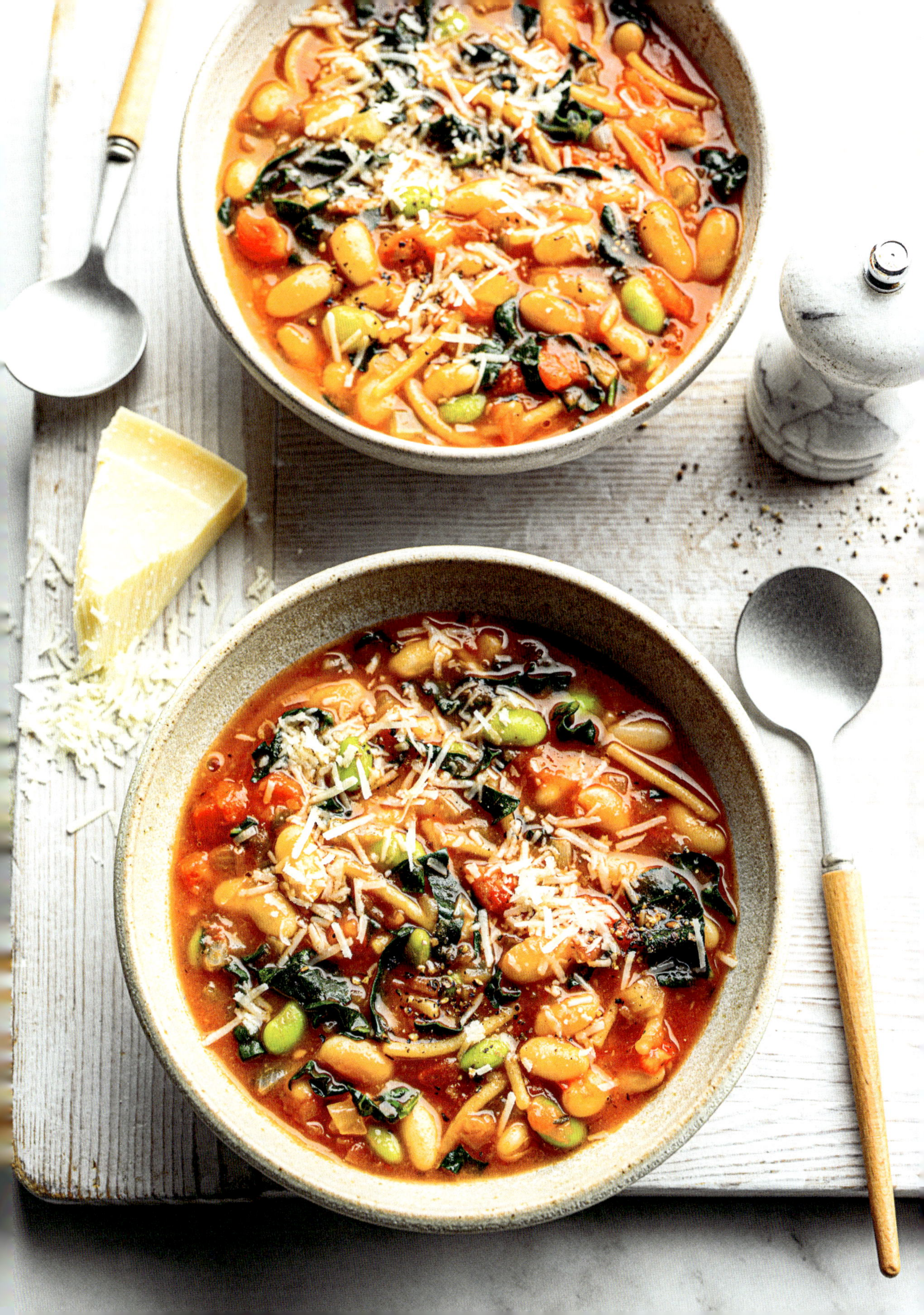

UNDER 300 CALORIES

PER SERVING | **297cals** | PROTEIN **22.5g** | CARBS **3g** | FIBRE **1g**

Almost-instant High-protein 'Pizza'

SERVES **1** | PREP **5** mins | COOK **10** mins

½ tbsp olive oil
3 thin slices of pointed/ sweetheart cabbage (cut through the centre to make a cross section)
2 large eggs, beaten with a pinch of salt
1 tbsp tomato purée
½ tsp dried oregano
3–4 anchovies
Handful of ready-grated mozzarella

This is an unusual pizza, as the base is made by cutting through the middle of a pointed cabbage. Once you have three thin slices through the circumference, they are placed one on top of the other in a frying pan to cook. The beaten egg drizzles through the cabbage, setting in the pan to make the base. It is then flipped to finish cooking, before adding the delicious toppings.

1. Place a frying or omelette pan over a medium heat. Drizzle with the olive oil then stack the slices of cabbage in the pan. Pour over the egg, being careful not to let the egg spread beyond the cabbage. Cook for about 5 minutes until firm, then turn over and cook for another 2 minutes on the other side.

2. Transfer the pizza base to a plate, then spread the tomato purée over the surface. Sprinkle with the oregano, top with anchovies and scatter over the cheese. Finally season with some black pepper.

GLUTEN FREE · NUT FREE

PER SERVING | 534cals | PROTEIN 31g | CARBS 20g | FIBRE 6g

UNDER 600 CALORIES

High-protein and Garlicky Cauliflower Cheese

SERVES 2 | PREP 5 mins | COOK 23 mins

1 small cauliflower, cut into small florets (about 550g)
1 tbsp olive oil
300g full-fat cottage cheese
40g garlic and herb cream cheese (I use Boursin)
100ml full-fat milk
1 tbsp chia seeds
50g Cheddar, grated

No-fuss creamy comfort food with a hint of garlic.

1. Preheat the oven to 200°C/180°C/Gas 6. You will need a 20cm square baking dish, or similar.

2. Tip the cauliflower florets on to a baking tray, drizzle with the olive oil and cook for about 8 minutes, shaking occasionally. When they've started to brown and are soft but al dente, remove from the oven and set aside.

3. Meanwhile, in a bowl or jug, mix together the cottage cheese, cream cheese, milk and chia seeds. Use a stick blender to blitz for about 30 seconds until smooth.

4. Transfer the florets to the baking dish and pour the cheese mixture over the top. Scatter over the grated Cheddar and roast in the oven for about 15 minutes, until heated through and browning in places.

VEGGIE | GLUTEN FREE | NUT FREE

UNDER 400 CALORIES

PER SERVING | **393cals** | PROTEIN **14g** | CARBS **11.5g** | FIBRE **5g**

Beetroot Salad with Puy Lentils, Goats' Cheese and Toasted Walnuts

SERVES **1** | PREP **10** mins

10–12 walnut halves, roughly chopped
Handful of baby spinach
1 cooked beetroot, cubed
15g soft goats' cheese
3 tbsp cooked Puy lentils (from a pouch or tin)
Drizzle of olive oil
Drizzle of balsamic vinegar

Such a classic combination and with lots of nutrient-rich ingredients.

1. Toast the nuts in a dry frying pan over a medium heat for about 2 minutes, until just fragrant. Keep an eye on them to make sure they don't burn. Set aside.

2. Place the spinach in a serving bowl. Top with the beetroot, goats' cheese and lentils.

3. Scatter over the toasted walnuts, then drizzle with the olive oil and balsamic vinegar to serve.

VEGGIE GLUTEN FREE

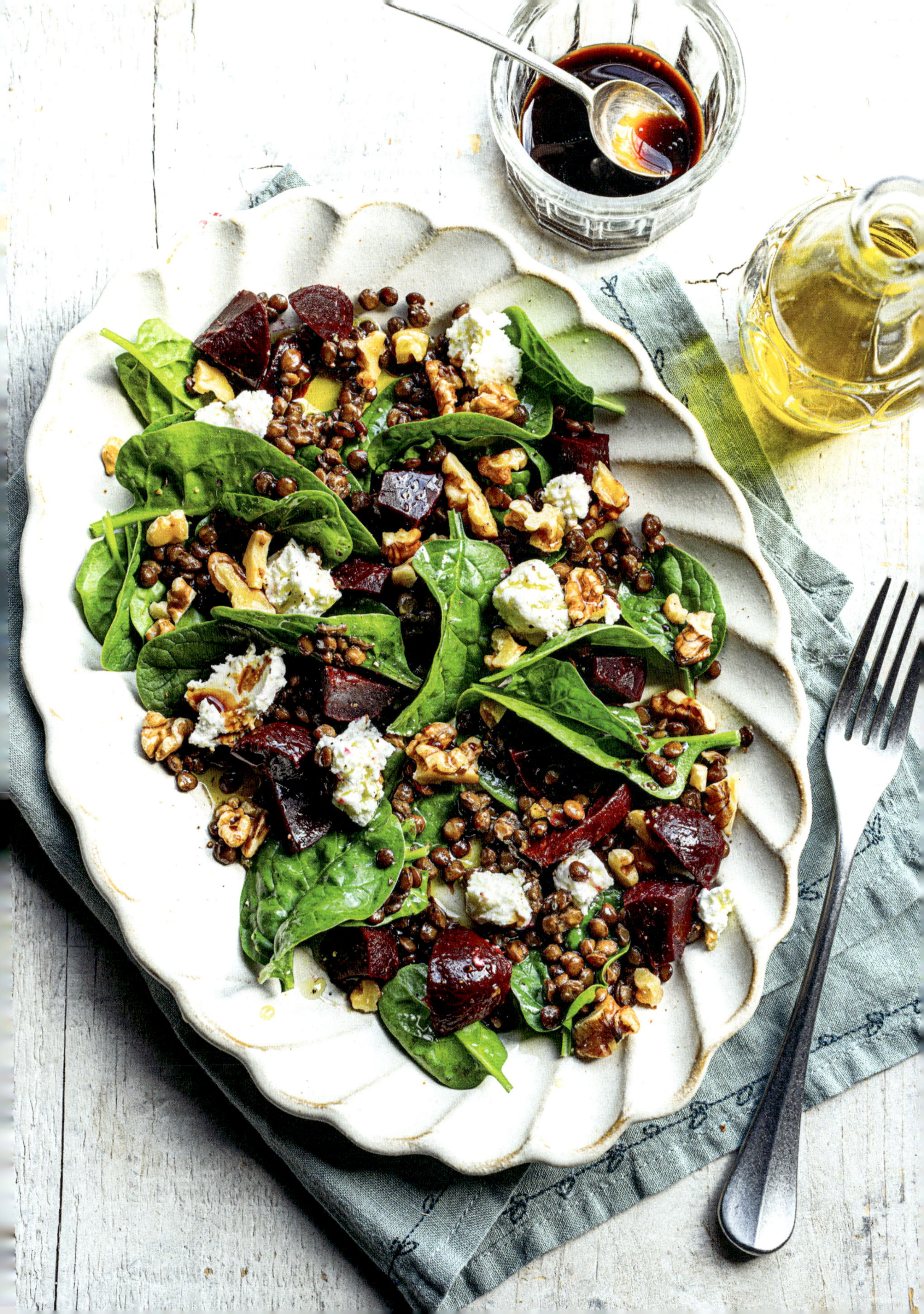

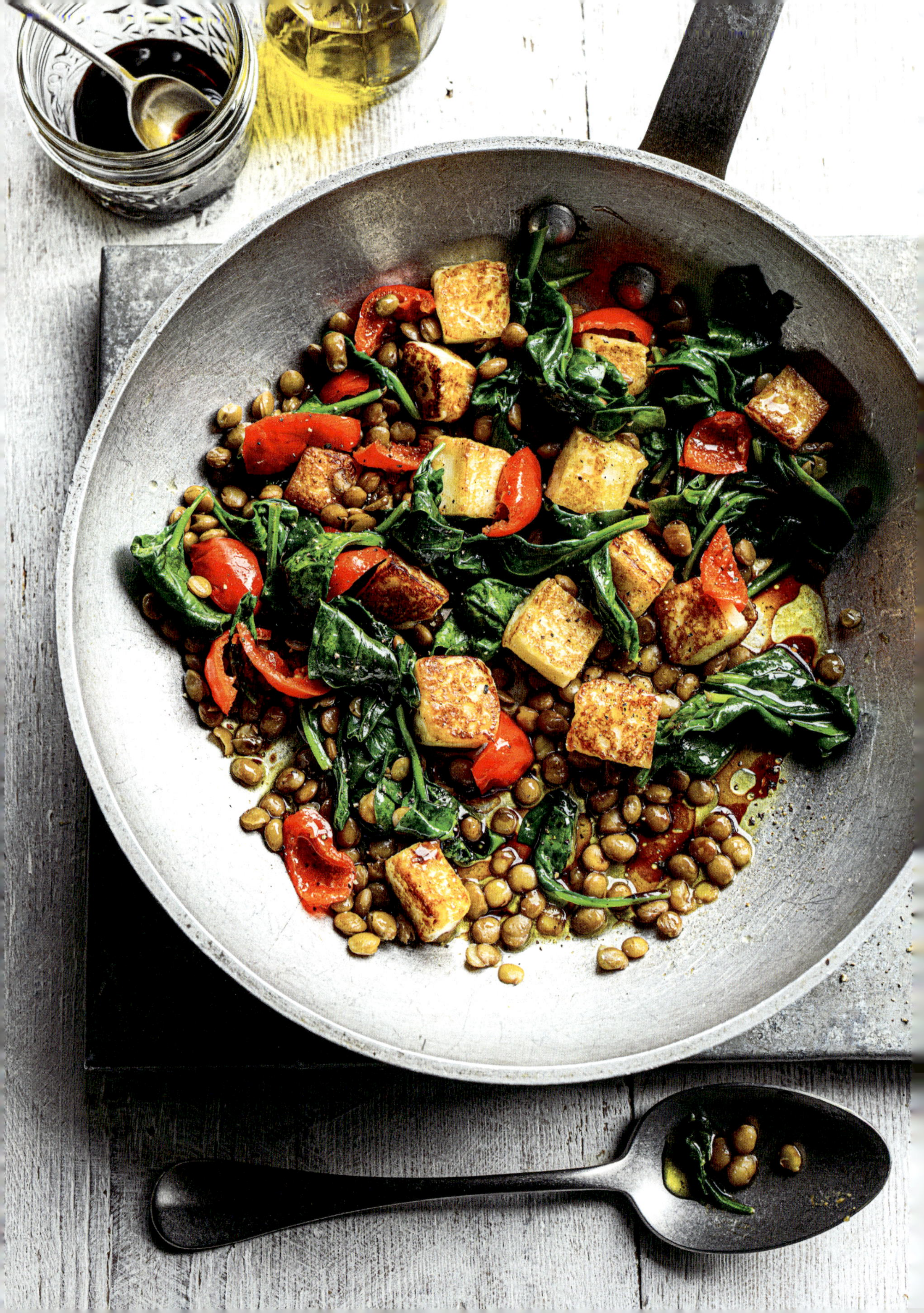

PER SERVING | **433cals** | PROTEIN **21g** | CARBS **20.5g** | FIBRE **5g**

UNDER 500 CALORIES

Warm Lentils and Halloumi

SERVES 1 | PREP 5 mins | COOK 7 mins

1 tbsp olive oil
50g halloumi, cut into small cubes
75g cooked green lentils (from a pouch or tin)
4 sweet piquanté peppers from a jar, roughly chopped
3 handfuls of baby spinach (about 100g)
Dash of balsamic vinegar
Dash of extra-virgin olive oil

The sweet piquanté peppers add a mildly spicy flavour, which contrasts well with the lentils and halloumi, and delivers a good balance of fibre and protein. Lentils are a great source of fibre.

1. Heat the olive oil in a frying pan over a medium heat. Add the halloumi cubes and fry for a couple of minutes.

2. Turn the halloumi, then add the lentils and peppers and cook for 3–4 minutes.

3. Finally, add the spinach and fry until wilted, then stir into the mix.

4. Tip into a serving bowl and finish with a dash of balsamic vinegar, a dash of extra-virgin olive oil and a pinch of black pepper.

VEGGIE GLUTEN FREE NUT FREE

BRUNCH WRAP 3 WAYS

You can make these the night before and keep them in the fridge, or eat half and keep the other half for later. Use a wholemeal or seeded wrap.

UNDER 400 CALORIES PER SERVING | 392cals

Chicken Avo

1 seeded or wholemeal wrap
1 tbsp hummus
100g cooked chicken
Large handful of baby spinach

1. Spread the wrap with the hummus, then top with the chicken. Season with salt and freshly ground black pepper, then scatter over the baby spinach leaves.

2. Fold the wrap over and cut in half to serve.

PROTEIN **39g** | CARBS **32g** | FIBRE **4g**

UNDER 400 CALORIES PER SERVING | 341cals

Smoked Salmon

1 seeded or wholemeal wrap
1 tbsp cream cheese
1 tsp pesto
50g smoked salmon slices
Lemon wedge, for squeezing
Handful of baby spinach or basil leaves

1. Spread the cream cheese and pesto over the wrap. Top with the smoked salmon and season with plenty of ground black pepper.

2. Squeeze over the lemon and top with the spinach or basil.

3. Fold the wrap over and cut in half to serve.

PROTEIN **20g** | CARBS **32g** | FIBRE **3g**

UNDER 500 CALORIES PER SERVING | 450cals

Cooked Breakfast

1 tsp olive oil or butter
1 egg, beaten
1 cooked sausage, sliced
2 grilled mushrooms, sliced
Handful of baby spinach

1. Place the oil or butter in a small omelette pan over a medium heat. Season the egg with salt and pepper, then pour into the pan. Swirl the egg out to the edges and cook for 1–2 minutes, then slide it out of the pan and on to the wrap.

2. Top with the slices of sausage and mushroom and the baby spinach leaves.

3. Fold the wrap over and cut in half to serve.

PROTEIN **23g** | CARBS **35g** | FIBRE **4.5g**

NUT FREE

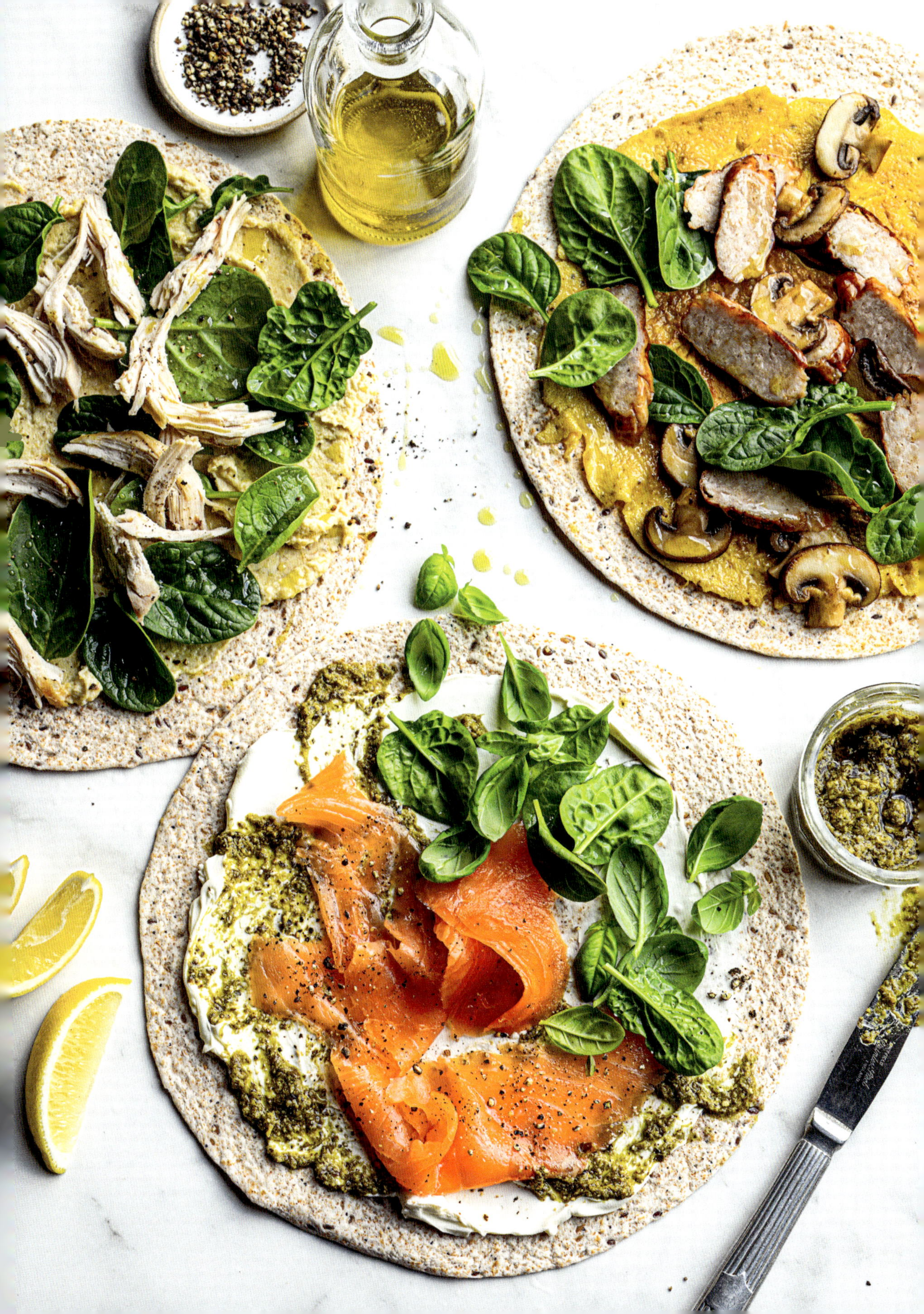

UNDER 300 CALORIES

PER SERVING | 250cals | PROTEIN 14g | CARBS 24g | FIBRE 4.5g

Lentil and Tomato Soup

SERVES 4 | PREP 10 mins | COOK 35 mins

1 tbsp olive oil
½ onion, diced
1 large garlic clove, diced (optional)
¼–½ tsp dried chilli flakes (optional)
½ tsp ground cumin (optional)
140g dried red lentils, rinsed
1 × 400g tin chopped tomatoes
1 vegetable stock cube
1 tbsp chia seeds
100g lardons

This is a classic combination for an excellent, mildly spiced soup. Red lentils melt into a creamy base, bringing both fibre and protein. Lentils are the unsung heroes of the store cupboard! You could finish this dish with a spoonful of full-fat Greek yoghurt to further boost the protein levels.

1. Place a saucepan over a medium–low heat and add the olive oil and onion. Cook for about 5 minutes, stirring occasionally.

2. Add all the remaining ingredients, except the lardons. Refill the tomato can twice with water and add this, too. Bring the mixture up to a boil, then reduce the heat and simmer gently for 30 minutes, topping up with extra water, if needed, until the lentils are cooked.

3. Meanwhile, fry the lardons in a pan over a medium heat until crispy.

4. Check the seasoning, then serve the soup in bowls scattered with 1 tablespoon of lardons per person.

GLUTEN FREE · NUT FREE · DAIRY FREE

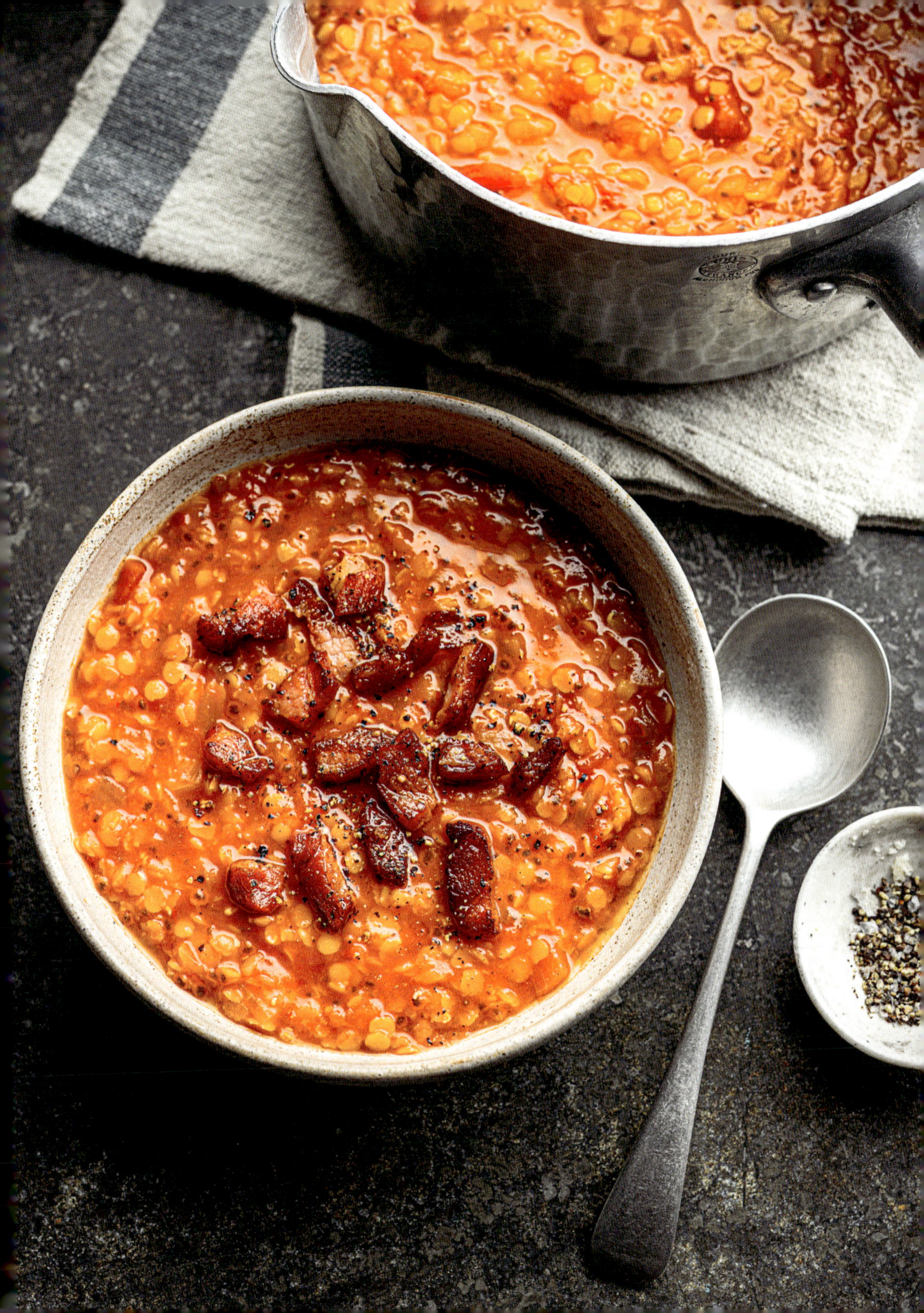

UNDER 100 CALORIES

PER SERVING | **25cals** | PROTEIN **5g** | CARBS **0.5g** | FIBRE **0.5g**

Healthy Gut Chicken Stock

MAKES	PREP	COOK
1 litre	**20** mins	**4** hours

475–500g chicken wings
1 carrot, roughly chopped
1 onion, diced
1 leek, sliced
1 large garlic clove, unpeeled, bashed or sliced in half
2 celery sticks, roughly chopped
1 bouquet garni (or 2 large bay leaves)
1 tbsp apple cider vinegar
3 black peppercorns

This is a classic recipe for delicious homemade stock – it will come in useful for soups and casseroles. Switch the veg according to what you have available. I keep random offcuts of discarded or leftover veg at the bottom of my fridge to dice and add to the pot when I make stock. You could also use the carcass left over after roasting a chicken, if you have one, rather than buying chicken wings.

1. Put the chicken wings and all the other ingredients in a large saucepan with a well-fitting lid. Pour in 1 litre of cold water and season with a generous pinch of salt.

2. Bring to the boil over a high heat, then reduce the heat, cover with a lid and simmer for about 2–4 hours, skimming the surface occasionally to remove any scum. Top up with more water, if needed.

3. Strain the liquid through a mesh sieve, pressing the bones and veg down with a masher to extract as much liquid as possible. Remove the meat from the chicken wings and add to the stock, or save to use for sandwiches or salads.

4. Leave the stock to cool and store in the fridge for up to 3–4 days, or freeze for up to 3 months.

GLUTEN FREE · NUT FREE · DAIRY FREE

PER SERVING | **32cals** | PROTEIN **3g** | CARBS **1.5g** | FIBRE **1.5g**

UNDER 100 CALORIES

Instant Miso Soup

SERVES **1** | PREP **1** min | COOK **5** mins

Soothing, simple and rehydrating. Add extra protein if you like, such as a small handful of cooked chicken or prawns.

½ tbsp miso paste
1 tbsp frozen edamame beans
Handful of baby spinach
Dash of sesame oil (optional)

1. Place 250ml water in a small saucepan. Bring up to the boil, then stir in the miso paste.

2. Add the edamame and spinach and return the soup to the boil. Reduce the heat and simmer gently for a few minutes.

3. Serve with a dash of sesame oil, if using.

VEGAN | GLUTEN FREE | NUT FREE | DAIRY FREE

UNDER 300 CALORIES

PER SERVING | **246cals** | PROTEIN **11g** | CARBS **30g** | FIBRE **9g**

White Bean Soup with Chorizo

SERVES **2** | PREP **5** mins | COOK **15** mins

90g chorizo sausage, skinned and diced (optional)
1 tbsp olive oil
½ small onion, roughly chopped
1 × 400g tin white beans (such as cannellini)
1 × 400g tin chopped tomatoes
1 vegetable stock cube
Handful of roughly chopped parsley leaves
3 tbsp Greek yoghurt (optional)

Easy, satisfying comfort food, topped up with protein from the diced chorizo, which adds a taste of Spain.

1. If using, place the chorizo in a saucepan over a medium heat. Fry until the chorizo releases the oil and becomes crispy. Remove the chorizo with a slotted spoon and set aside. Discard the oil.

2. Add the olive oil and onion to the same pan and place over a medium–low heat. Cook for 4–5 minutes, until the onion is softened.

3. Add the beans and their liquid, tomatoes and the stock cube, stir well, and bring up to the boil. Reduce the heat, cover with a lid and simmer for 10 minutes, adding a splash of water, if needed, to loosen.

4. Serve the soup in deep bowls, sprinkled with parsley and scattered with the crispy chorizo, if using, or topped with a large tablespoon of Greek yoghurt, if you prefer.

GLUTEN FREE · NUT FREE

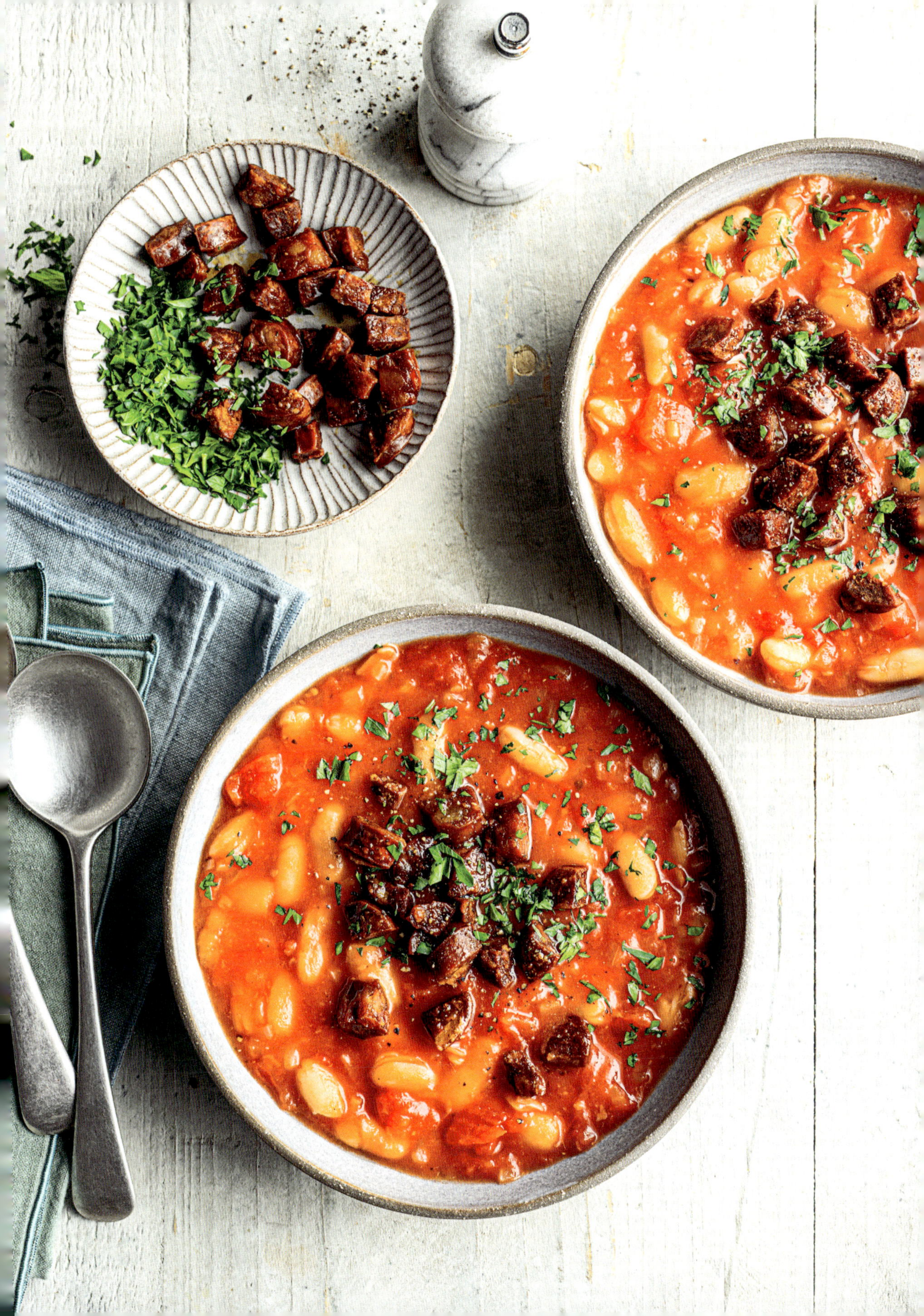

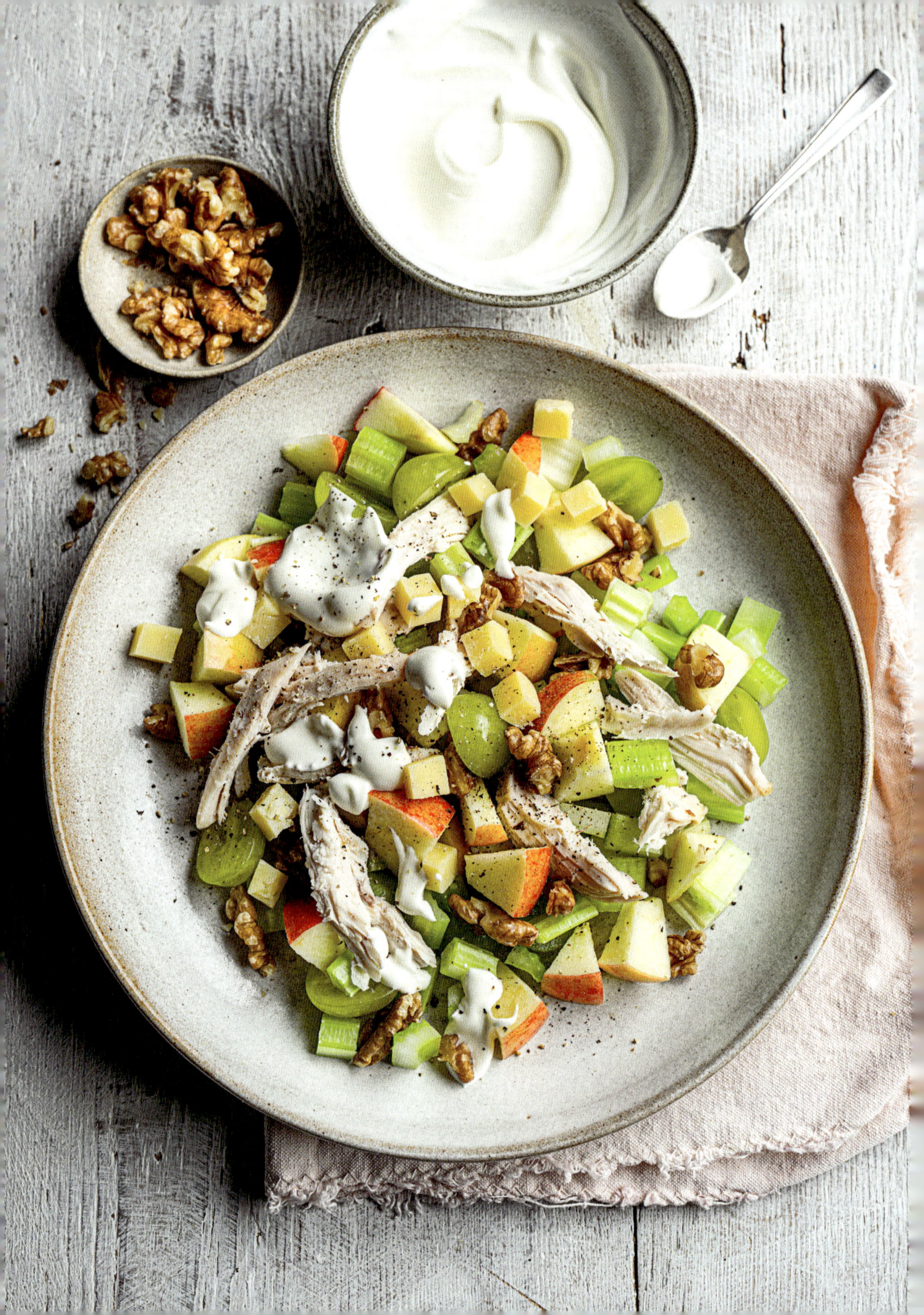

PER SERVING | **375cals** | PROTEIN **24g** | CARBS **10g** | FIBRE **2.5g**

UNDER 400 CALORIES

Waldorf Chicken Salad

SERVES 1 | PREP 15 min

This classic salad is crunchy and refreshing, with chicken, grapes and a creamy dressing. It makes a light but satisfying meal.

2 celery sticks, halved lengthways and finely chopped
6 green grapes, halved
1 small apple, cored and chopped into cubes
15g Cheddar, cut into cubes
Juice of ½ lemon
55g cooked chicken, chopped or shredded
4 walnut halves, roughly chopped

For the dressing
1 heaped tsp mayonnaise
1 heaped tbsp plain yoghurt

1. Tip the celery, grapes, apple and cheese into a serving bowl.

2. Squeeze in the lemon juice (this will stop the apple browning, and brighten the flavour), then top with the chicken and walnuts. Season with a pinch of salt and pepper.

3. To make the dressing, mix the ingredients in a small jug, then spoon over the salad to serve.

GLUTEN FREE

UNDER 600 CALORIES

PER SERVING | **500cals** | PROTEIN **24g** | CARBS **21g** | FIBRE **9g**

Pepper Pots

SERVES 2 | PREP 7 mins | COOK 30 mins

2 red peppers
1 tbsp olive oil
100g mushrooms, chopped
½ red onion, chopped
6 cherry tomatoes, halved
1 tbsp capers (plus a little caper juice)
100g Puy lentils (from a pouch or tin)
1 tsp dried mixed herbs
16 walnut halves, roughly chopped
2 eggs
1 tbsp grated Parmesan

Colourful juicy stuffed peppers, full of Mediterranean flavours, rich in fibre and protein from the eggs and lentils.

1. Preheat the oven to 200°C/Fan 180°C/Gas 6, and line a small baking tin or dish with non-stick baking paper or foil.

2. Begin by slicing the top off the red peppers just about 2cm under the stem, reserving the tops as a lid. Clear the seeds from the main body of the peppers.

3. Using your hands, rub ½ teaspoon of the oil on the outside of the peppers to coat. Sit them upright snugly in the prepared dish and bake them in the oven for 8–10 minutes.

4. Meanwhile, place the remaining olive oil in a large frying pan over a medium heat. Add the mushrooms and onion and cook for 7–8 minutes. Stir in the tomatoes, capers and their juice, lentils, herbs, walnuts and a pinch of salt and pepper, and cook for another 5 minutes.

5. Remove the peppers from the oven and spoon the lentil mixture into them, dividing it equally. Return the stuffed peppers to the oven, still upright, and bake for 10 minutes.

6. Take the dish out of the oven again and make a dent in the filling with the back of a spoon. Crack an egg into each one. Scatter with the Parmesan and put the lids back on. Return them to the oven for a final 5 minutes.

GLUTEN FREE

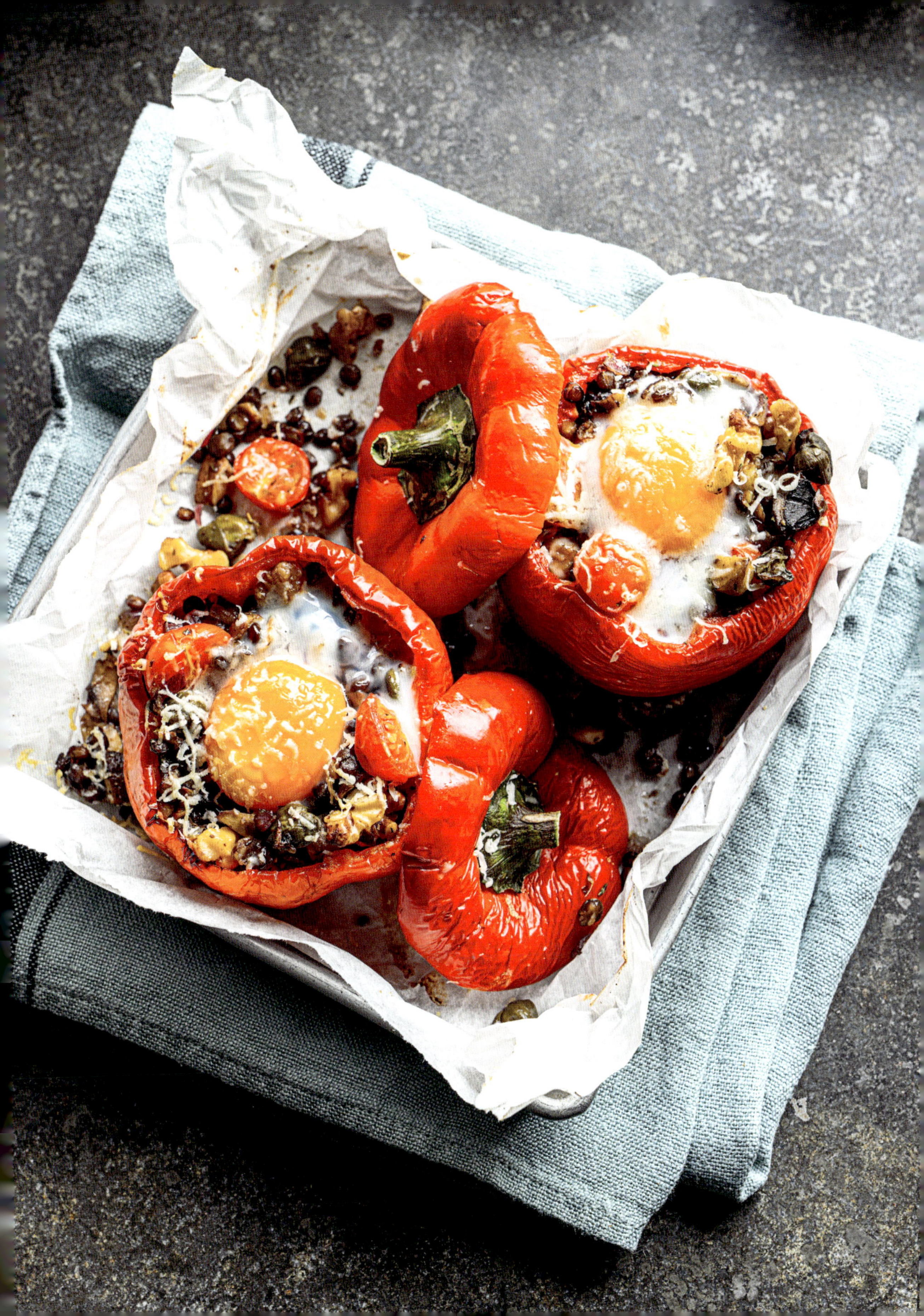

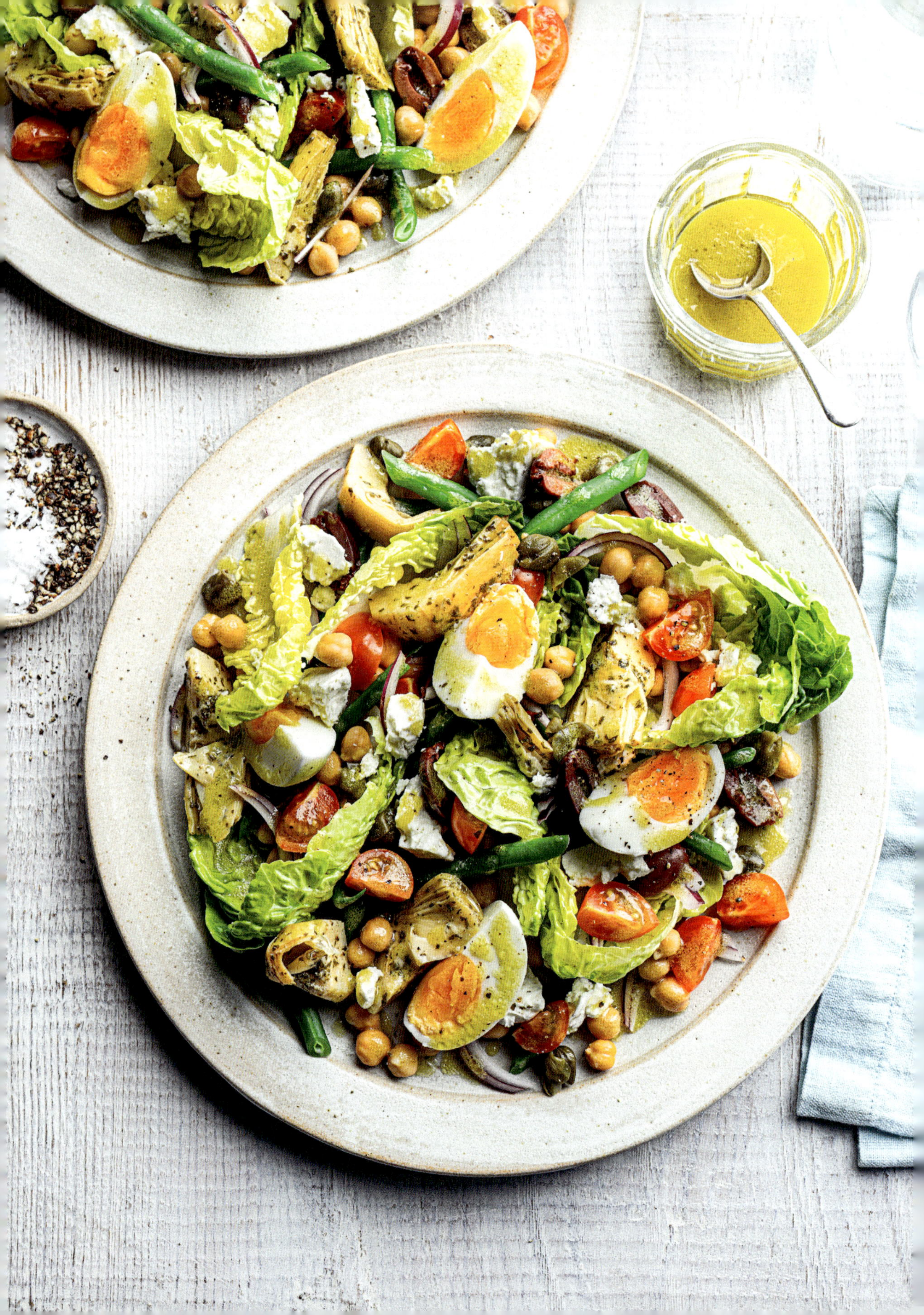

PER SERVING | 520cals | PROTEIN 24g | CARBS 33g | FIBRE 15g

UNDER 600 CALORIES

Chickpea Niçoise

SERVES 2 | PREP 20 mins | COOK 1 min

2 handfuls of green beans (fresh or frozen)
2 Little Gem lettuces, leaves separated and torn if large
1 × 400g tin chickpeas, drained
½ red onion, finely sliced
10 cherry tomatoes, quartered, or 2 ripe tomatoes, cut into wedges
2 tbsp (about 12) pitted black olives
6 artichoke hearts from a jar, halved
2 hard-boiled eggs, quartered
2 tbsp capers, drained
25g feta, crumbled

For the dressing
1 tsp Dijon mustard
1 tbsp apple cider vinegar
2 tbsp extra-virgin olive oil

This classic French salad always feels special, and is full of flavour. It's also easy to assemble. Although it is traditionally made with tuna, here I have used chickpeas and feta for a delicious meat-free alternative.

1. Boil or steam the green beans in a centimetre of water, just very briefly for 1 minute until soft but with bite, and drain.

2. Divide the lettuce leaves between two bowls, then top with the chickpeas, onion, tomatoes, olives, green beans and artichoke hearts. Finish with the eggs, capers and feta.

3. To make the dressing, whisk together all the ingredients, except the honey or maple syrup, if using, until it emulsifies and thickens.

4. Drizzle the dressing over the salad, then season with a generous pinch of salt and pepper.

VEGGIE | GLUTEN FREE | NUT FREE

UNDER 400 CALORIES

PER SERVING | **340cals** | PROTEIN **46g** | CARBS **4g** | FIBRE **2g**

Chicken, Anchovy and Egg Salad

SERVES 2 | PREP 10 mins

4 large handfuls of baby spinach
4 large handfuls of rocket leaves
4 spring onions, chopped (or 2 tbsp chopped cornichons)
200g cooked chicken, chopped or shredded
2 hard-boiled eggs, quartered
8 anchovies, chopped

For the dressing
1 tbsp pesto
3 tbsp plain yoghurt

As well as delivering a good hit of omega 3 from the anchovies, the delicious umami taste gives it an extra layer of flavour. Plain yoghurt works best for the dressing – Greek yoghurt is too thick.

1. Divide the spinach and rocket between two bowls.

2. Top with the spring onions, chicken, eggs and anchovies, dividing the ingredients equally between the two bowls. Season generously with black pepper.

3. To make the dressing, mix the ingredients in a small jug, then spoon over the salad to serve.

GLUTEN FREE | NUT FREE

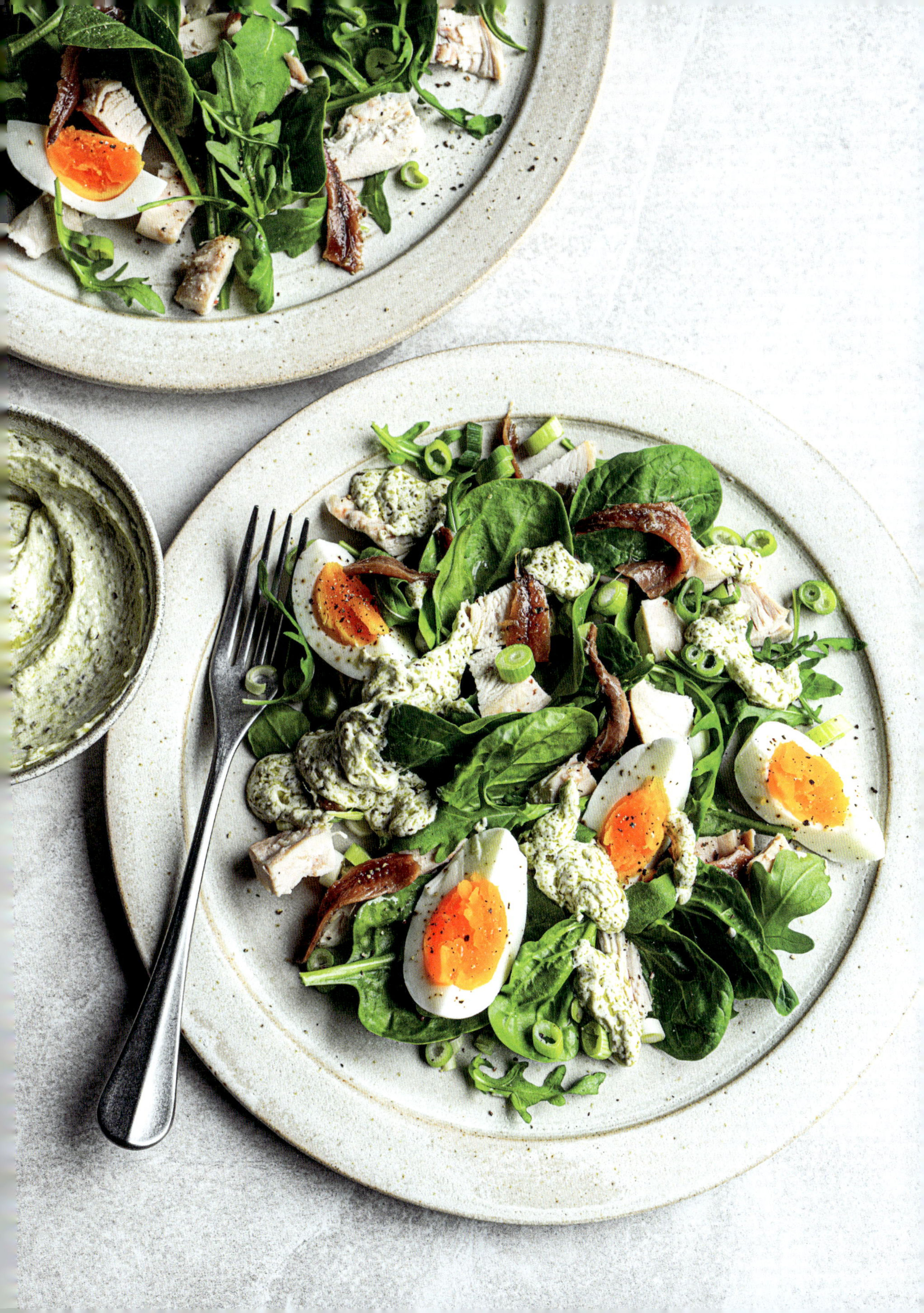

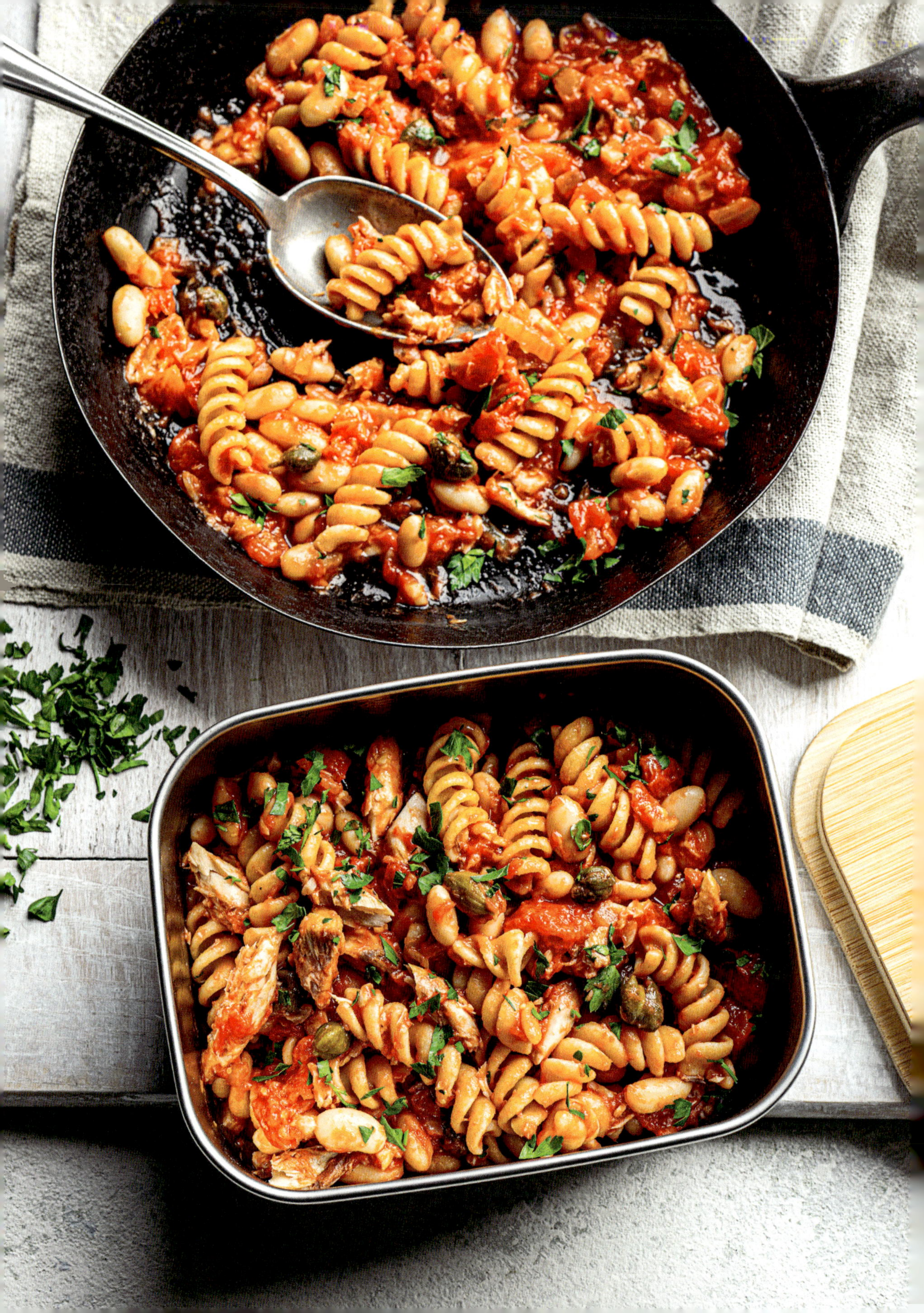

PER SERVING | **376cals** | PROTEIN **19g** | CARBS **33g** | FIBRE **8.5g**

UNDER 400 CALORIES

Dan's Fish and Pasta Lunch Box

SERVES 2 | PREP 10 mins | COOK 22 mins

50g dried wholemeal pasta
1 tbsp olive oil
½ medium onion, diced
1 garlic clove, diced
½ × 400g tin chopped tomatoes
1 × 125g tin mackerel, drained
½ × 400g tin cannellini beans, drained
1 tbsp capers
Large handful of parsley or rocket leaves, chopped

My son Dan is an enthusiastic and creative cook, and I loved this flavourful dish. Quick and easy, using tinned mackerel, which boosts omega 3, all the ingredients can be found in your store cupboard.

1. Cook the pasta in boiling salted water, according to the packet instructions. Drain and set aside, reserving a cup of the pasta cooking water.

2. Meanwhile, place the oil and onion in a frying pan and cook over a low heat for 4–5 minutes. Add the garlic and fry for another minute.

3. Add the chopped tomatoes, mackerel, cannellini beans and capers, and mix well. Simmer for 5 minutes to heat through.

4. Tip in the drained pasta and stir over the heat, adding a splash of the reserved pasta cooking water, if needed, to loosen.

5. Serve in two bowls, sprinkled with the chopped parsley or rocket.

NUT FREE | DAIRY FREE

UNDER 500 CALORIES

PER SALMON SERVING	PER CHICKEN SERVING
426cals	**468cals**
PROTEIN 33g	PROTEIN 24.5g
CARBS 10g	CARBS 6g
FIBRE 4g	FIBRE 4.5g

Protein Salads in Jars

SERVES 1 | PREP 15 mins

SALMON AND EGG SALAD
50g smoked salmon slices, cut into pieces
1 hard-boiled egg, quartered
2 tbsp cooked Puy lentils (from a pouch or tin)
Handful of Seedy Sprinkles **(see page 39)**
8 sugar snap peas, roughly chopped
4 cherry tomatoes, halved
2 handfuls of salad leaves

For the dressing
½ tsp Dijon mustard
2 tsp apple cider vinegar
1 tbsp extra-virgin olive oil
½ tsp honey (optional)

CHICKEN AVOCADO SALAD
50g roast chicken, shredded or chopped
2 tbsp cooked quinoa (from a pouch)
1 tbsp chopped almonds
¼ avocado, chopped
Handful of cooked broccoli florets
2 handfuls of baby spinach

For the creamy pesto dressing
1 tbsp pesto
1 tbsp plain yoghurt
1 tbsp extra-virgin olive oil

Each of these two recipe suggestions serves 1 person. Making salad in a jar keeps it from falling apart on the way to work, and it looks so inviting with the colourful layers. They are bound to become a favourite, and you can adapt as you like. Find a few jars with a secure lid and off you go; it'll save you money as well.

1. Spoon the dressing into the base of a 500ml jar.

2. Add the layer of protein (salmon, egg and lentils, or chicken and quinoa), which is a barrier between the dressing and the more delicate leaves.

3. Top with the seeds or nuts for texture, then add the vegetables, cooked or raw, and finish with leaves or herbs. Screw on the lid.

4. To serve, tip the jar upside down, give it a good shake and empty on to a plate for perfectly dressed salad.

GLUTEN FREE

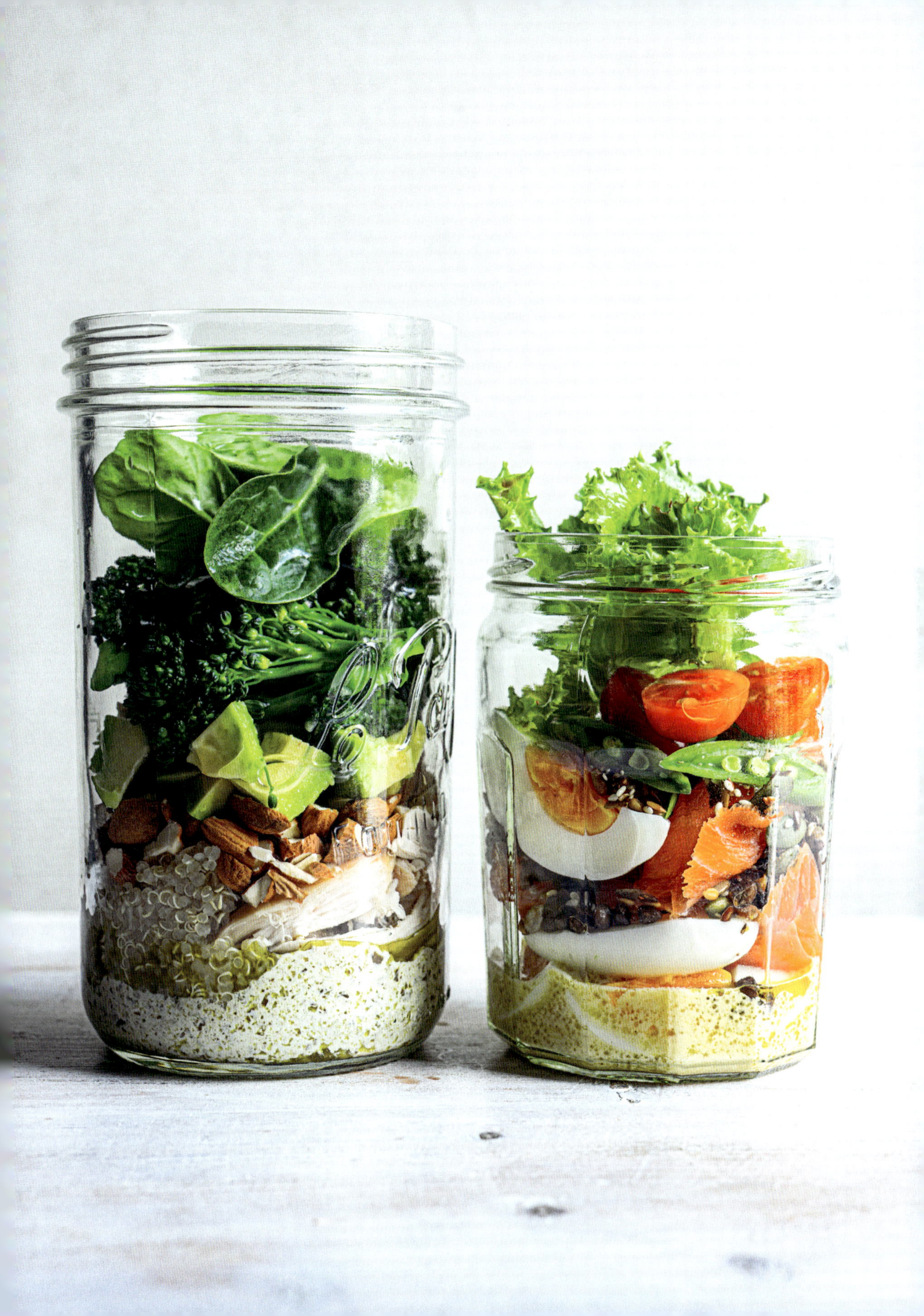

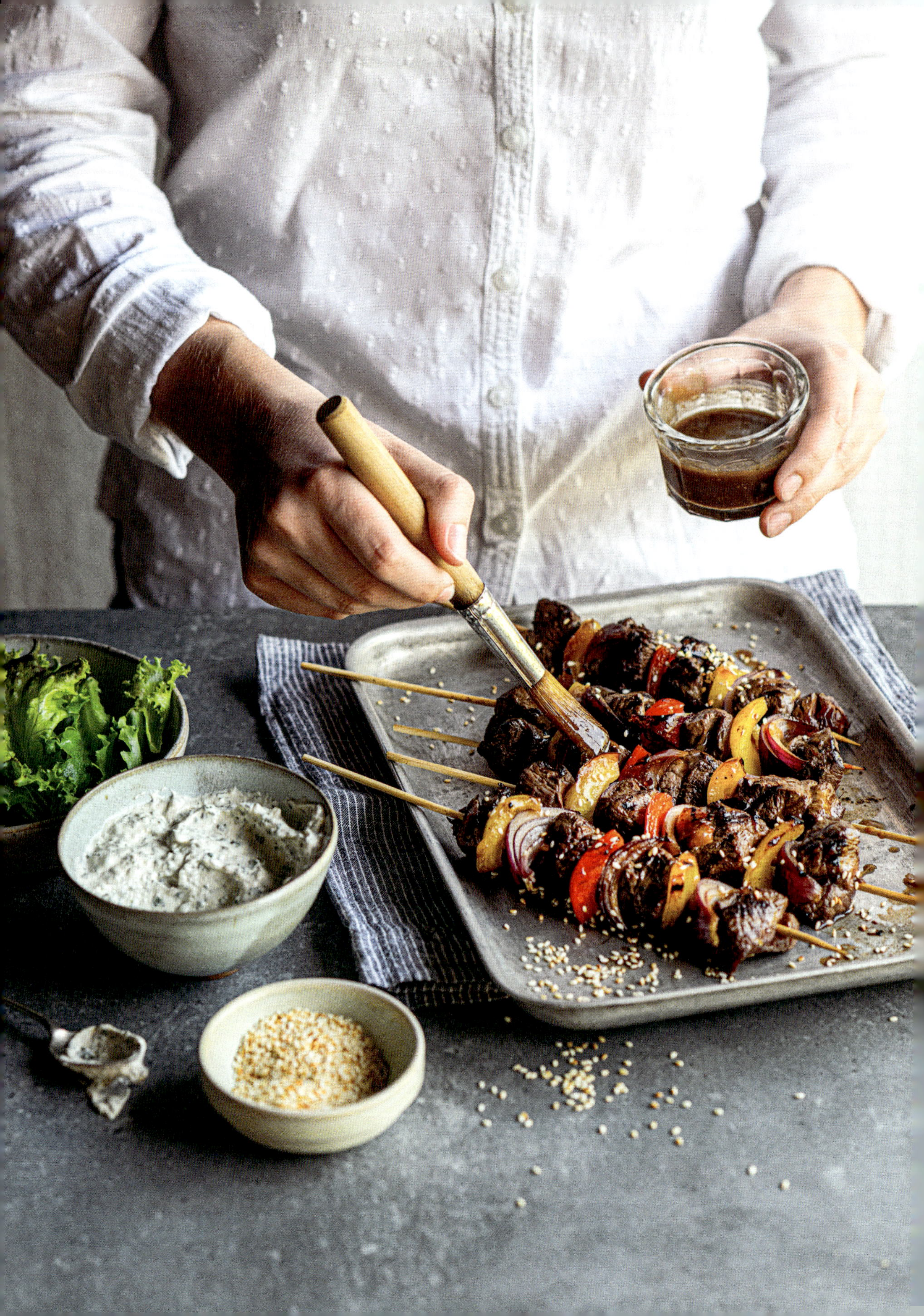

Pork, Lamb and Beef

UNDER 400 CALORIES

PER SERVING | **307cals** | PROTEIN **10g** | CARBS **10g** | FIBRE **6g**

Chorizo, White Bean and Avocado Salad

SERVES **2** | PREP **5** mins | COOK **4** mins

50g chorizo sausage, skinned and cut into small dice
75g mixed salad leaves
75g drained tinned or jarred cannellini beans, rinsed
40g red cabbage, shredded
¼ small red onion, diced
1 small avocado, peeled, destoned and cut into small chunks
1 tbsp extra-virgin olive oil
Juice of ½ lemon

Everything you want from a salad – protein, fibre and lots of fresh veg. This makes a complete light meal, but you could also serve it with a slice of crusty wholemeal bread. The diced cooked chorizo is crisp, garlicky and golden, almost like smoky crispy croutons but without the carbs.

1. Place the chorizo in a dry frying pan over a medium heat. When the oil starts to release from the chorizo, turn the heat down slightly and cook for 3–4 minutes, stirring occasionally, until golden and crisp. Remove from the heat and set it aside.

2. Arrange the salad leaves on a serving dish and top with the beans, cabbage, onion and avocado.

3. In a small jug, mix together the olive oil and lemon juice with a pinch of salt and pepper. Pour the dressing over the salad, then scatter over the crispy chorizo to serve.

GLUTEN FREE · NUT FREE · DAIRY FREE

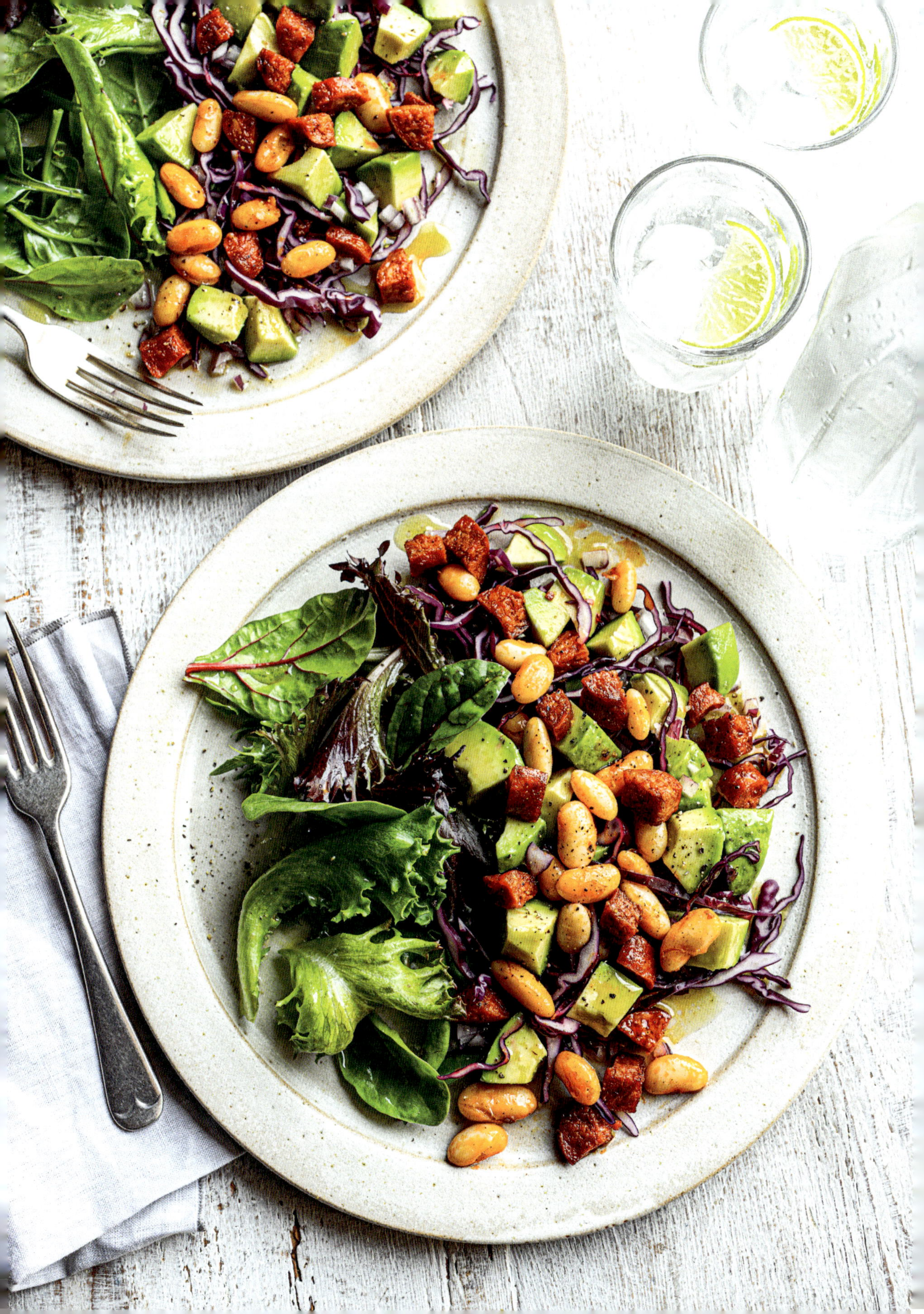

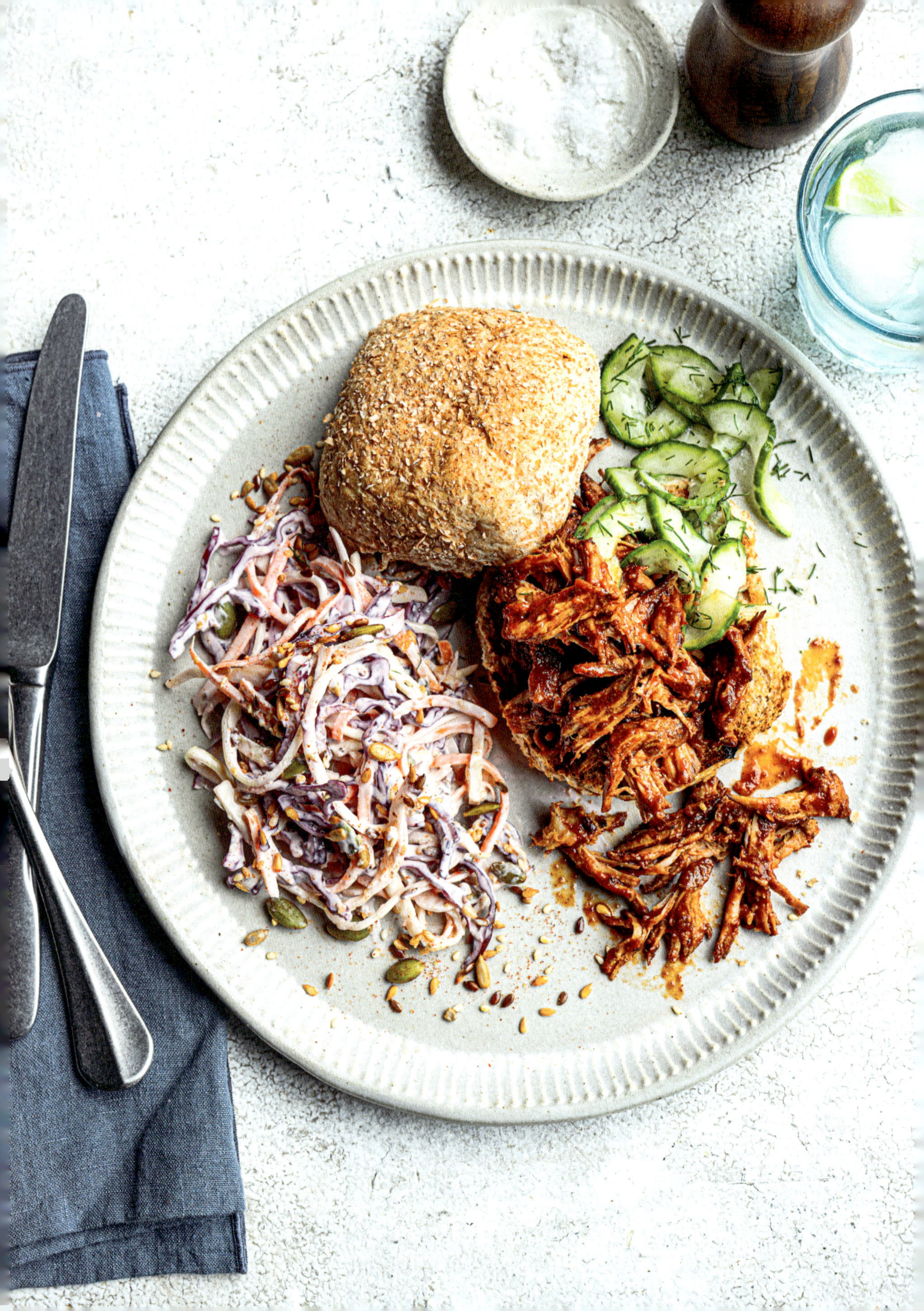

PER SERVING | **237cals** | PROTEIN **33g** | CARBS **6g** | FIBRE **0.5g**

UNDER 300 CALORIES

Cheat's Pulled Pork

SERVES 4 | PREP 65 mins | COOK 70 mins

2 tbsp tomato purée
2 tbsp balsamic vinegar or apple cider vinegar
1 tbsp runny honey
2 large garlic cloves, minced
1 tbsp ground cumin
1–2 tsp chipotle chilli flakes
1 tsp smoked paprika
4 pork shoulder steaks (about 600g total weight)
1 tbsp olive oil
4 small wholemeal buns or 2 wholemeal pitta breads (optional)

This is a speedy version of classic pulled pork, using pork steaks rather than a shoulder joint, which takes longer to slow cook. Here, the sticky, smoky pork is served in a wholemeal pitta or bun with slaw, but you could serve it in a lettuce leaf wrap.

1. Mix the tomato purée, vinegar, honey, garlic, cumin, chilli flakes and smoked paprika in a bowl. Add 3–4 tablespoons of water and season well with salt and pepper. Add the pork and turn to coat well in the sauce. Cover and marinate in the fridge for about 1 hour.

2. Preheat the oven to 170°C/Fan 150°C/Gas 3½.

3. Heat the olive oil in a large frying pan over a medium–high heat. Lift the pork steaks out of the dish and into the pan. Cook for 5 minutes, turning once, until browned and slightly blackened in places. Transfer any remaining marinade from the dish to a small saucepan.

4. Transfer the pork to a roasting tin in an even layer, then pour in 150ml water. Cover the tin with foil and cook in the preheated oven for 1 hour, or until the pork is tender. Leave to rest for 15 minutes, covered in the tin.

5. Lift the pork out of the tin and shred with 2 forks or your fingers into strips. Place the pork in a bowl. Pour any juices from the tin into the pan with the leftover marinade, then cook over a medium heat for 5–7 minutes, until reduced and thickened. Pour the sauce over the pork and turn to coat in the sauce.

6. Serve the pork in a wholemeal bun with Seedy Slaw (see page 231) and Quick Pickled Cucumber (see page 222), if you like.

GLUTEN FREE | NUT FREE | DAIRY FREE

UNDER 400 CALORIES

PER SERVING | **375cals** | PROTEIN **31g** | CARBS **15g** | FIBRE **5g**

Keema Bowls

SERVES **4** | PREP **10** mins | COOK **45** mins

2 tbsp olive oil
1 onion, finely chopped
500g minced pork
2 garlic cloves, minced
4cm piece of fresh root ginger, peeled and finely grated
1 heaped tbsp mild curry powder
3 tomatoes, finely chopped
100g cooked Puy lentils (from a pouch or tin)
150g frozen peas
4 tbsp full-fat Greek yoghurt
Pinch of nigella seeds or cumin seeds (optional)

This lightly spiced pork mince dish contains Puy lentils as well as the more usual peas for a fibre and protein boost. You could serve it with a wholemeal flatbread or brown rice. Any leftovers will happily keep in the fridge for up to 3 days (or you can freeze them). Simply add a splash of water when reheating.

1. Heat the olive oil in a large sauté pan over a medium heat. Add the onion, turning the heat down slightly, and cook for 8 minutes, until softened. Add the mince and cook for 10 minutes, breaking it down with a fork until browned all over. Stir in the garlic and ginger, then cook for 1 minute. Add the curry powder and cook for 1 minute.

2. Pour in 250ml water and stir in the tomatoes. Season with salt and pepper, and bring to a simmer. Cook, part-covered and stirring occasionally, for 15 minutes.

3. Stir in the lentils and peas and cook for another 10 minutes, until the mince is tender and the peas are heated through.

4. Serve the keema in bowls topped with some Tomato, Mint and Cucumber Salad (see page 234), or simple chopped tomatoes, and a good spoonful of yoghurt. Finish with a pinch of nigella or cumin seeds, if you like.

GLUTEN FREE | NUT FREE

PER SERVING | 367cals | PROTEIN 41g | CARBS 16g | FIBRE 6g

UNDER 400 CALORIES

Spanish Pork and Chorizo Stew

SERVES 4 | PREP 10 mins | COOK 47 mins

1 tbsp olive oil
600g pork shoulder steaks, trimmed of excess fat and cut into bite-sized chunks
1 large onion, thinly sliced
1 large red pepper, deseeded and cut into chunks
60g chorizo sausage, skinned and diced
3 large garlic cloves, finely chopped
1 tbsp tomato purée
300ml chicken stock
1 × 400g tin white beans, such as cannellini or butter beans, drained
Handful of chopped parsley, to serve

Rich and smoky from the paprika and chorizo, this has a wonderful Mediterranean flavour. This stew is a nice example of pairing protein (pork) and fibre (beans), which are one of the easiest sources of quality fibre.

1. Heat the oil in a flameproof casserole over a medium heat. Add the pork and cook for 7 minutes, turning occasionally, until browned all over. Add the onion, red pepper and chorizo, and cook for another 5 minutes.

2. Add the garlic and cook briefly, then stir in the tomato purée and pour in the chicken stock. Season with salt and pepper, and bring the sauce up to the boil. Reduce the heat, partially cover with a lid, and simmer for 30 minutes.

3. Stir in the beans and cook for a final 5 minutes, until the pork is tender and the sauce has reduced and thickened. Serve sprinkled with parsley.

GLUTEN FREE | NUT FREE | DAIRY FREE

UNDER **400** CALORIES

PER SERVING | **335cals** | PROTEIN **36g** | CARBS **17g** | FIBRE **4g**

Hoisin Pork Lettuce Wraps

SERVES **2** | PREP **25** mins | COOK **6** mins

A healthier twist on the usual: pork replaces duck, and crisp lettuce leaves are used instead of pancakes to make a tasty, light meal.

1 tbsp light soy sauce
2 tbsp hoisin sauce
300g pork loin steaks, trimmed of any fat and cut into thin strips
2 tsp olive oil
8 large Little Gem lettuce leaves
1 carrot, cut into matchsticks
1 snack cucumber, cut into matchsticks
2 spring onions, shredded
2 tsp toasted sesame seeds

1. Mix together the soy sauce and hoisin sauce in a bowl. Add the pork and turn until coated. Set aside for at least 15 minutes to marinate.

2. Heat the oil in a frying pan over a medium heat. Add the pork and cook for 3 minutes on one side, until golden. Spoon any remaining marinade from the bowl over the pork, then turn it over and cook for another 3 minutes, until cooked through. Remove from the heat, cover, and leave to rest for 5 minutes.

3. Meanwhile, prepare the vegetables and arrange them on a serving plate.

4. To assemble the wraps, place a few strips of carrot, cucumber and spring onion on each lettuce leaf, top with a few pieces of pork, and finish with a sprinkling of sesame seeds.

AIR-FRYER TIP

Prepare the pork as Step 1. Preheat the air fryer to 180°C, if needed. Cook the pork for 10 minutes, turning once, until cooked through. Serve as above.

NUT FREE

DAIRY FREE

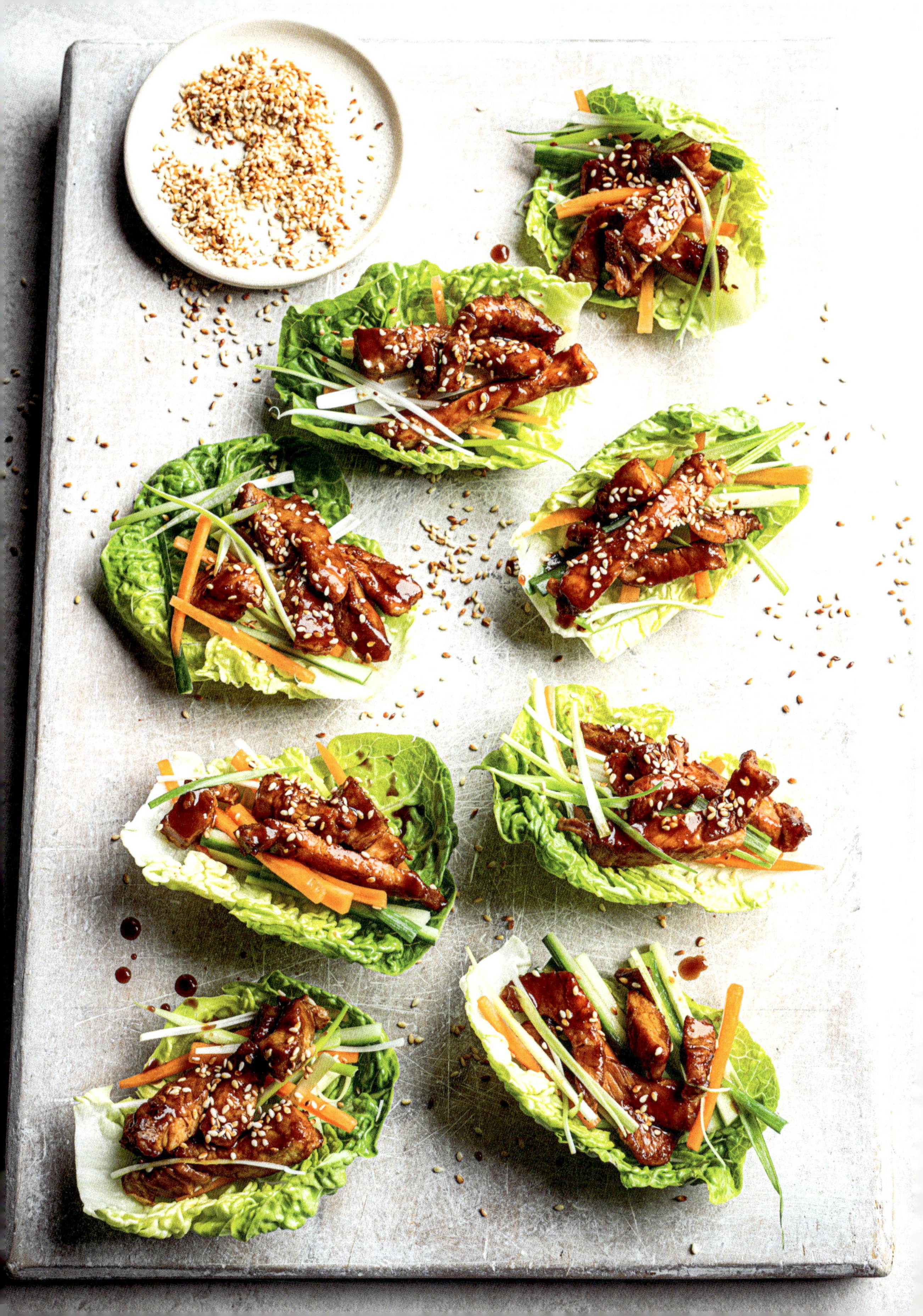

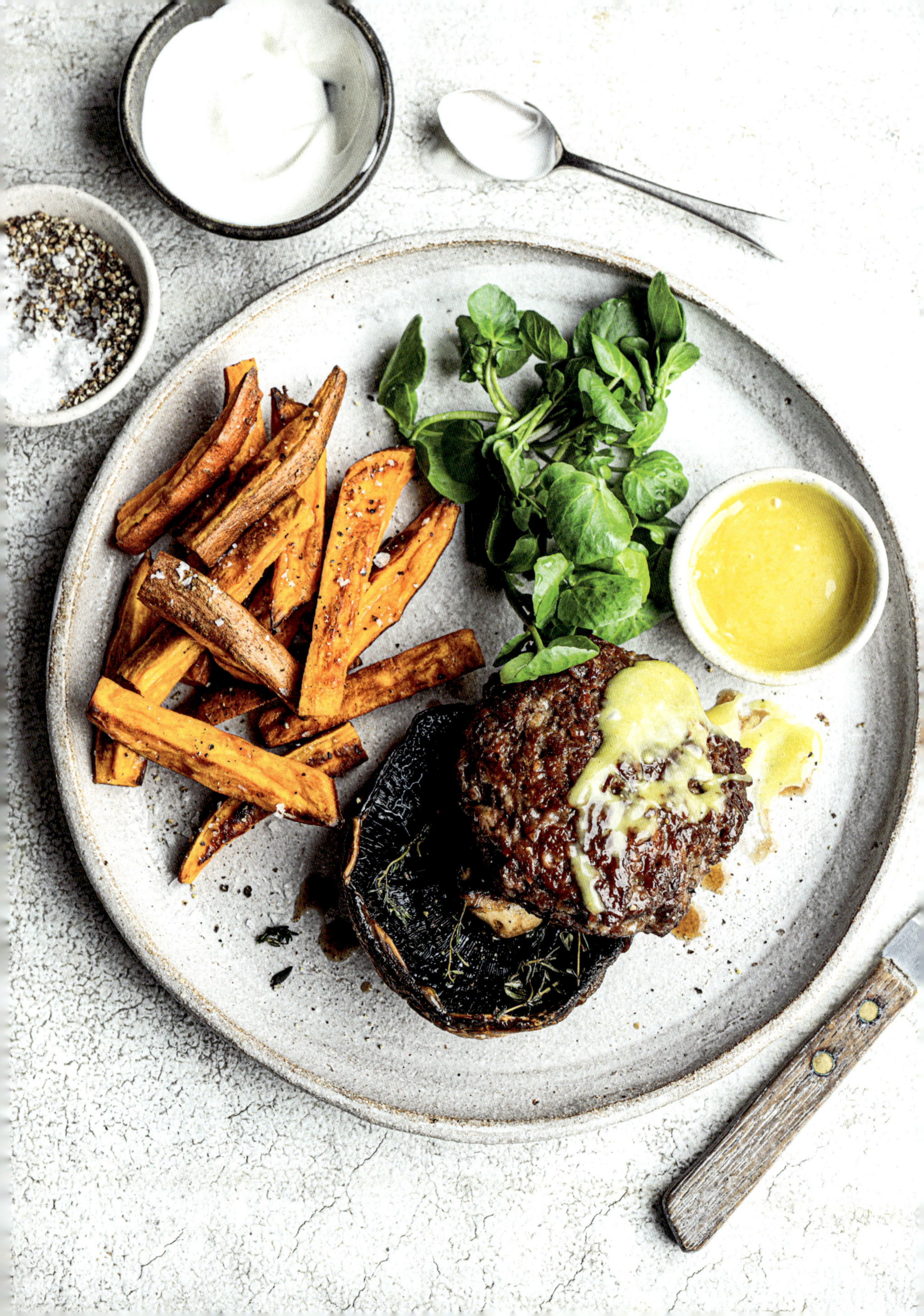

PER SERVING | **322cals** | PROTEIN **32g** | CARBS **2g** | FIBRE **0.5g**

UNDER 400 CALORIES

Venison Burgers with Mushroom 'Buns'

SERVES 2 | PREP 30 mins | COOK 15 mins

250g venison mince
25g mature Cheddar, finely grated
1 tsp garlic granules
2 Portobello mushrooms
4 sprigs of thyme or ½ tsp dried thyme
1½ tbsp olive oil
1 tbsp mayonnaise or full-fat Greek yoghurt
½ tsp runny honey
1 tsp English mustard
Handful of watercress or rocket leaves

Venison is healthier and more sustainable than beef, with more protein, iron, B vitamins and essential omega 3, and it has 40 per cent less fat than beef. A large mushroom replaces the usual carb-heavy bun in this recipe. A little grated Cheddar is also added to the mince to enhance the flavour and keep the burgers succulent, since venison is low in fat and can dry out during cooking. Serve the burgers with Sweet Potato Chips (see page 238).

1. Put the mince, Cheddar and garlic granules in a bowl. Season with salt and pepper, then mix with your hands until combined. Shape the mince mixture into 2 burgers, then chill in the fridge for 20 minutes. Preheat the oven to 200°C/Fan 180°C/Gas 6.

2. Put the mushrooms in a small baking dish on top of the thyme sprigs, and brush the caps with 1 tablespoon of the olive oil. (If using dried thyme instead of fresh, sprinkle it over the caps.) Add a splash of water to the dish, season the mushrooms, then cook in the oven for 12–15 minutes, turning once, until tender.

3. Meanwhile, heat a frying pan over a medium heat. Brush the burgers with the remaining oil and cook in the frying pan for 4–5 minutes on each side, until golden on the outside and cooked through. Leave to rest on a warm plate for 3–5 minutes.

4. Mix together the mayonnaise or yoghurt, honey and mustard.

5. To serve, put a mushroom on each serving plate and top with the burgers. Finish with a spoonful of the honey-mustard sauce and serve with watercress or rocket alongside.

AIR-FRYER TIP

Preheat the air fryer to 180°C, if needed. Prepare the venison burgers as Step 1, then place in the air fryer, drizzle each with 1 teaspoon of oil, and cook for 15–20 minutes, turning once. After a few minutes, add the mushrooms and cook for 12–15 minutes, turning once. Serve with the honey-mustard sauce as above.

GLUTEN FREE | NUT FREE

UNDER 400 CALORIES

PER SERVING | **383cals** | PROTEIN **28g** | CARBS **2.5g** | FIBRE **1g**

Harissa Lamb Kofta with Lemony Mint Yoghurt

SERVES 4 | PREP 45 mins | COOK 8 mins

500g minced lamb
40g ground almonds
2 garlic cloves, minced
1 heaped tbsp harissa paste
150g full-fat Greek yoghurt
Juice of ½ lemon
3 tbsp finely chopped mint leaves
1 tbsp olive oil
Lemon wedges, to serve

These simple koftas use harissa paste to add a gentle heat and flavour. Kofta often contain breadcrumbs or flour to bind them, which increases their refined carb content. Instead, I've used ground almonds, which keeps the carbs low and boosts the protein. Serve them with this delicious lemony mint yoghurt and a salad. On a non-fasting day, add 2–3 tablespoons of quinoa or brown rice.

1. Place the mince, ground almonds, garlic and harissa in a bowl. Season with salt and pepper, then mix with your hands until combined.

2. Divide the mixture into 12 portions (about 45g each) and, using wet hands, shape each one into a sausage-shaped kofta about 6cm long. Cover and refrigerate for 30 minutes.

3. Meanwhile, combine the yoghurt, lemon juice and mint in a bowl and mix well.

4. Heat the oil in a frying pan over a medium heat. Add the kofta and cook in batches for 7–8 minutes, turning occasionally, until golden and cooked through.

5. Serve the kofta with the lemony mint yoghurt, a green salad and lemon wedges alongside.

AIR-FRYER TIP

Prepare the kofta as Steps 1–2. Preheat the air fryer to 180°C, if needed. Brush the kofta with a little oil and cook (you may need to do this in batches) for 12–15 minutes, turning once, until golden and cooked through. Serve with the lemony mint yoghurt as above.

GLUTEN FREE | DAIRY FREE

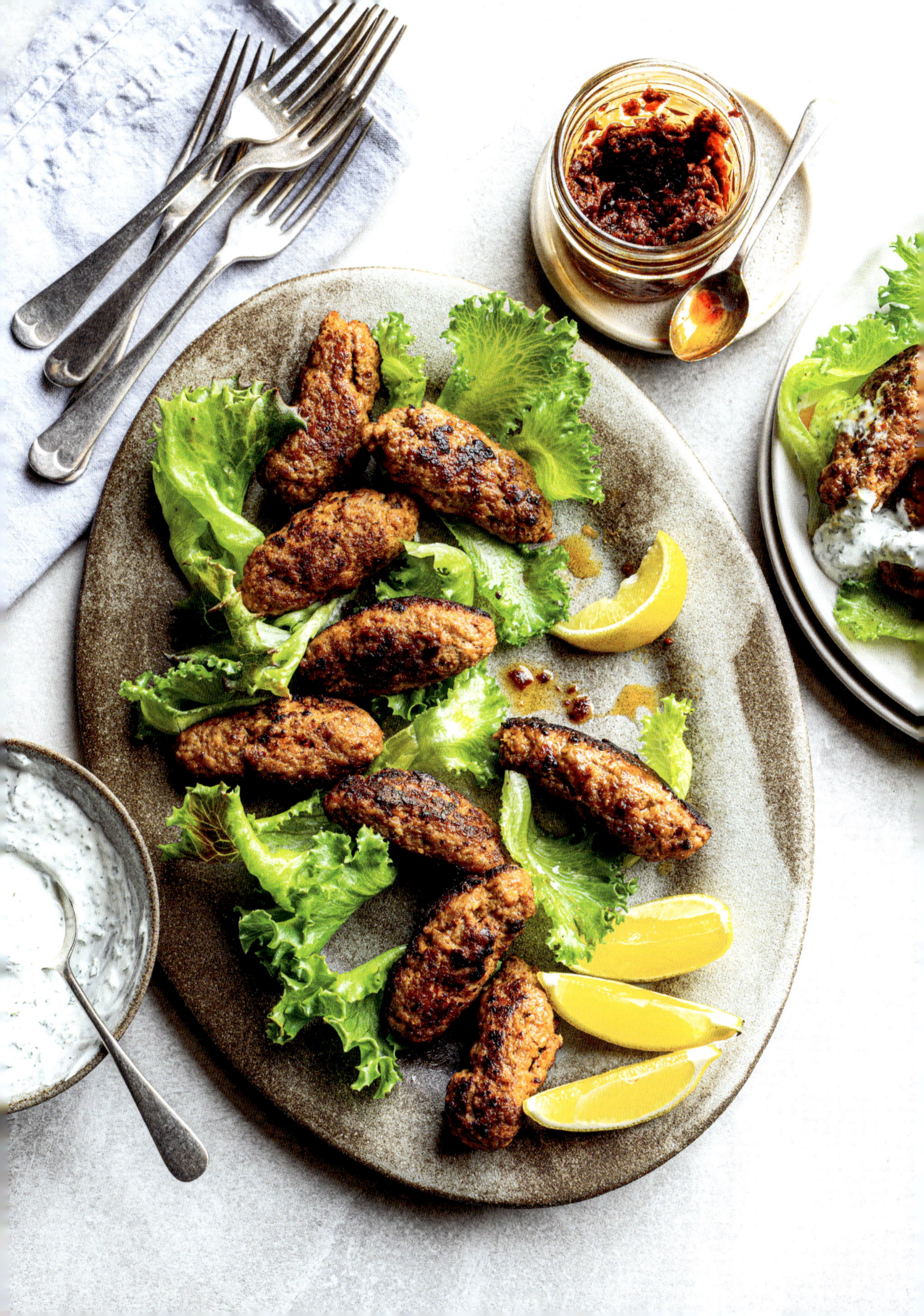

UNDER 400 CALORIES

PER SERVING | **340cals** | PROTEIN **28g** | CARBS **8g** | FIBRE **3g**

Mediterranean Roast Lamb

SERVES 2 | PREP 10 mins | COOK 20 mins

1½ tbsp olive oil
2 sprigs of rosemary
2 garlic cloves, peeled and halved
2 lamb loin chops (about 180g total weight)
6 tomatoes, halved
1 courgette, cut into batons
8 pitted black olives

Tomatoes, courgettes, olives and fresh rosemary are classic flavours with lamb. Here, they come together to make a simple and light roast. Serve it with rocket leaves or steamed greens like kale. You could also add a few baby new potatoes to the roasting tin.

1. Mix ½ tablespoon of the olive oil in a dish with 1 sprig of the rosemary and the halved garlic cloves. Season with salt and pepper, then add the lamb and turn to coat in the seasoned oil. Leave to marinate in the fridge for 1 hour, if time allows.

2. Preheat the oven to 200°C/Fan 180°C/Gas 6.

3. Put the tomatoes and courgette in a roasting tin. Add the remaining oil and rosemary sprig, season and roast in the oven for 5 minutes.

4. Meanwhile, remove the lamb from the fridge. Place a frying pan over a high heat and, when hot, turn the heat down to medium and add the lamb. Sear the lamb for 5 minutes, turning once, until browned and golden. Transfer the lamb to the roasting tin with the tomatoes and courgette, add the olives, then roast the lamb for 12–15 minutes, until cooked but still a little pink in the middle.

5. Remove the lamb and set aside, covered, to rest for 5 minutes. Turn off the oven and leave the tomatoes, courgette and olives to keep warm. Serve the lamb with the tomatoes and courgette and a spoonful of Mint Yoghurt Sauce (see page 242), if liked, on the side.

GLUTEN FREE · NUT FREE · DAIRY FREE

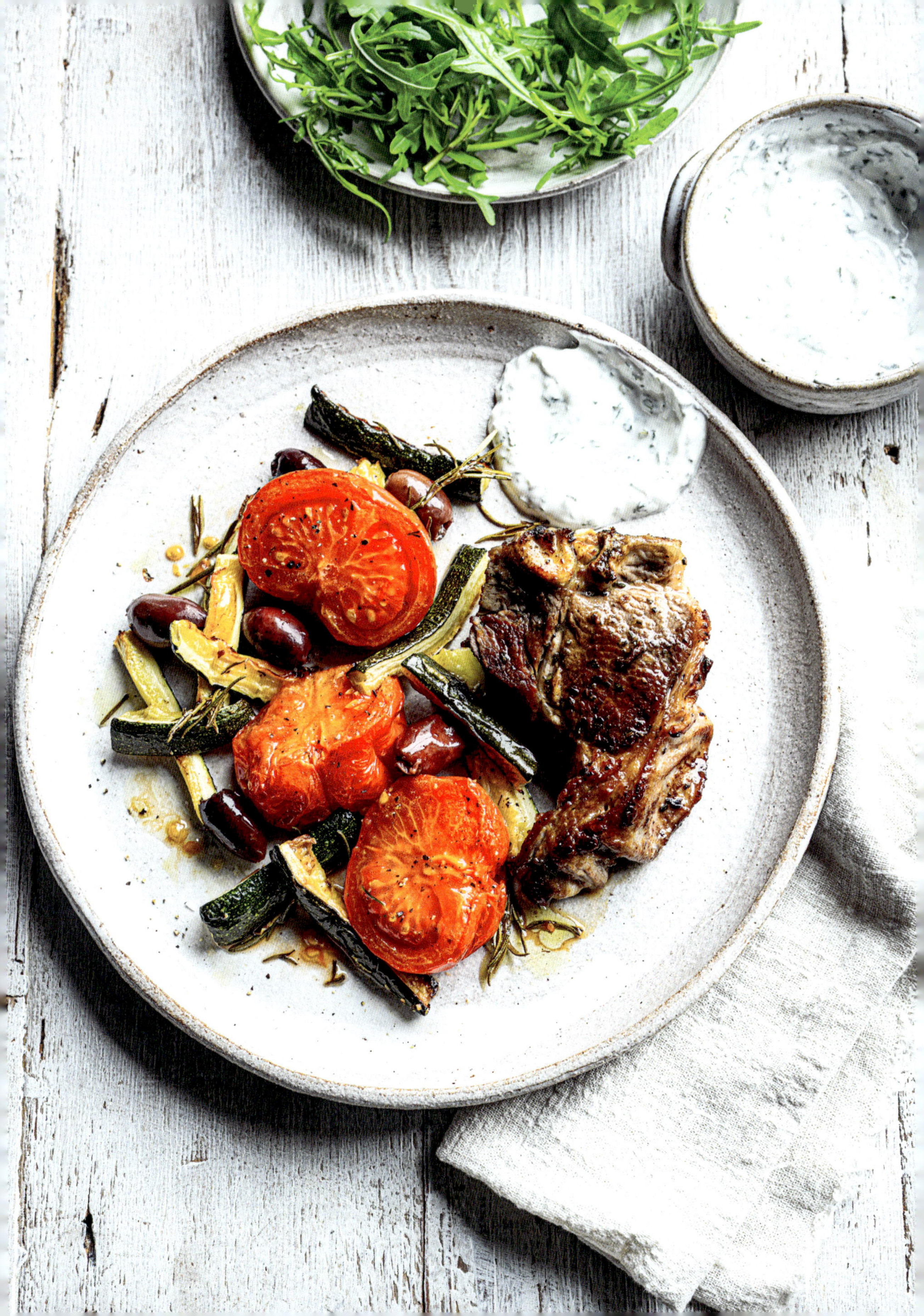

UNDER 500 CALORIES

PER SERVING | 414cals | PROTEIN 27g | CARBS 16g | FIBRE 5g

Garlicky Meatballs with Tomato and White Beans

SERVES 4 | PREP 20 mins | COOK 30 mins

2 tbsp olive oil
1 small onion, finely chopped
1 × 400g tin chopped tomatoes
1 tsp dried thyme
1 × 400g tin cannellini beans, drained
1 bay leaf (optional)
400g minced beef
1 garlic clove, minced
1 egg
Handful of pitted olives (about 20)

Super easy to make and ideal for the family. Serve with steamed greens. On a non-fast day, add Sweet Potato Chips (see page 238) or 2–3 tablespoons of quinoa.

1. Place a large frying pan over a low heat. Add half the oil and half the onion and cook gently for 5 minutes until softened.

2. Stir in the tinned tomatoes, half the thyme, the beans and the bay leaf, if using. Cook over the gentle heat for 20–25 minutes, adding a splash of water to loosen, if needed.

3. Meanwhile, make the meatballs. In a bowl, combine the mince, garlic and egg with the remaining onion and thyme, plus a generous pinch of salt and black pepper. Mix together, then form into 8–10 smallish meatballs with clean hands.

4. Place a separate frying pan over a medium heat. Add the remaining oil and the meatballs and fry them, turning occasionally, for about 6–8 minutes, until browned.

5. Tip the meatballs into the tomato sauce and continue to heat gently for another 5 minutes, to ensure the meatballs are cooked through.

GLUTEN FREE · NUT FREE · DAIRY FREE

PER SERVING | **505cals** | PROTEIN **36g** | CARBS **19g** | FIBRE **10g**

UNDER **600** CALORIES

Beany Beef Bourguignon

SERVES **4** | PREP **40** mins | COOK **105** mins

400g stewing beef, cut into 5cm cubes (I use diced braising steak)
1 tsp sea salt
1 tsp freshly ground black pepper
1 tbsp olive oil
1 large onion, finely chopped
100g lardons, pancetta or bacon
330g chestnut mushrooms
12 shallots, peeled and left whole
1 large carrot, sliced
2 garlic cloves, diced
2 tbsp chia seeds
1 × 400g tin cannellini beans (or another white bean)
1 × 750ml bottle red wine
2 large bay leaves (optional)
1 tsp dried thyme or fresh thyme leaves
Handful of chopped parsley leaves, to garnish

This is a slight variation on the traditional rich and hearty French beef stew with bacon, mushrooms and carrots, along with an inexpensive bottle of red wine. We also slip in some white beans, adding fibre and a creaminess to the dish.

1. Season the beef with the salt and ground black pepper, and set aside for 30 minutes at room temperature.

2. Preheat the oven to 170°C/Fan 150°C/Gas 3½.

3. Add the oil to a large flameproof casserole and place over a medium heat. Add the onion, lardons and mushrooms and fry for about 10–15 minutes, until browned and crisp. Remove with a slotted spoon and transfer to a plate.

4. Turn up the heat, add the beef and fry for about 5 minutes, turning occasionally, until brown. Transfer to the plate with the lardons and mushrooms.

5. Reduce the heat, stir in the shallots and carrot and cook for about 10 minutes, stirring occasionally. Add the garlic and cook for 1 minute. Stir in the chia seeds, beans and their liquid, wine, bay leaves, if using, and thyme. Stir to incorporate all the brown bits at the bottom of pot, then return the beef, lardons and mushrooms to the casserole, cover with a lid, and transfer to the preheated oven. Cook for about 1 hour 15 minutes, until the beef is very tender.

6. Serve sprinkled with parsley.

GLUTEN FREE | NUT FREE | DAIRY FREE

UNDER 300 CALORIES

PER SERVING | **275cals** | PROTEIN **37g** | CARBS **7g** | FIBRE **2g**

Steak Tagliata

SERVES 2 | PREP 10 mins | COOK 6 mins

1 × 300g thick good-quality steak, such as sirloin, ribeye or rump, at room temperature
2 tsp extra-virgin olive oil
75g rocket leaves
3 tomatoes, deseeded and diced
2 tsp balsamic vinegar
20g Parmesan, pared into thin shavings

The success of this classic Italian dish relies on good-quality ingredients, particularly the steak. The rich meat is contrasted with the sharp balsamic glaze and the peppery rocket, alongside the Parmesan. Serve it with long-stem broccoli and Sweet Potato Chips (see page 238) on the side, if you like.

1. Brush both sides of the steak with half of the oil and season with salt and pepper.

2. Heat a frying pan over a medium–high heat. When the pan is hot, turn the heat down slightly and cook the steak for 2½–3 minutes on each side, until browned on the outside and still slightly pink inside. Remove to a warm plate, cover, and leave to rest for 10 minutes.

3. When ready to serve, place the rocket leaves on a serving dish. Slice the steak on the diagonal against the grain and place it on top of the rocket, spooning over some of the pan juices, if you like. Scatter over the tomatoes, then drizzle with the balsamic and the remaining olive oil. Finish with a sprinkling of Parmesan, then season and serve straight away.

GLUTEN FREE | NUT FREE

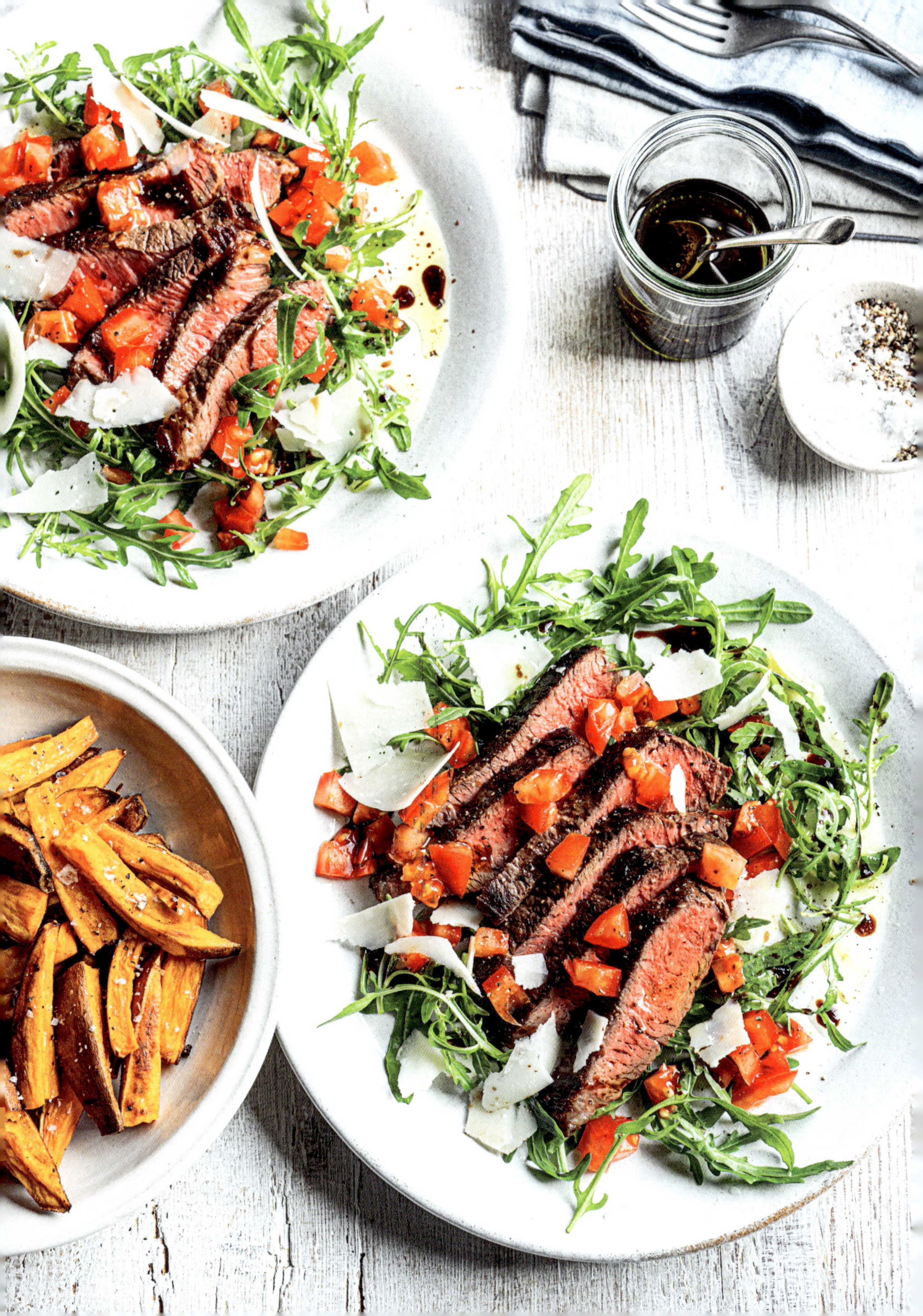

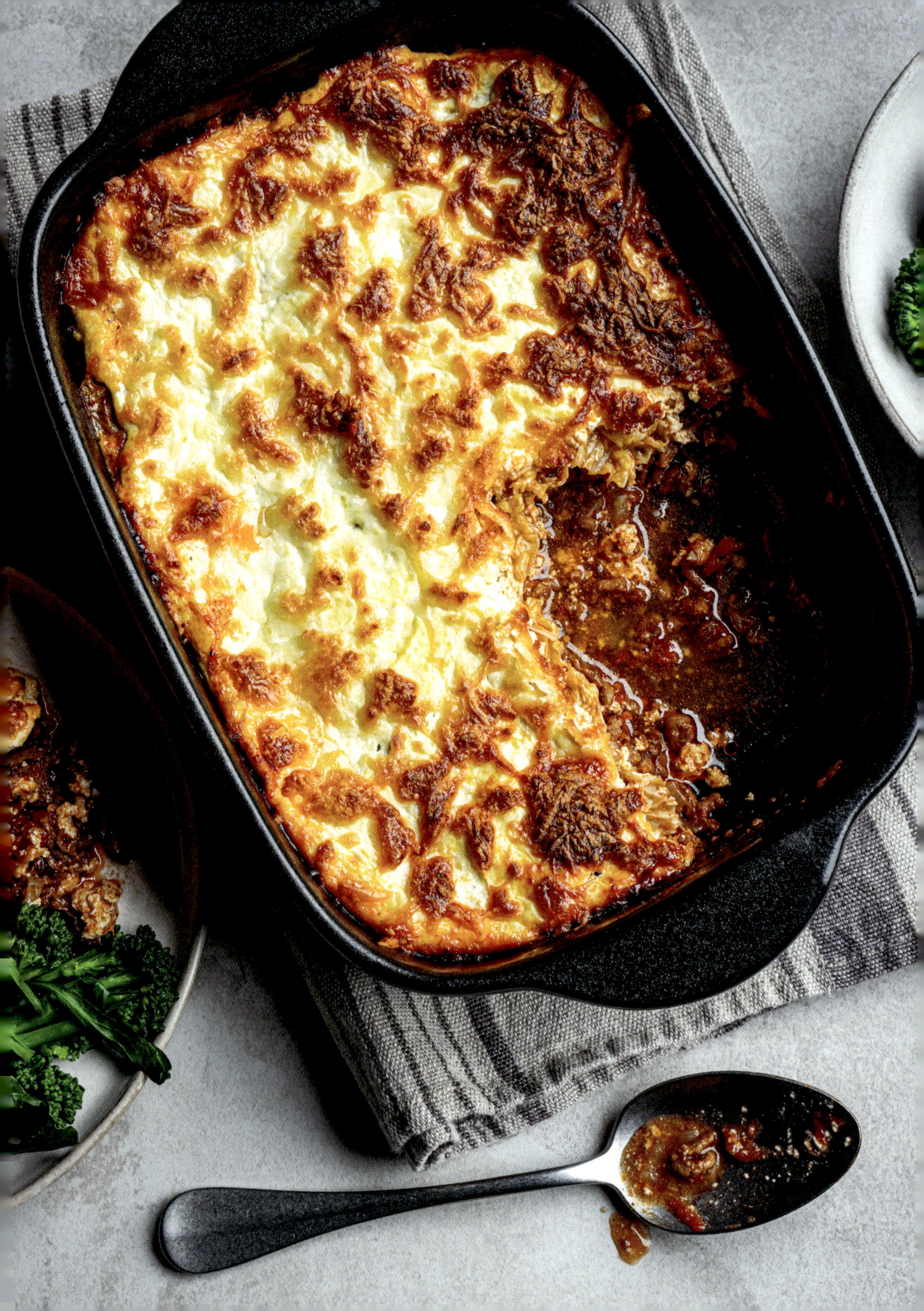

PER SERVING | **546cals** | PROTEIN **44g** | CARBS **7g** | FIBRE **3g**

UNDER 600 CALORIES

No-pasta Lasagne

SERVES 4 | PREP 15 mins | COOK 70 mins

1 tbsp olive oil
1 onion, finely chopped
1 celery stick, finely chopped
500g minced beef (about 12 per cent fat)
2 garlic cloves, finely chopped
1 tsp dried thyme
1 tbsp tomato purée
1 × 400g tin chopped tomatoes
150ml beef stock
1 tbsp chia seeds
4 large Savoy cabbage leaves
350g ricotta
1 egg, lightly beaten
30g Parmesan, finely grated
Large pinch of freshly grated nutmeg
125g grated mozzarella

Savoy cabbage leaves make an excellent and juicy low-carb alternative to pasta sheets in this recipe, while the twist on the béchamel sauce features a mixture of cheeses and a pinch of nutmeg.

1. Preheat the oven to 200°C/Fan 180°C/Gas 6. You will need a roughly 23 × 16cm baking dish.

2. Heat the oil in a saucepan over a medium–high heat. Add the onion, celery and beef, and cook for 10 minutes, until the mince is browned and the onion is soft. Add the garlic and thyme and cook for 1 minute, then stir in the tomato purée.

3. Tip the tomatoes, stock and chia seeds into the pan and bring it to the boil. Turn down the heat, part-cover with a lid, and simmer for 30 minutes, stirring occasionally, until reduced and thickened. Season with salt and pepper.

4. Meanwhile, cut each cabbage leaf in half down the middle, removing the thickest part nearest the stalk, then cut in half again. Spread the cabbage leaves out, placing them flat in a large steamer basket, set over a pan of simmering water. Steam for 3–4 minutes, until tender, then refresh under cold running water. Drain well and pat dry. Set aside.

5. In a bowl, mix together the ricotta, egg, Parmesan and nutmeg. Season with salt and pepper.

6. To assemble the lasagne, spoon half the beef into the bottom of the dish in an even layer. Top with four pieces of the cabbage, then place another piece of cabbage on top of each one. Spoon half the ricotta mixture on top, spreading it out in an even layer. Top with the remaining beef and another double layer of cabbage. Spread the remaining ricotta mixture on top, then finish with the mozzarella. Bake in the oven for 35–40 minutes, until golden on top.

GLUTEN FREE · NUT FREE

UNDER 300 CALORIES

PER SERVING | **290cals** | PROTEIN **37g** | CARBS **11g** | FIBRE **4g**

Sesame Beef Skewers

SERVES 2 | PREP 80 mins | COOK 12 mins

- 1 × quantity Soy and Sesame Dressing (see page 243)
- 2 garlic cloves, minced
- 300g sirloin steak, trimmed of excess fat, cut into 2cm chunks
- 1 small red pepper, deseeded and cut into 2cm pieces
- 1 small orange pepper, deseeded and cut into 2cm pieces
- 1 large red onion, halved and cut into thin wedges
- 2 tsp olive oil
- 2–3 tbsp Herby Tahini Dressing (see page 241, optional)
- 1 tsp toasted sesame seeds (optional)

Simple, colourful and full of flavour, these kebabs can be grilled, barbecued or air-fried. If using wooden skewers, soak them in cold water for at least 30 minutes to prevent them from burning during cooking. Serve with a mixed leaf salad or coleslaw (see page 231).

1. Pour the dressing into a rectangular dish, long enough for your skewers to fit. Stir in the garlic and season with pepper. Add the steak, peppers and the onion and stir to coat in the marinade. Leave in the fridge, covered, for 1 hour.

2. Preheat the grill (or barbecue) to high. Thread the steak and veg onto 6 skewers. Place them on a grill pan and brush with some of the remaining marinade.

3. Drizzle with oil and grill for 10–12 minutes, turning every 3 minutes or so, and brushing with more marinade, until cooked and golden in places. Leave to rest for a couple of minutes.

4. Serve the skewers with a leafy salad and the tahini yoghurt dressing on the side, and sprinkled with sesame seeds, if using.

AIR-FRYER TIP

Preheat the air fryer to 190°C. Marinate and assemble the skewers as in Steps 1–2. Drizzle with oil and cook for 8–10 minutes, turning occasionally and brushing with more marinade. Serve as above.

NUT FREE | DAIRY FREE

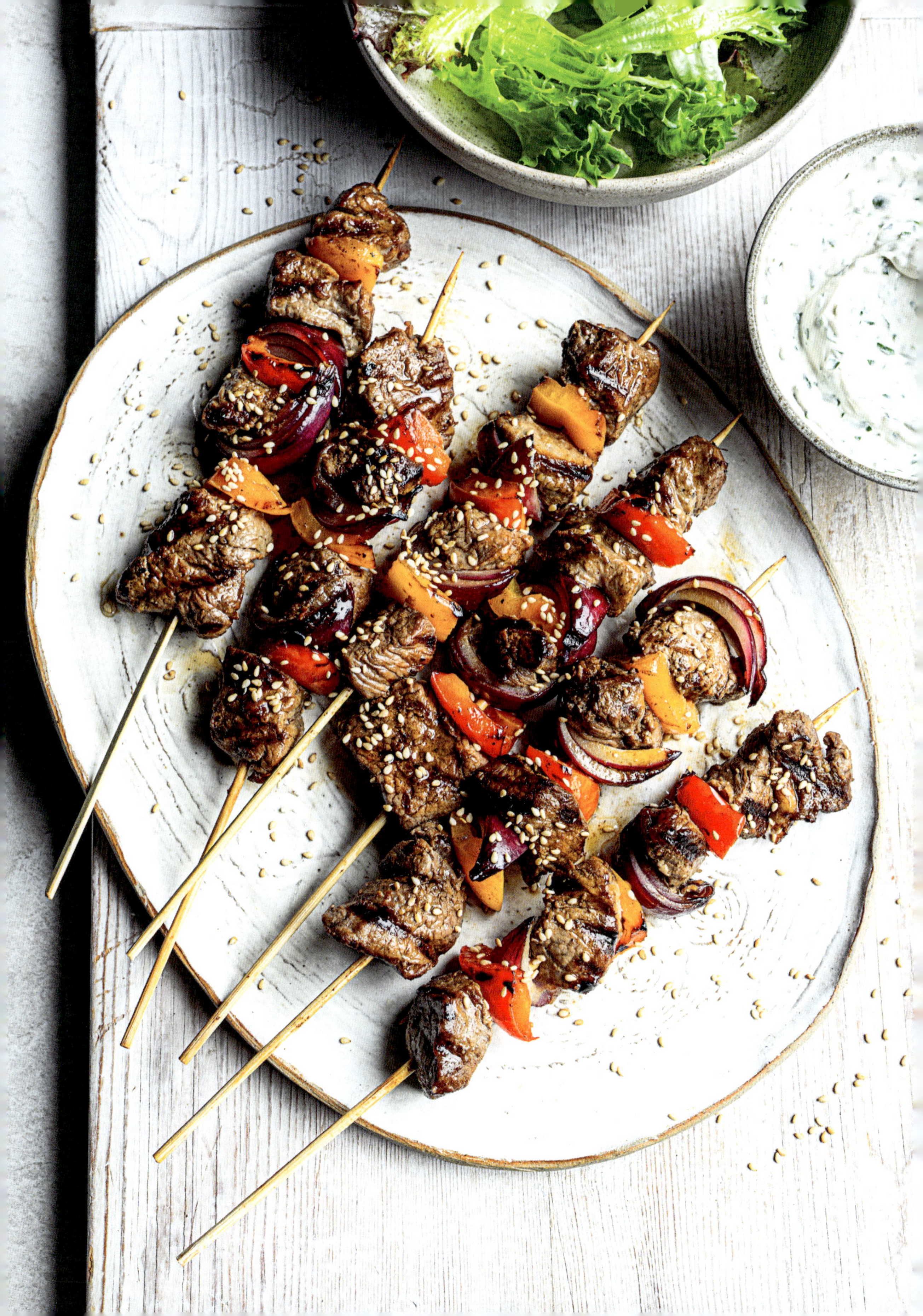

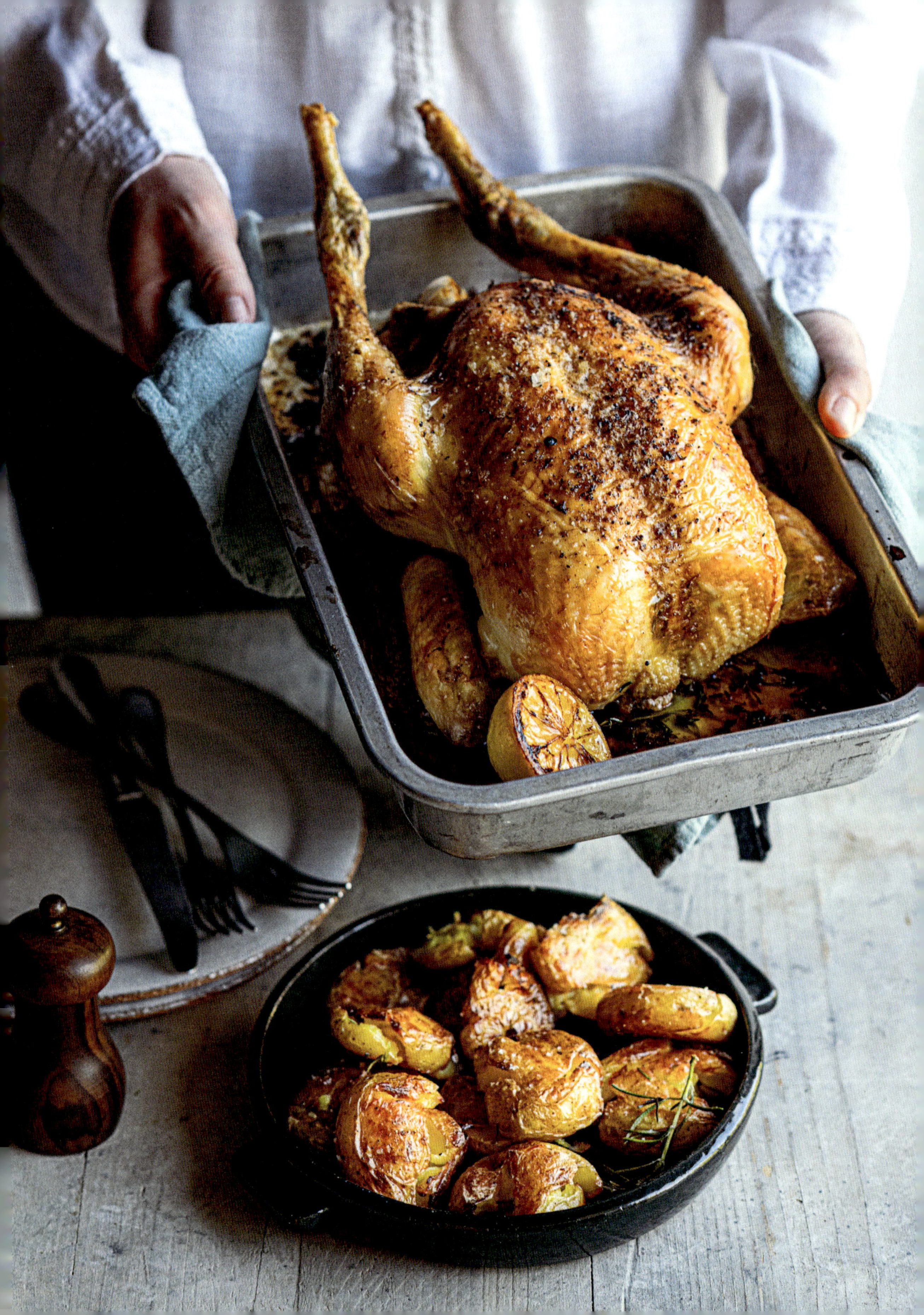

Chicken and Turkey

UNDER 500 CALORIES

PER SERVING | 402cals | PROTEIN 31g | CARBS 12g | FIBRE 4g

Chicken Korma

SERVES 4 | PREP 40 mins | COOK 30 mins

This is one of the nation's favourites. We serve it with cauliflower rice, which is low carb and has plenty of fibre, but you could also opt for a small amount of brown rice.

500g skinless, boneless chicken thighs
4 tbsp full-fat Greek yoghurt
2cm piece of fresh root ginger, peeled and diced
3 onions
¼–½ chilli, or 1 tsp dried chilli flakes, to taste
4 garlic cloves, peeled
2 tbsp neutral oil
1 tbsp turmeric powder
1 tbsp garam masala
½ tsp ground black pepper
1 × 400ml tin reduced-fat coconut milk
3–4 tbsp ground almonds
Handful of coriander leaves, roughly chopped, to garnish
1 lime, cut into wedges (optional)

1. Score the chicken flesh, then place in a large bowl with the yoghurt and ginger. Turn to coat well, then cover and leave to marinate for 30–60 minutes.

2. Roughly chop 2 of the onions, then place in a food processor with the chilli, garlic and a little water to loosen, and blend to a paste.

3. Heat the oil in a large frying pan or wok over a medium heat. Finely chop the remaining onion and tip into the pan with the garlic and chilli paste, turmeric, garam masala, black pepper and a generous pinch of salt, and fry for about 4–5 minutes, stirring occasionally.

4. Pour in the coconut milk and add the marinated chicken. Bring to a boil, then reduce the heat, cover with a lid and simmer gently for 30 minutes.

5. Stir in the ground almonds and simmer for another 10 minutes, until cooked through.

6. Serve with fresh coriander sprinkled over the top, and some more sliced chilli and wedges of lime, if you like.

GLUTEN FREE

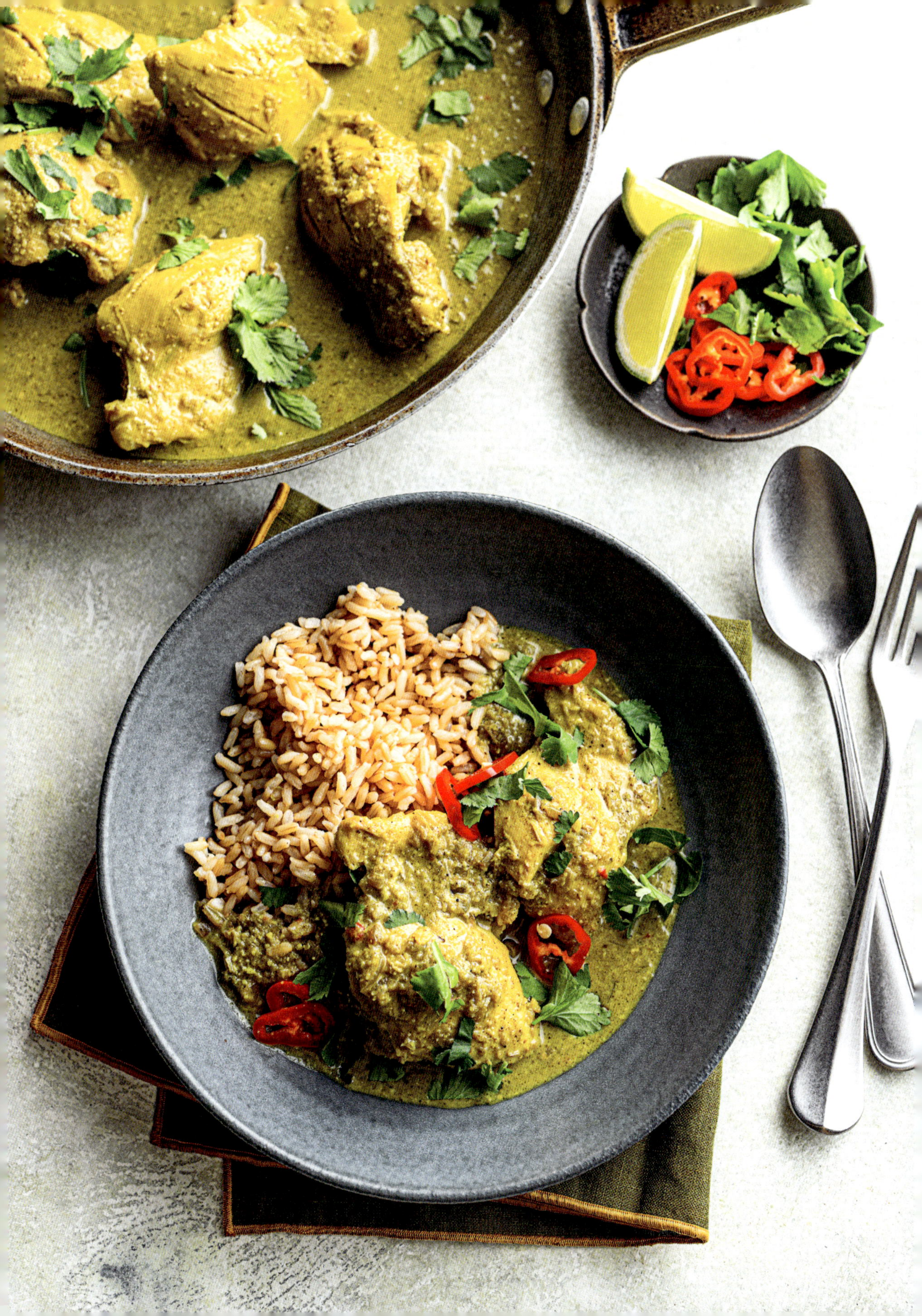

UNDER 500 CALORIES

PER SERVING | **416cals** | PROTEIN **34g** | CARBS **17g** | FIBRE **10g**

Thai-style Red Chicken Curry

SERVES 4 | PREP 25 mins | COOK 30 mins

1 tbsp coconut oil or olive oil
1 onion, diced
500g skinless, boneless chicken thighs, cut into large pieces
1 × 400g tin black beans, drained and rinsed
1 × 190g jar red Thai curry paste
1 × 400ml tin reduced-fat coconut milk
4cm piece of fresh root ginger, peeled and grated
4 pak choi, sliced
Large bunch of coriander, leaves roughly chopped, to garnish

This is one of my favourite, go-to family recipes, full of creamy aromatic flavour – mixing sweet, exotic and umami spices, yet so easy to assemble. It also delivers a good balance of protein and fibre to keep you satiated. Serve with 2–3 tablespoons of brown rice per person or some wholegrain noodles.

1. Heat the oil in a large saucepan over a medium heat. Add the onion and fry for about 5 minutes.

2. Increase the heat, add the chicken and fry for a further 5 minutes.

3. Season generously with salt and black pepper, then add all the remaining ingredients, apart from the coriander. Bring to a boil, then reduce the heat, cover with a lid and simmer gently for about 20 minutes, until the chicken is cooked through.

4. Sprinkle with fresh coriander to serve.

GLUTEN FREE · NUT FREE · DAIRY FREE

PER SERVING | **414cals** | PROTEIN **44g** | CARBS **31g** | FIBRE **9g**

UNDER **500** CALORIES

Moroccan-spiced Chicken Stew

SERVES **4** | PREP **20** mins | COOK **40** mins

2 tbsp olive oil
2 tbsp ras el hanout
1 large onion, diced
600g skinless, boneless chicken thighs, cut into large pieces
1 × 400g tin chopped tomatoes
1 × 400g tin chickpeas, drained
100g dried red lentils
4 dried apricots, diced
4cm piece of fresh root ginger, peeled and diced (optional)
Handful of coriander leaves, to garnish

This is one of my favourite easy and flavourful recipes – you literally throw all the ingredients together and let it simmer away gently covered by a well-fitting lid. This is a lovely example of pairing protein (chicken) and fibre (chickpeas and lentils).

1. In a large flameproof casserole with a well-fitting lid, warm the oil over a medium heat. Stir in the ras el hanout and fry for a couple of minutes.

2. Add all the remaining ingredients, except the coriander, then fill one of the empty tins with water, and add this to the casserole too. Bring the mixture to the boil, then reduce the heat, cover with a lid and simmer gently for 40 minutes, stirring occasionally. If the dish looks a bit dry, add some more water.

3. Sprinkle with chopped coriander and serve with steamed greens and cauli rice, or a small portion of brown rice or quinoa.

GLUTEN FREE | NUT FREE | DAIRY FREE

UNDER 400 CALORIES

PER SERVING | **318cals** | PROTEIN **33g** | CARBS **18g** | FIBRE **8g**

Mediterranean One-pan Chicken with Roasted Garlic

SERVES **2** | PREP **10** mins | COOK **40** mins

This summery chicken dish is all cooked together in one pan – easy and fuss-free. Serve with your favourite green veg on the side.

3–4 skinless, boneless chicken thighs, depending on size
3 carrots, halved and cut into batons
1 onion, cut into thick wedges
1 tbsp olive oil
1 tsp dried thyme
2 sprigs of rosemary, halved
1 lemon, halved
3 large garlic cloves, unpeeled
8 cherry tomatoes

1. Preheat the oven to 200°C/Fan 180°C /Gas 6.

2. Put the chicken, carrots and onion in a large roasting tin. Drizzle with the oil, sprinkle with the thyme, and season with salt and pepper. Turn everything to coat in the oil mixture, then tuck the rosemary under the chicken and add the lemon halves and garlic cloves to the tin.

3. Roast the chicken and vegetables for 20 minutes, then turn the carrots and onion, baste the chicken, and add the tomatoes. Return the tin to the oven for another 15–20 minutes, until the chicken is cooked through.

4. Spoon the chicken, carrots, onion and tomatoes onto serving plates. Remove the rosemary sprigs and squeeze the lemon halves and soft garlic out of its skin into the tin. Mash the garlic into the juices in the tin and serve with the chicken.

AIR-FRYER TIP

Preheat the air fryer to 180°C, if needed. Prepare the chicken and vegetables as Step 2. Add to the air fryer (you may need to do this in batches) and cook for 20 minutes. Baste the chicken, then add the tomatoes and cook for another 5–8 minutes, until the chicken is cooked through.

GLUTEN FREE | NUT FREE | DAIRY FREE

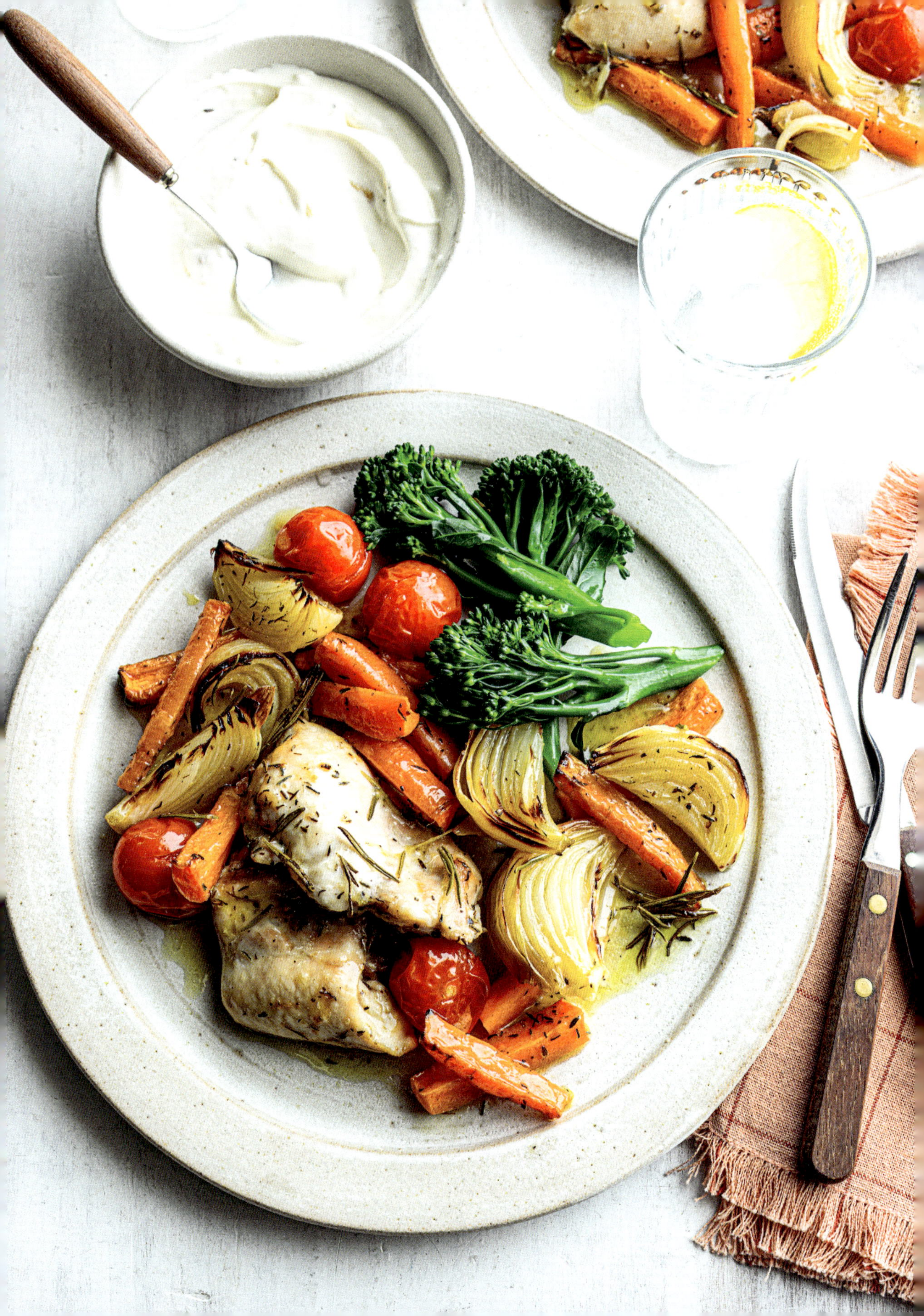

UNDER 300 CALORIES

PER SERVING | **241cals** | PROTEIN **43g** | CARBS **4g** | FIBRE **1g**

Ginger and Spring Onion Poached Chicken

SERVES 2 | PREP 10 mins | COOK 6 mins

2 × 175g skinless, boneless chicken breasts
6cm piece of fresh root ginger, sliced diagonally (save 1cm to add to the dressing)
3 spring onions, green and white parts separated
4 tsp light soy sauce
1½ tsp toasted sesame oil
1½ tsp rice vinegar or apple cider vinegar
½ cucumber
1 tsp toasted sesame seeds

Poaching is an excellent way to cook chicken simply and without fuss, and is a classic soothing comfort food. The poaching liquid is delicately flavoured with ginger and spring onion, and the chicken comes with smashed cucumber and a ginger and soy dressing. Ginger is excellent for calming the digestive system and can even ease nausea.

1. Place the chicken breasts in a saucepan and pour in enough water to just cover, about 500ml. Add the sliced ginger and the white part of the spring onions. Bring to a boil, then reduce the heat and simmer, partially covered, for 6 minutes or until the chicken is just cooked through. Remove from the heat and leave the chicken in the poaching liquid for 4–5 minutes.

2. Meanwhile, mix together the soy sauce, sesame oil and vinegar in a small pan. Peel and finely grate the reserved ginger and add to the pan. Warm everything through for 1 minute.

3. With the end of a rolling pin, bash the cucumber slightly to break the skin, then roughly chop into chunks.

4. Transfer the chicken breasts from the poaching liquid onto a board, then slice each one diagonally. Place them into shallow serving bowls, then spoon the warm dressing over the top. Slice the green part of the spring onion and sprinkle over the chicken with the sesame seeds. Serve with the smashed cucumber on the side.

NUT FREE
DAIRY FREE

PER SERVING | **412cals** | PROTEIN **40g** | CARBS **29g** | FIBRE **6g**

UNDER **500** CALORIES

Chicken Curry Traybake

SERVES **2** | PREP **10** mins | COOK **30** mins

1 × 400g tin chopped tomatoes
100g drained tinned chickpeas
100g cooked quinoa
1 tbsp olive oil
1–2 tbsp mild curry paste of your choice
2 garlic cloves, minced
3–4 skinless, boneless chicken thighs, depending on size, roughly chopped
Handful of coriander leaves
Mint Yoghurt Sauce (see page 242), to serve (optional)

This protein- and fibre-rich meal couldn't be easier to make; you simply mix everything together in a roasting tin and bung it in the oven. Serve it with green vegetables or salad, if you like.

1. Preheat the oven to 200°C/Fan 180°C/Gas 6.

2. Tip the chopped tomatoes, chickpeas, quinoa, olive oil, curry paste and garlic into a roasting tin and mix well. Season with salt and pepper, then stir in the chicken pieces until combined.

3. Cook in the preheated oven for 30 minutes, turning the chicken halfway, until it is cooked through.

4. Sprinkle with coriander and serve with the Mint Yoghurt Sauce, if using.

GLUTEN FREE | NUT FREE | DAIRY FREE

UNDER 400 CALORIES

PER SERVING | 352cals | PROTEIN 36g | CARBS 23g | FIBRE 7g

Chicken and Black Bean Traybake

SERVES 2 | PREP 10 mins | COOK 35 mins

- 4 tsp olive oil
- 1 tsp ground cumin
- ½ tsp smoked paprika
- ½ tsp dried oregano
- 3–4 skinless, boneless chicken thighs, depending on size
- 150g sweet potato, skin on, cut into 1cm chunks
- 100g drained tinned black beans, rinsed
- 60g tinned no-sugar or salt sweetcorn
- Handful of coriander leaves, to finish (optional)

This is a lovely Mexican-inspired, one-pan meal. It serves two people, but you can easily double the quantity to serve four, if you prefer. It provides a good mix of protein and fibre – and lots of flavour. Serve it with some Roasted Garlic Mayo (see page 241) or Guacamole (see page 243).

1. Preheat the oven to 200°C/Fan 180°C /Gas 6.

2. Mix together half the olive oil with the cumin, smoked paprika and oregano in a shallow dish, then season with salt and pepper. Add the chicken thighs and turn to coat them in the flavourings. Place the chicken in a large roasting tin, spooning over any remaining marinade from the bowl.

3. Place the sweet potato chunks in a bowl, drizzle over the remaining oil, season, and toss until combined. Tip the sweet potato into the tin with the chicken, then spread everything out evenly. Roast in the oven for 20 minutes.

4. Remove the tin from the oven, baste the chicken with any juices in the pan and turn the sweet potatoes, then add the black beans and sweetcorn. Return the tin to the oven and cook for another 15 minutes, until the chicken is golden and cooked through and the sweet potato is tender.

5. Serve scattered with coriander, if you like, and a spoonful of your choice of sauce on the side.

AIR-FRYER TIP

Preheat the air fryer to 180°C, if needed. Prepare the chicken and sweet potato as Steps 2–3. Add the chicken and sweet potato to the air fryer (you may need to do this in batches) and cook for 15 minutes. Baste the chicken and turn the potato, then add the corn and beans and cook for another 5–10 minutes, until the chicken is cooked through. Serve as above.

GLUTEN FREE | NUT FREE | DAIRY FREE

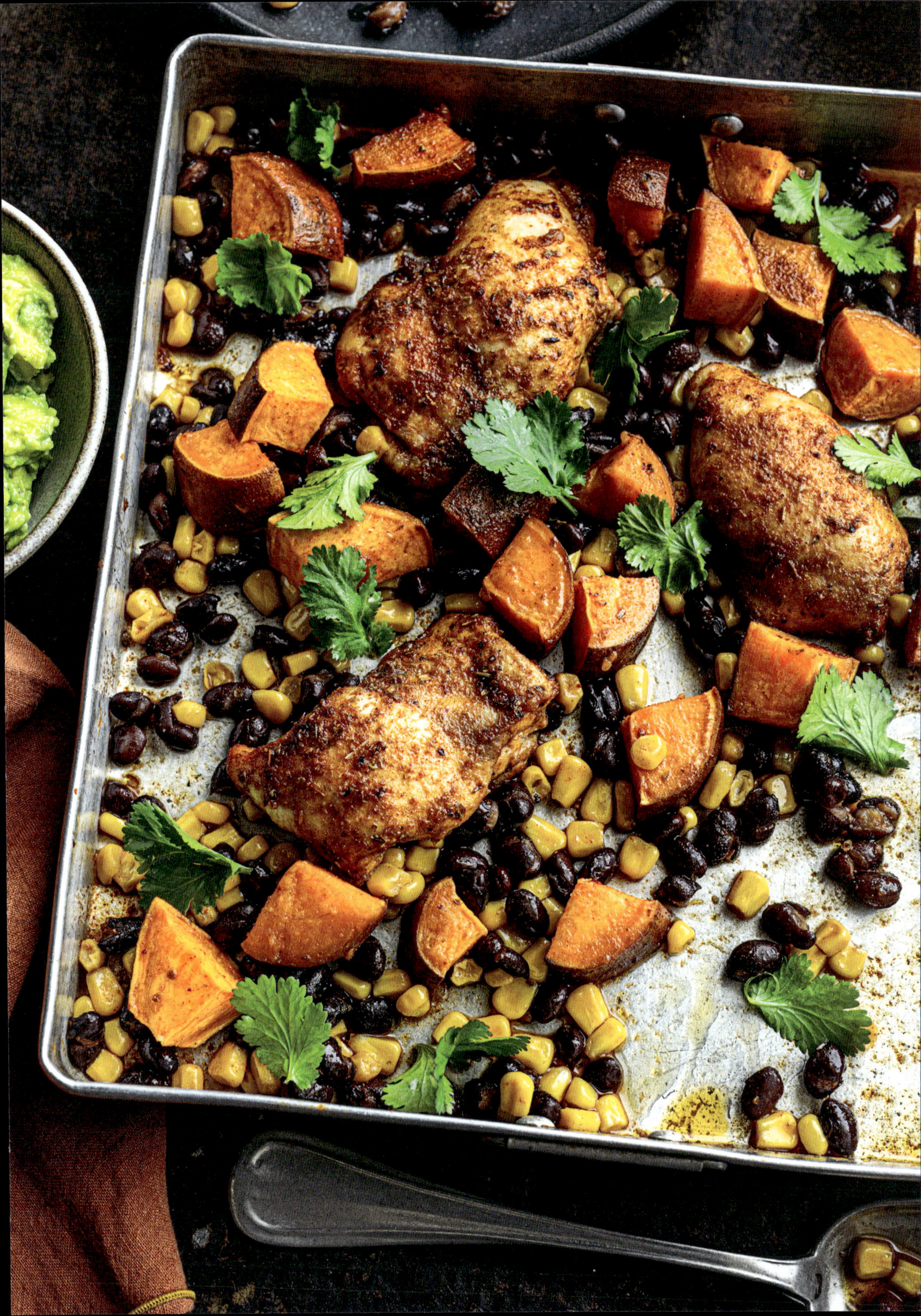

UNDER **600** CALORIES

PER SERVING | **541cals** | PROTEIN **54g** | CARBS **29g** | FIBRE **11g**

Chicken Poke Bowls

SERVES **1** | PREP **15** mins

50g cooked quinoa (from a pouch)
60g cooked edamame beans (podded weight)
1 carrot, finely sliced or grated
1 snack cucumber, diced
1 spring onion, sliced diagonally
125g cooked chicken, shredded
1 tsp light soy sauce
1 tsp sesame oil (optional)
2 tsp Seedy Sprinkles (see page 39) or toasted mixed seeds
2 tbsp full-fat Greek yoghurt
1–2 tsp sriracha

This version of the Hawaiian favourite is a great way to use up leftover roast chicken. You can use the chicken cold or reheat it in a little soy sauce and sesame oil. The fresh ingredients can be varied depending on what you have in the fridge, but this recipe makes a good starting point.

1. Place the quinoa in a serving bowl, top with the edamame, carrot, cucumber and spring onion, placing them in individual piles. Add the chicken, then drizzle the soy sauce and sesame oil, if using, over the top. Sprinkle with the seeds.

2. Mix the yoghurt and sriracha together in a small bowl, then spoon into the middle of the bowl to serve.

NUT FREE

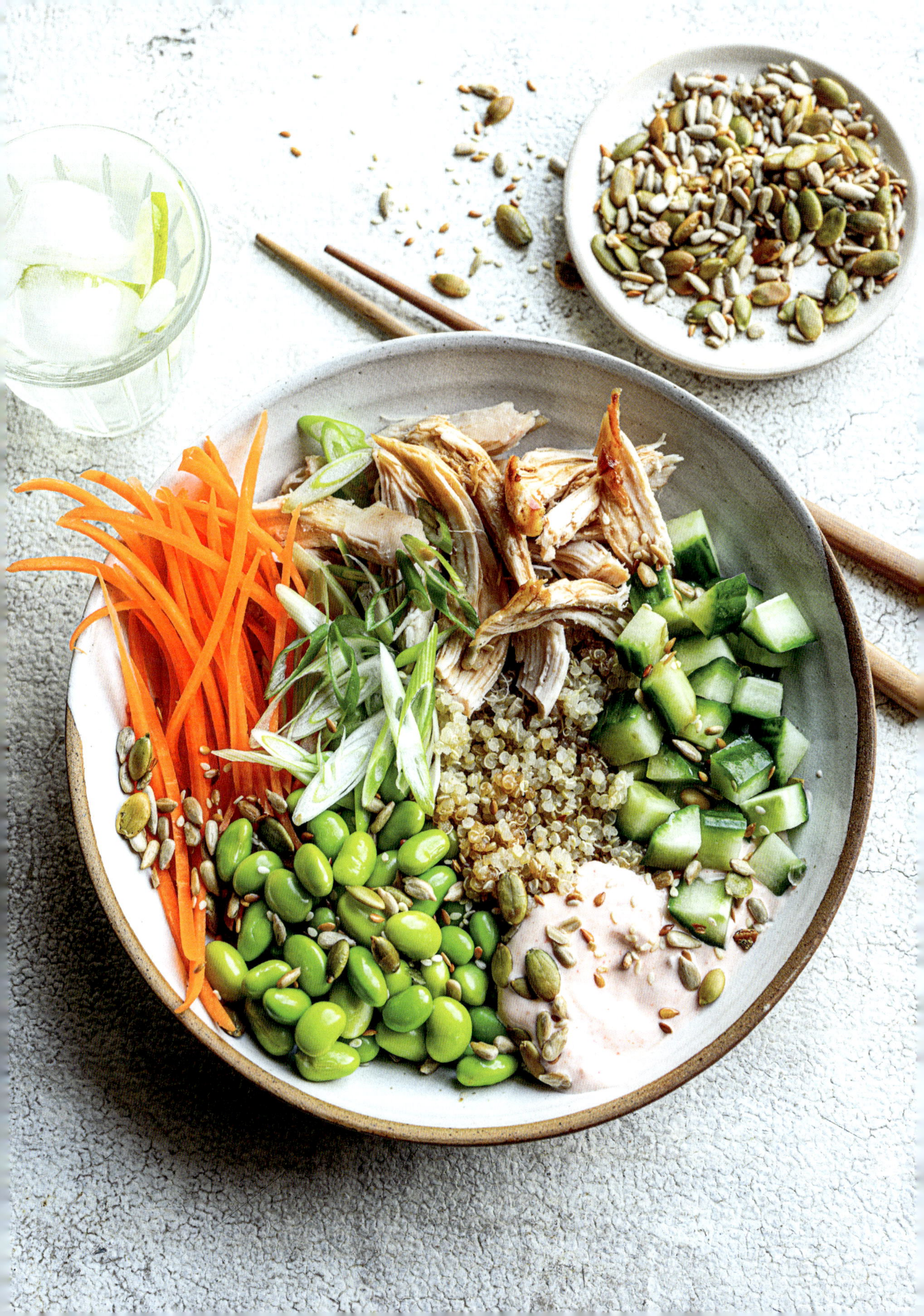

UNDER 400 CALORIES

PER SERVING | **331cals** | PROTEIN **61g** | CARBS **8g** | FIBRE **1g**

Korean-style Baked Chicken

SERVES **2** | PREP **70** mins | COOK **20** mins

1 tbsp gochujang paste
1 tsp rice vinegar or apple cider vinegar
1 tsp light soy sauce
1 tsp runny honey
2 tsp sesame oil
1 lime
3 large skinless, boneless chicken thighs, each cut into 3 pieces
2 handfuls of crispy shredded lettuce, such as Iceberg
2 spring onions, shredded

The Korean spice paste gochujang packs a punch and adds a glossy, sticky glaze to these chicken bites. Serve as a light meal with cauliflower rice or cooked brown rice and Seedy Slaw (see page 231).

1. Mix together the gochujang, vinegar, soy sauce, honey, sesame oil and the juice of ½ lime in a large bowl. Add the chicken and turn to coat. Cover and marinate in the fridge for 1 hour, or longer if time allows.

2. When ready to serve, preheat the oven to 200°C/Fan 180°C/Gas 6. Line a baking tray with non-stick baking paper.

3. Place the chicken pieces, spaced slightly apart, on the tray and spoon over some of the marinade. Bake for 15–20 minutes, turning halfway and spooning over more of the marinade, until cooked through and glossy.

4. Place the shredded lettuce on a large serving plate and top with the chicken. Finish with a sprinkling of spring onions, with the remaining lime cut into wedges to serve.

AIR-FRYER TIP

Preheat the air fryer to 180°C, if needed. Prepare the chicken as Step 1. Put the chicken in the air fryer and cook for 10–12 minutes, turning halfway and spooning over more of the marinade, until cooked through and glossy. Serve as above.

NUT FREE | DAIRY FREE

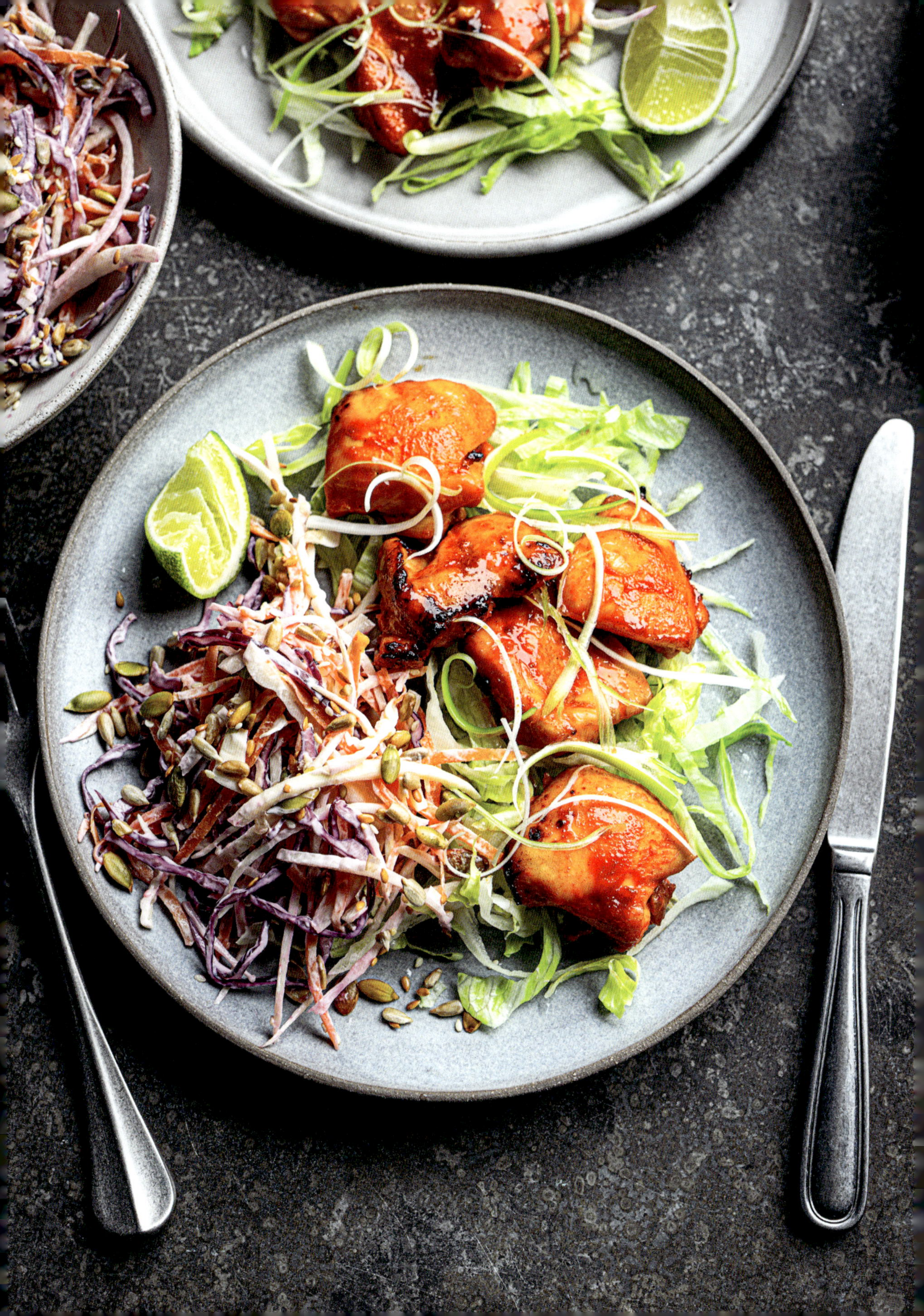

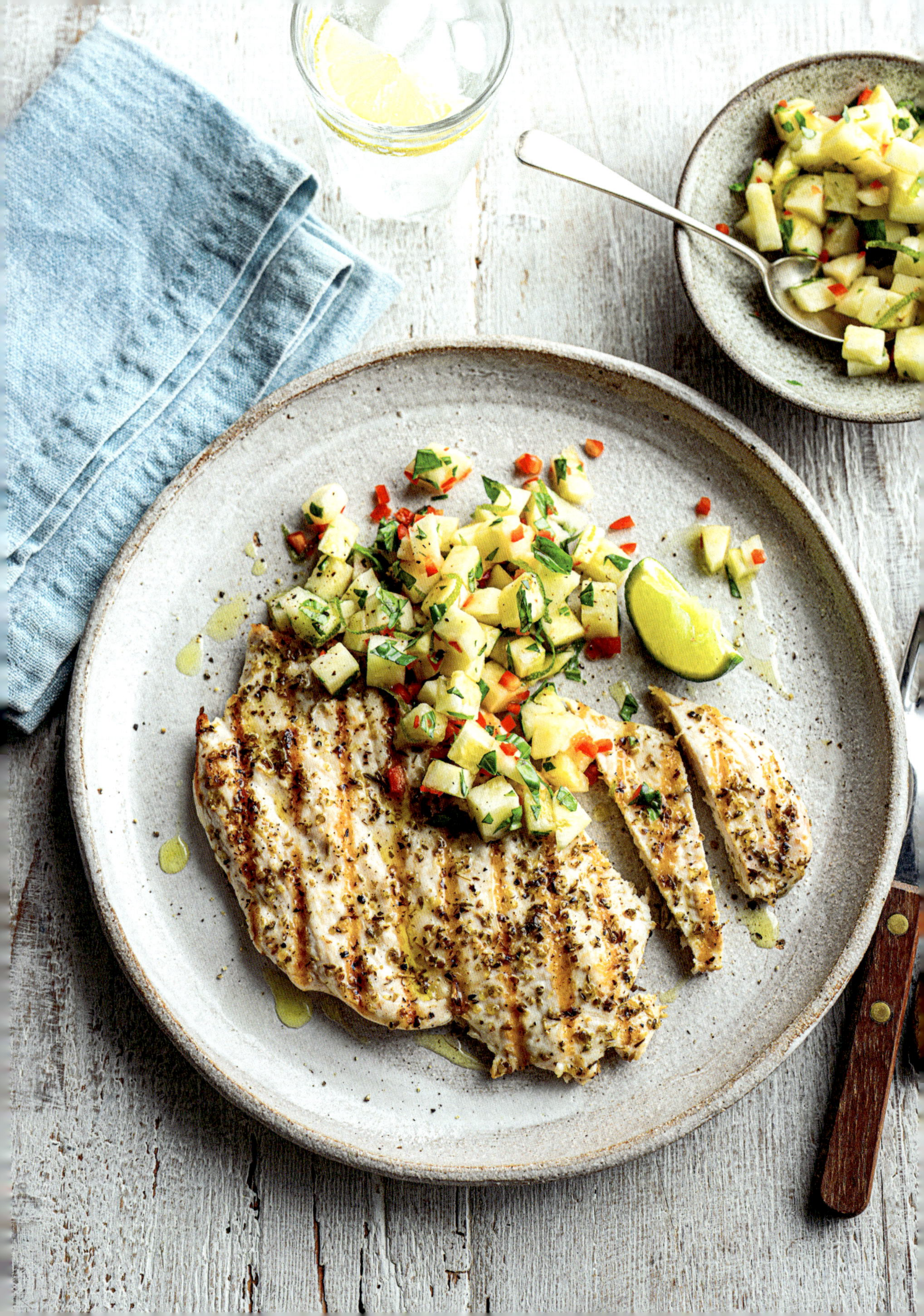

PER SERVING | **240cals** | PROTEIN **42g** | CARBS **6g** | FIBRE **1g**

UNDER 300 CALORIES

Chargrilled Chicken with Pineapple Salsa

SERVES 2 | PREP 10 mins | COOK 6 mins

2 × 175g skinless, boneless chicken breasts
2 tsp olive oil
1 tsp dried oregano
120g pineapple, diced (fresh or canned in natural juice)
½ mild red chilli, diced, or a pinch of dried chilli flakes
6 basil leaves, roughly chopped
Juice of ½ lime

When losing weight, you sometimes crave fruity and juicy foods. Here is an option that shouldn't spike sugars as it's part of a meal. Light and nutritious, this takes minutes to make, but packs in the flavour. The chicken is cooked on a ridged griddle pan, which gives it its signature chargrilled flavour, though you can always pan-fry, if that's easier. The salsa adds a zingy freshness. You can add some tinned black beans to the salsa to boost the fibre count, if you like.

1. Put the chicken breasts between 2 sheets of cling film and flatten with the end of a rolling pin or meat mallet until about 1–1.5cm thick all over.

2. Mix together the olive oil and oregano in a shallow dish. Season with salt and pepper, then add the chicken and turn to coat both sides in the olive oil mixture.

3. Heat a dry griddle pan over a medium–high heat, add the chicken and turn the heat down slightly. Cook the chicken for 5–6 minutes, turning once, until golden and cooked through. Remove from the pan and leave to rest briefly while you make the salsa.

4. Mix together the pineapple, chilli, basil and lime juice in a bowl. Serve the salsa alongside the chicken.

AIR-FRYER TIP

Preheat the air fryer to 190°C, if needed. Prepare the chicken as in Steps 1–2, then cook for 8–10 minutes, turning halfway, until golden and cooked through. Serve as above.

GLUTEN FREE | NUT FREE | DAIRY FREE

UNDER 400 CALORIES

PER SERVING | **360cals** | PROTEIN **55g** | CARBS **0g** | FIBRE **0g**

Lemon and Thyme Roast Chicken

SERVES **4** | PREP **10** mins | COOK **80** mins

3 tbsp olive oil
1 large lemon, halved
1.5kg whole chicken, at room temperature
4 sprigs of thyme
2 bay leaves (optional)
1 garlic bulb, halved horizontally through the middle
½ chicken stock pot or cube
10g butter

Nothing beats a good roast chicken, and this one is flavoured with the classic combination of lemon, thyme and garlic. This is similar to the recipe Michael loved to make for the family. It comes with a light gravy and is perfect with a few crispy Smashed New Potatoes (see page 236) and lots of green veg. It also works well served cold with a leafy green salad.

1. Preheat the oven to 200°C/Fan 180°C /Gas 6.

2. Mix the olive oil with the juice of ½ lemon and season well with salt and pepper. Slash the skin of the remaining half of the lemon and stuff it into the cavity of the chicken with half of the thyme sprigs, bay leaves, if using, and the garlic halves. Brush the seasoned oil all over the chicken. Set the chicken on a rack over the remaining sprigs of thyme in a medium roasting tin, then pour 250ml water into the bottom of the tin.

3. Roast the chicken for about 1 hour 20 minutes, basting it every 20 minutes or so, until the skin is crisp and golden and the juices run clear when the thickest part of the thigh is pierced with a sharp knife. Pour a little extra water into the tin, if it starts to dry out. Place the chicken on a warm plate, cover with foil and leave to rest for 15 minutes.

4. Meanwhile, make a light gravy. Pour the juices from the roasting tin into a saucepan, scraping up any bits stuck in the bottom of the tin. Let the juices settle, then spoon off and discard the fat that has risen to the top. Add 200ml water to the juices in the pan and bring it to the boil. Stir in the chicken stock pot or cube and the butter and cook for a few minutes until reduced and thickened slightly. Season to taste, if needed.

5. Carve the chicken and serve with potatoes, green veg and the light gravy.

GLUTEN FREE NUT FREE

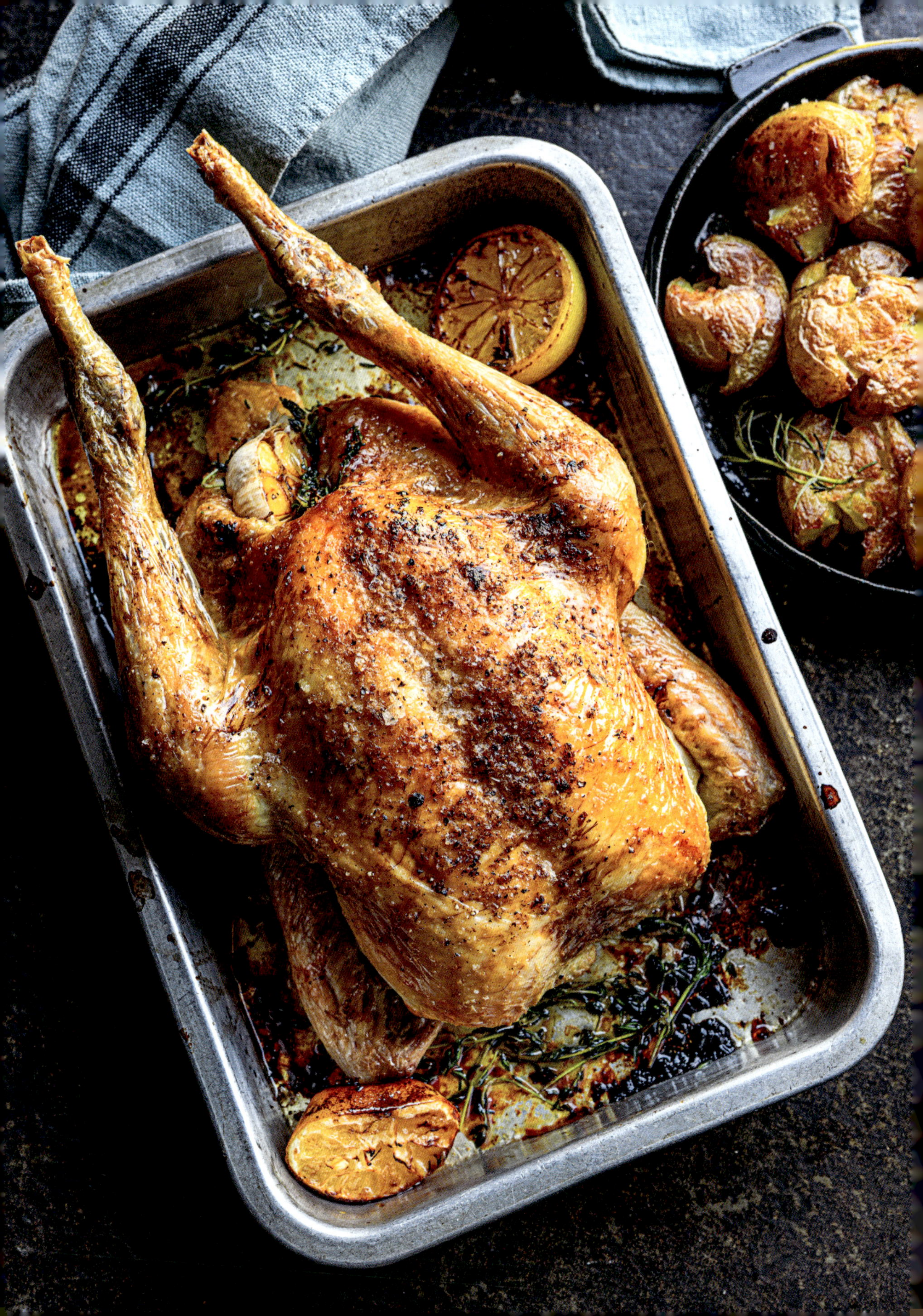

UNDER 400 CALORIES

PER SERVING | **371cals** | PROTEIN **29.7g** | CARBS **36.0g** | FIBRE **13.9g**

Quick Chicken Stew

SERVES 2 | PREP 10 mins | COOK 20 mins

2 tsp extra virgin olive oil
½ onion, finely diced
1 carrot, diced
2 celery stalks, diced
2 garlic cloves, minced
1 tsp ground cumin
½ tsp turmeric
Dried chilli flakes (optional)
1 × 400g tin chopped tomatoes
1 × 400g tin canned lentils, drained and rinsed
100g cooked chicken, shredded
40g spinach leaves

A much-loved recipe from the Fast 800 programme. You could add a side of mashed sweet potato or butternut on a non-fast day, or top with mashed potato and a sprinkle of cheese for a family-friendly pie. If you don't have pre-cooked chicken, substitute for 140g of raw diced chicken and add at the same time as the garlic – brown the meat before adding the spices and continuing on.

1. Heat the olive oil in a saucepan over a medium heat. Add the onion, carrot and celery and sauté for 2–3 minutes until it starts to soften. Add the minced garlic and cook for another minute until fragrant.

2. Stir in the cumin, turmeric and chilli flakes (if using). Cook for about 30 seconds, stirring constantly, to toast the spices.

3. Add the tomatoes and lentils and mix well. Stir in the cooked chicken breast and bring the mixture to a gentle simmer. Reduce the heat to low, cover with a lid and let it simmer for 5–7 minutes. If the stew becomes too thick for your liking, add a splash of water to reach your desired consistency.

4. Stir in the spinach during the last minute of cooking to wilt. Season to taste and serve with a crunchy green salad or steamed low calorie non-starchy vegetables.

GLUTEN FREE · NUT FREE · DAIRY FREE

PER SERVING | **260cals** | PROTEIN **27g** | CARBS **17.5g** | FIBRE **6.5g**

UNDER 300 CALORIES

Turkey Chilli

SERVES 6 | PREP 10 mins | COOK 40 mins

- 1 tbsp olive oil
- 1 onion, finely chopped
- 500g minced turkey (about 7 per cent fat)
- 2 garlic cloves, finely chopped
- 1 tsp dried oregano
- 1 tsp smoked paprika
- ½–1 tsp chilli powder, to taste
- 1 tbsp ground cumin
- 1 × 400g tin chopped tomatoes
- 350ml beef or chicken stock
- ½ tbsp unsweetened cocoa powder
- 1 × 400g tin black beans or kidney beans, drained and rinsed
- 1 × 400g tin green lentils, drained
- 8 sweet piquanté peppers from a jar, chopped
- Greek yoghurt, to serve (optional)

Taste-wise, you can't really tell the difference between this chilli made with turkey mince and one made with beef mince, but it is much quicker to cook and more economical to buy. This makes a big pot of chilli, which can be portioned up and stored in the fridge for up to 3 days, or frozen for longer.

1. Heat the oil in a saucepan over a medium heat. Add the onion and cook for 5 minutes, until softened.

2. Turn up the heat, add the turkey mince and cook for 5 minutes, breaking it up with a spatula, until browned. Reduce the heat, then stir in the garlic, oregano and spices.

3. Pour in the tinned tomatoes and stock and bring to the boil. Stir in the cocoa powder, beans, lentils and piquanté peppers. Season with salt and pepper, then reduce the heat and simmer for 30 minutes, partly covered with a lid, stirring occasionally, until reduced and thickened.

4. Serve topped with a tablespoon of yoghurt per person, if using.

GLUTEN FREE | DAIRY FREE

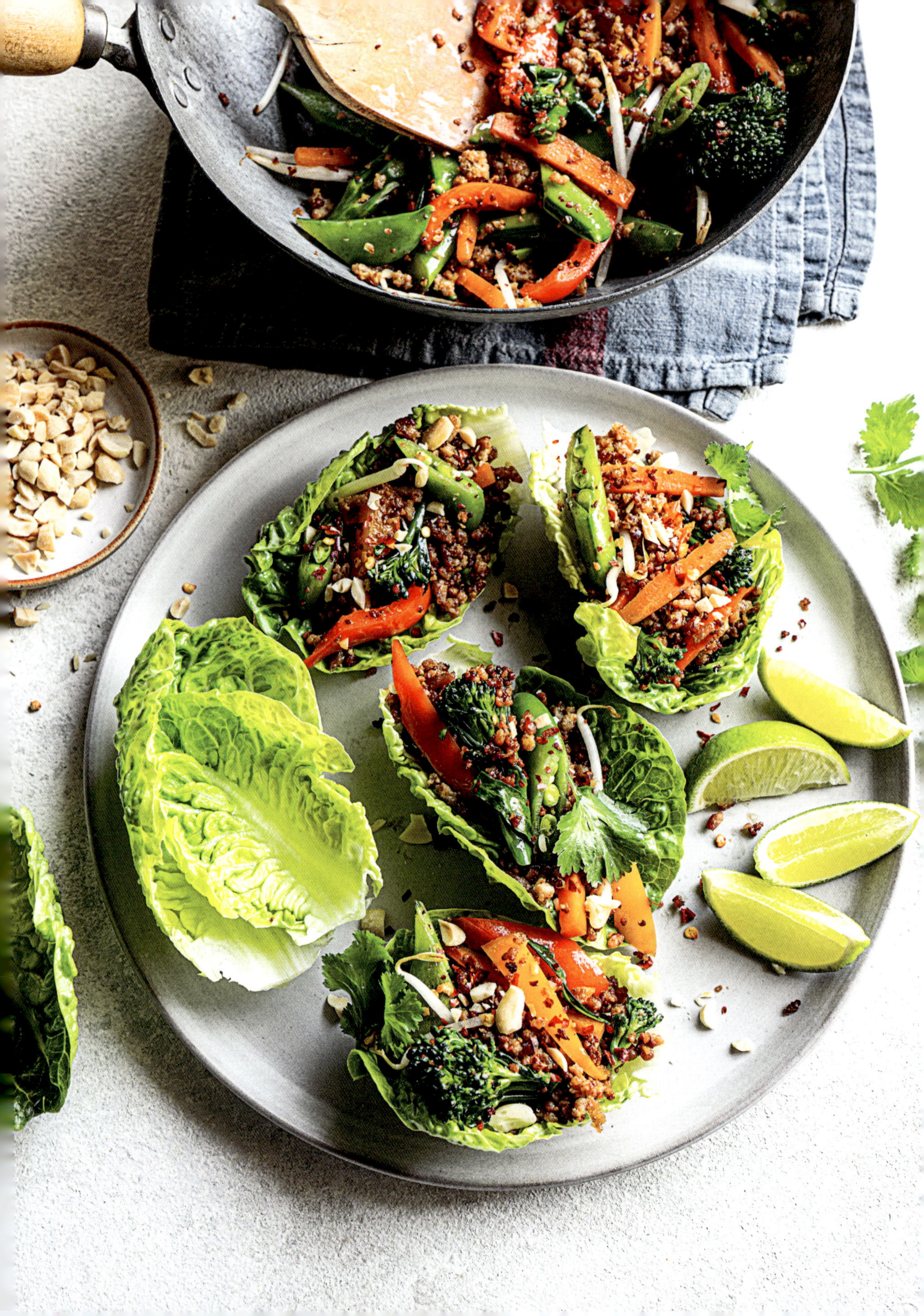

PER SERVING | **250cals** | PROTEIN **26.5g** | CARBS **8g** | FIBRE **3.5g**

UNDER 300 CALORIES

Turkey Larb

SERVES 4 | PREP 15 mins | COOK 20 mins

1 tbsp neutral oil
400g turkey mince (about 7 per cent fat)
1 stick of lemongrass, bashed
2.5cm piece of fresh root ginger, peeled and finely chopped
2 large garlic cloves, finely chopped
400g mixed vegetables for stir-frying
1 tbsp fish sauce or reduced-salt light soy sauce
1 Little Gem lettuce, leaves separated
25g unsalted roasted peanuts, roughly chopped
½ tsp chilli flakes, or to taste
Handful of chopped coriander leaves (optional)
1 lime, cut into wedges, to serve

There are many iterations of the popular Thai minced meat 'salad', but this twist abandons the usual chicken for turkey mince, which is juicy, nutritious and more affordable. With lots of brightly coloured added veg, this stir-fry brings freshness and nutritional value wrapped in a crunchy lettuce leaf. You could serve it with a small portion of cooked brown rice or noodles, if you like.

1. Heat the oil in a large frying pan or wok over a medium–high heat. Add the turkey and stir-fry for 10 minutes, until browned all over. Add the lemongrass, ginger and garlic and stir-fry for another 5 minutes, adding a splash of water, if needed.

2. Tip in the mixed vegetables and stir-fry for another 3 minutes, until softened slightly. Add the fish sauce and turn until combined. Pick out the lemongrass, then season with salt and pepper to taste.

3. To serve, arrange the lettuce leaves over a serving plate and spoon the mince mixture on top. Scatter over the peanuts, chilli and coriander leaves, if using. Serve with wedges of lime for squeezing over.

DAIRY FREE

UNDER 400 CALORIES

PER SERVING | **388cals** | PROTEIN **41g** | CARBS **24g** | FIBRE **4g**

Crispy Turkey Tacos

SERVES 2 | PREP 15 mins | COOK 16 mins

300g turkey breast, cut into strips or slices
1 tbsp fajita spice mix
1 tbsp olive oil
1 red pepper, deseeded and sliced
1 onion, cut into thin wedges
1 courgette, cut into batons
4 crisp corn tacos
1 Little Gem lettuce, shredded
20g mature Cheddar, grated (optional)
½ lime, cut into wedges

Turkey is an excellent alternative to chicken and more affordable, too. Lightly spiced with plenty of vegetables, stuffed into a crispy corn taco – what's not to like? You could top it with a spoonful of Guacamole (see page 243). Spice mixes are perfect for adding a burst of flavour without buying lots of individual spices.

1. Mix together the turkey, fajita spices and olive oil in a bowl. Season with salt and pepper and set aside to marinate for 30 minutes or overnight in the fridge, if time allows.

2. Heat a large, dry sauté pan over a medium–high heat. Add the red pepper, onion and courgette, turn down the heat and cook for 10 minutes, turning once or twice, until softened and blackened in places. (This will give the tacos a slightly smoky flavour.)

3. Add the turkey to the pan, along with any oil and spices from the bowl, and cook for 5–6 minutes, turning occasionally, until cooked through.

4. Warm the tacos following the instructions on the packet.

5. To serve, place some shredded lettuce in the bottom of each taco, then top with the turkey and vegetable mixture. Scatter over the grated cheese, if using, and serve with wedges of lime for squeezing over.

AIR-FRYER TIP

Preheat the air fryer to 180°C, if needed. Prepare the turkey as step 1. Place the vegetables in an even layer in the air fryer, drizzle with oil and season. Air fry for 10 minutes, then turn the vegetables, and add the turkey fajita mixture. Turn until everything is combined, then air fry for another 10–12 minutes, until the turkey is cooked through and the vegetables are tender.

GLUTEN FREE | NUT FREE

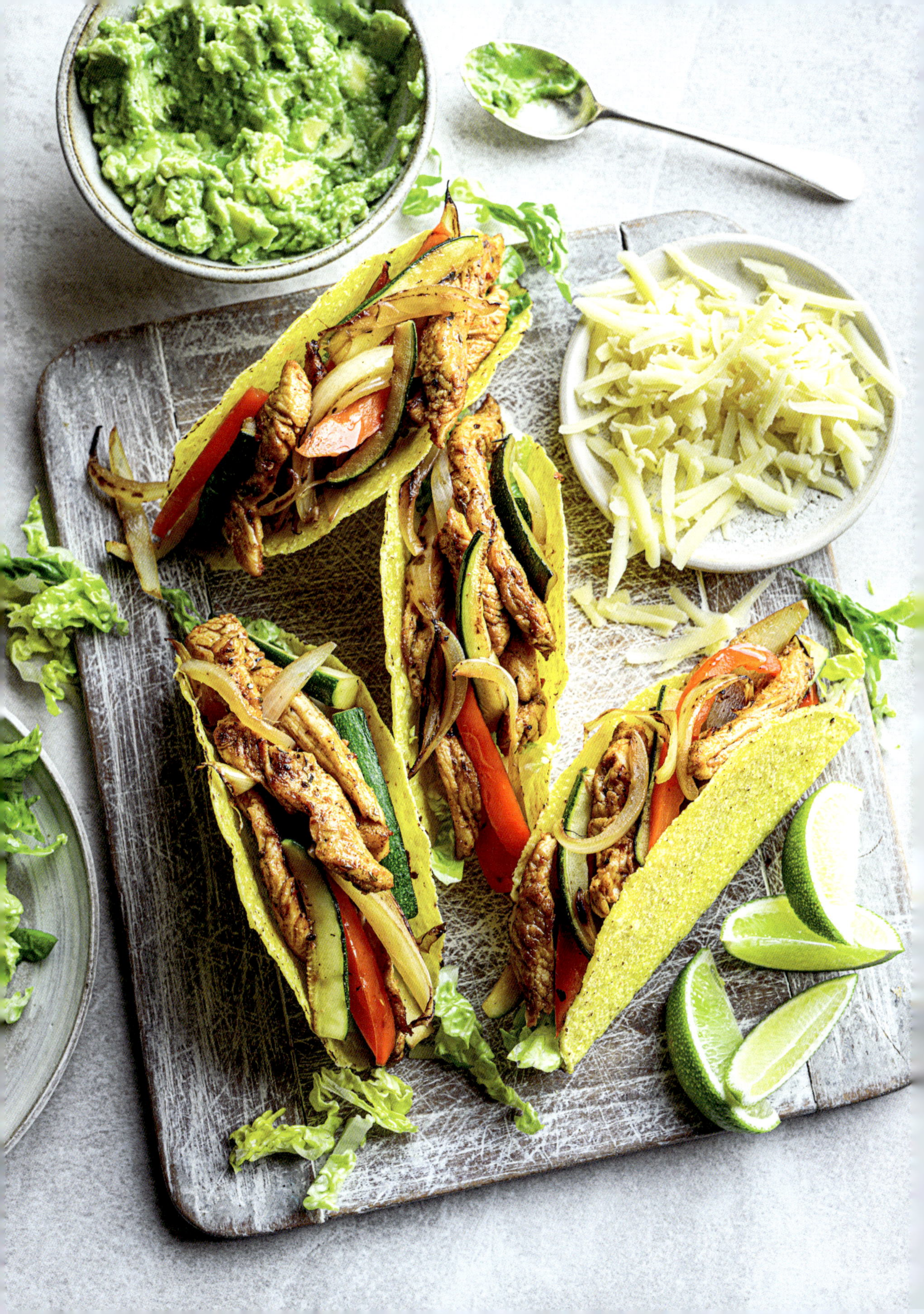

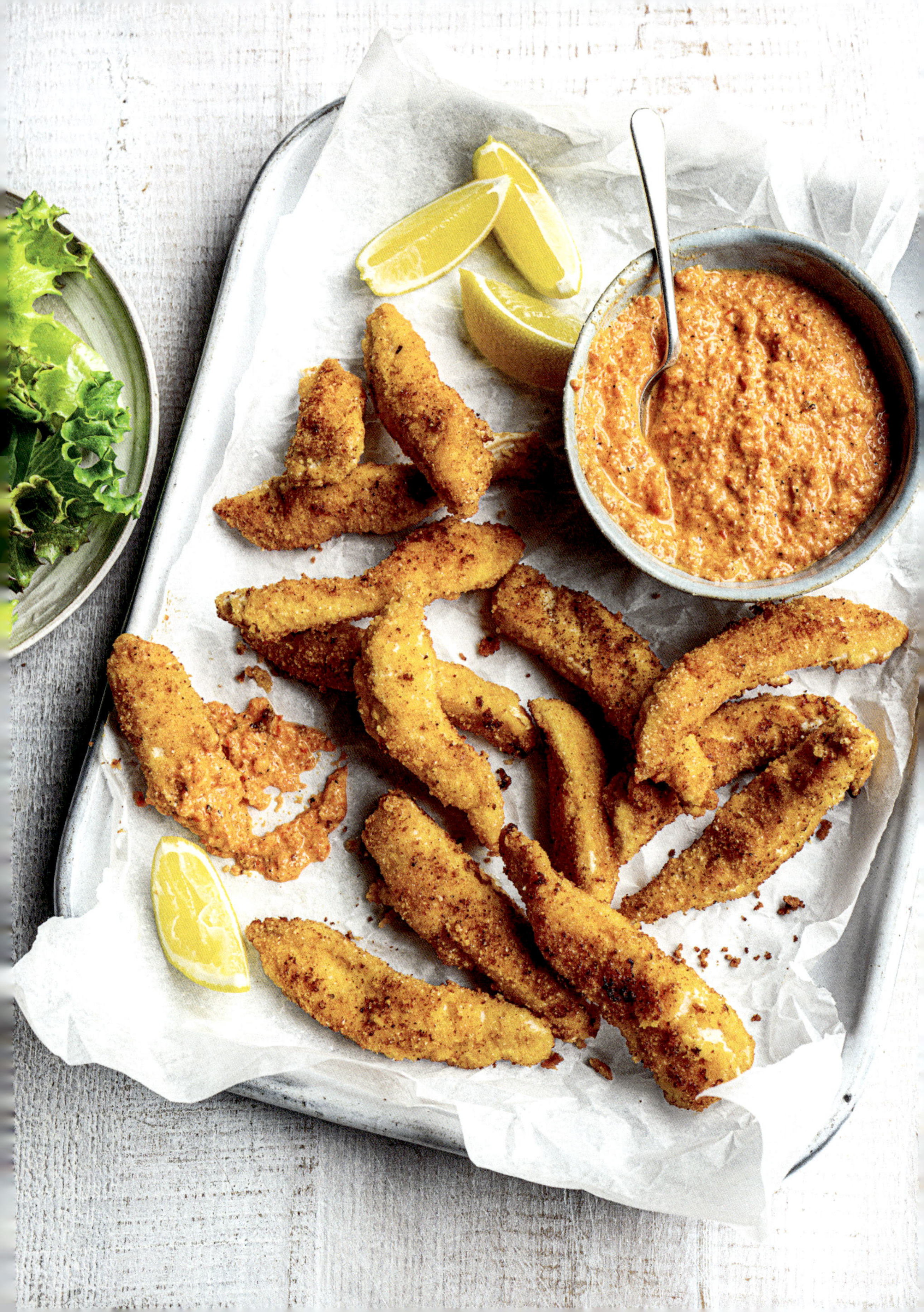

PER SERVING | **590cals** | PROTEIN **54g** | CARBS **7.5g** | FIBRE **4g**

UNDER 600 CALORIES

Turkey Goujons with Red Pepper Dip

SERVES 2 | PREP 15 mins | COOK 7 mins

These crispy, golden turkey strips have a slightly cheesy almond crust to boost protein. **See pages 239–43 for a wonderful selection of other dips and dressings.**

80g ground almonds
20g Parmesan, finely grated
½ tsp smoked paprika
1 egg
5 tsp extra-virgin olive oil
300g turkey breast, cut into strips or slices
2 large roasted red peppers from a jar, drained
1 garlic clove, minced
1 lemon, halved

1. Put 50g of the ground almonds in a shallow bowl with the Parmesan and paprika. Season with salt and pepper, and mix well.

2. Using a fork, whisk the egg in a separate shallow bowl until lightly beaten.

3. When ready to cook, heat 3 teaspoons of the olive oil in a large frying pan over a medium heat. Dip the turkey strips, one at a time, into the beaten egg, then into the ground almond mixture, until evenly coated. Add to the pan and cook for 6–7 minutes, turning once, until crisp and golden.

4. Meanwhile, to make the red pepper dip, blend the red peppers with the remaining ground almonds and olive oil, the garlic and the juice of ½ lemon until a coarse, thick purée. Season with salt and pepper.

5. Cut the remaining lemon half into wedges and serve with the turkey goujons and the dip on the side.

AIR-FRYER TIP

Preheat the air fryer to 180°C, if needed. Prepare the turkey as Steps 1–3. Using a pastry brush, dab the oil over the turkey goujons (or you could use an oil spray), then place them in the air fryer. Cook for 10–12 minutes, turning once, until crisp and cooked through.

GLUTEN FREE

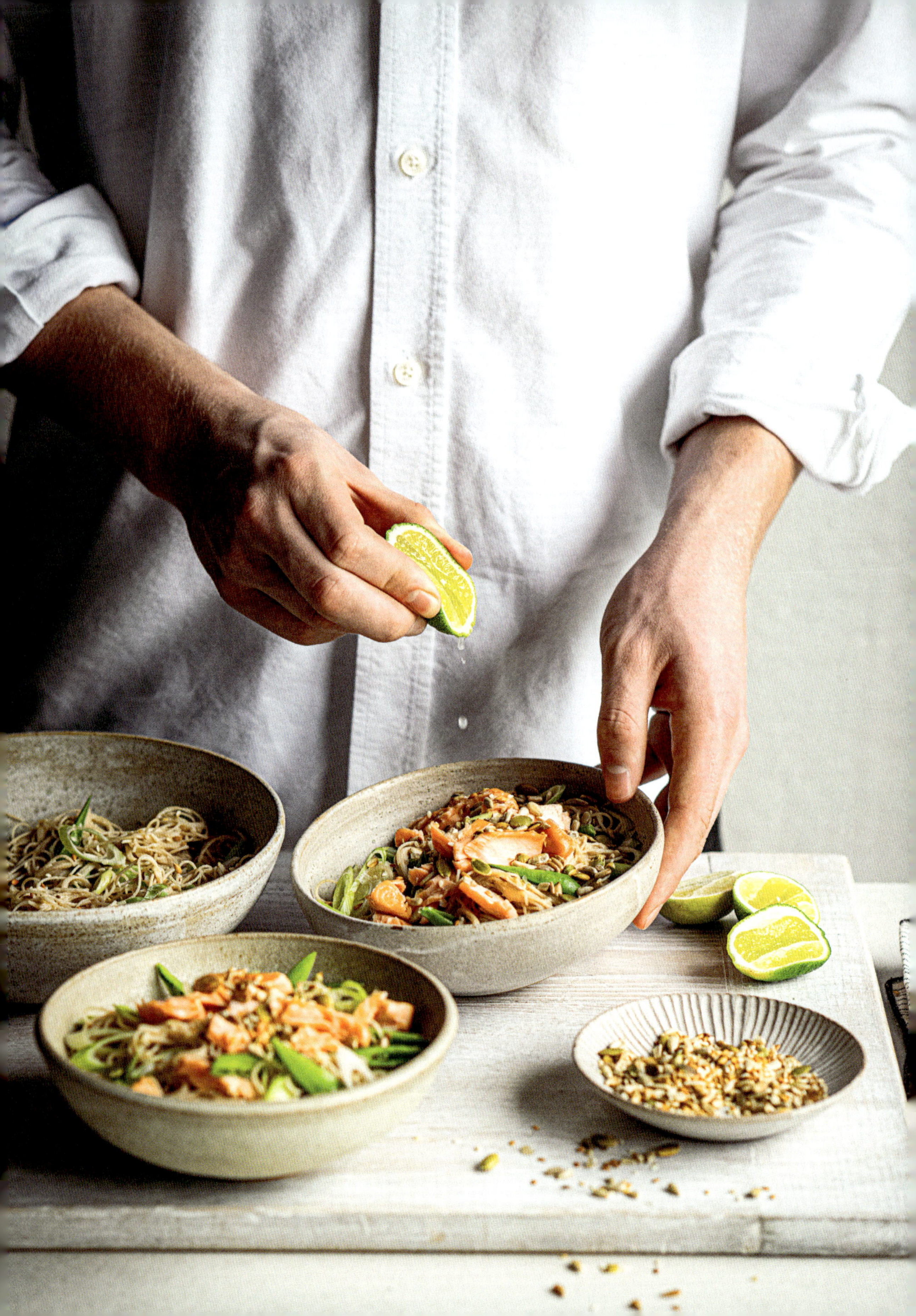

Fish and Seafood

UNDER 500 CALORIES

PER SERVING | **406cals** | PROTEIN **31g** | CARBS **30g** | FIBRE **3g**

Trout Noodle Salad with Miso Dressing

SERVES **2** | PREP **10** mins | COOK **5** mins

60g thin brown rice noodles or egg noodles
2 tsp white miso
2 tsp light soy sauce
1 tsp rice vinegar or apple cider vinegar
2 tbsp tahini
1–2 spring onions, thinly sliced diagonally
65g sugar snap peas, thinly sliced diagonally
2 cooked pink trout fillets, skin removed, broken into large flakes
2 tbsp Soy Seed Sprinkles (see page 39)

The noodles can be served while still warm or left to cool in this simple, Asian-inspired salad. It makes the perfect take-to-work lunch. You could top the noodles with cooked strips of chicken or pork, or cubes of smoked tofu. I like to use trout, as it is generally more sustainable than salmon.

1. Cook the noodles in boiling water according to the packet instructions. Drain and tip into a bowl.

2. Meanwhile, mix the miso, soy sauce, vinegar and tahini with 2–3 tablespoons of water to make a dressing. Pour the dressing over the cooked noodles and toss to coat.

3. Add the sugar snap peas and spring onions and mix well.

4. Divide the noodles and vegetables between two shallow serving bowls. Top with the trout and seeds to serve.

NUT FREE · DAIRY FREE

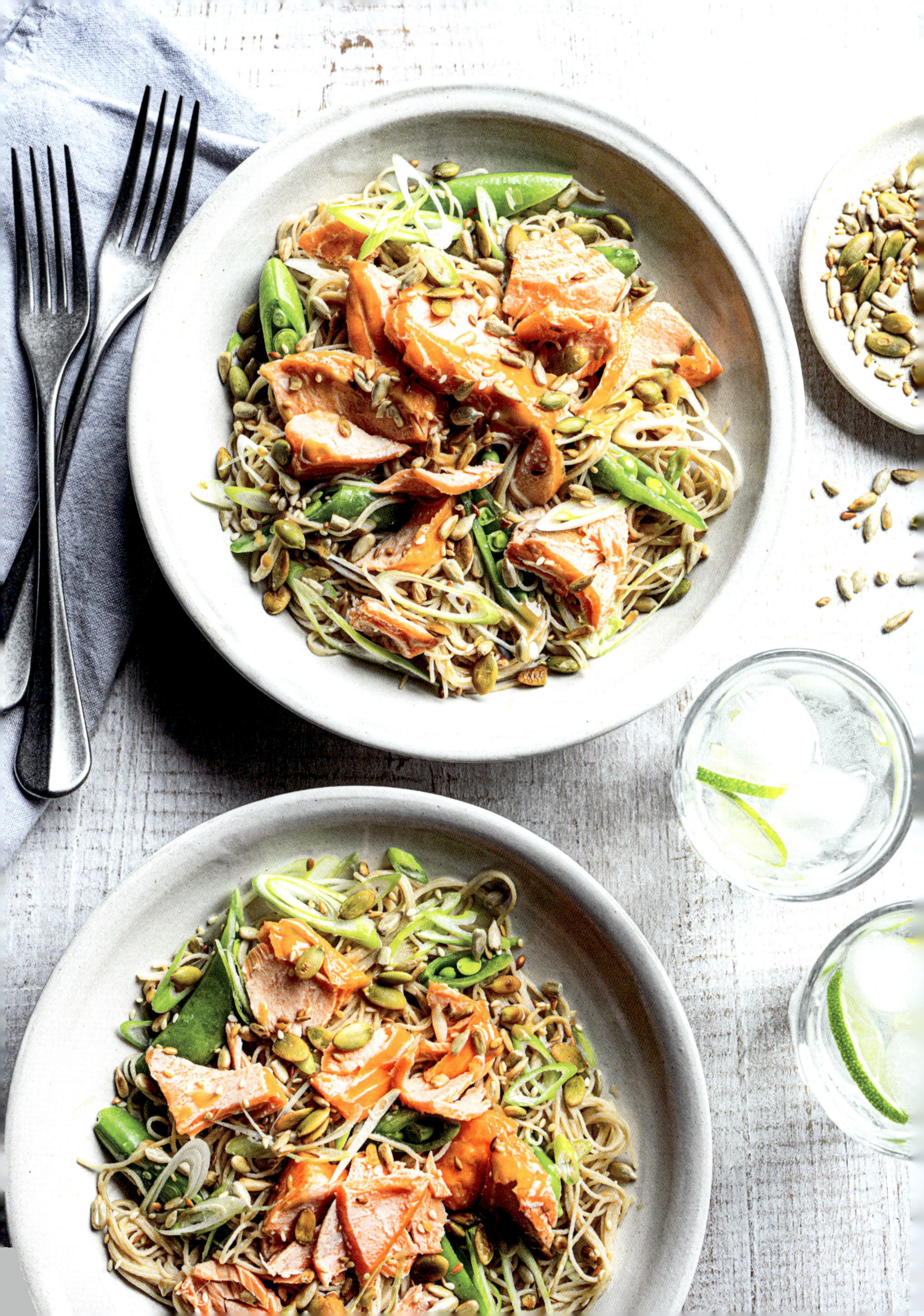

UNDER 300 CALORIES

PER SERVING | **253cals** | PROTEIN **21g** | CARBS **1g** | FIBRE **0.5g**

Sea Bass with Crispy Ginger

SERVES **2** | PREP **10** mins | COOK **6** mins

1 tbsp olive oil
2.5cm piece of fresh root ginger, peeled and cut into matchsticks
2 sea bass fillets (about 100g each)
2 tsp light soy sauce
1 tsp toasted sesame oil
1 spring onion, thinly sliced diagonally
1 mild red chilli, deseeded and thinly sliced diagonally, or a pinch of chilli flakes (optional)
1 tsp toasted sesame seeds
Handful of watercress, to serve

Thin slivers of crispy fried fresh ginger make a flavourful topping for these fillets of sea bass, and are also beneficial for digestion. You could use other white fish, such as sea bream or plaice. Serve with pak choi or other steamed greens and, on a non-fast day, some brown rice or noodles.

1. Heat the oil in a large frying pan over a medium heat. Add the ginger and cook, turning frequently, for 4–5 minutes, until crisp and starting to darken. Lift the ginger out with a slotted spoon onto a sheet of kitchen paper to drain. Set aside.

2. Season the sea bass fillets with salt and pepper, then add them to the same pan, skin-side down. Cook for 4–5 minutes, until the skin is crisp, then turn over and cook for another 30–60 seconds, until just cooked through.

3. Using a spatula, lift the fish onto serving plates and drizzle over the soy sauce and sesame oil. Top with the crispy ginger, spring onion and chilli, if using. Finish with a sprinkling of sesame seeds and serve with watercress on the side.

NUT FREE | DAIRY FREE

PER SERVING | **391cals** | PROTEIN **23g** | CARBS **24g** | FIBRE **10g**

UNDER 400 CALORIES

No-cook Prawn Burrito Bowls

SERVES 1 | PREP 15 mins

50g cooked quinoa (from a pouch)
½ tsp chia seeds (optional)
1 tsp extra-virgin olive oil
1 tsp apple cider vinegar
90g cooked peeled king prawns
50g drained tinned black beans, rinsed
2 Little Gem lettuce leaves, shredded
4 cherry tomatoes, quartered
½ avocado, sliced
2 tbsp Quick Pickled Pink Onions (see page 222)
1 × quantity Creamy Hot Sauce (see page 242), to serve (optional)

This is perfect for when you don't fancy cooking and just want something quick, fresh and tasty. It's more of an 'assembly' meal, meaning the ingredients are just assembled before serving. This can easily be adapted to suit what you have to hand in the fridge.

1. Put the quinoa and chia seeds, if using, in a shallow serving bowl. Add the olive oil and vinegar, then toss to coat.

2. Place the prawns, black beans, lettuce, tomatoes, avocado and pickled onions in individual small piles on top of the quinoa.

3. Pour the creamy hot sauce in the middle of the bowl, if using, and serve straight away.

GLUTEN FREE | NUT FREE | DAIRY FREE

UNDER **400** CALORIES

PER SERVING | **324cals** | PROTEIN **24g** | CARBS **12g** | FIBRE **1g**

Crab, Spinach and Coconut Bowl

SERVES **2** | PREP **10** mins | COOK **30** mins

1 banana shallot, roughly chopped
2.5cm piece of fresh root ginger, peeled and roughly chopped
1 mild red chilli, deseeded or ½ tsp chilli flakes, plus extra to serve (optional)
1 tbsp neutral oil
½ tsp turmeric powder
1 stick of lemongrass, bashed
2 lime leaves (optional)
1 × 400ml tin reduced-fat coconut milk
1 tbsp light soy sauce or fish sauce
50g frozen leaf spinach
80g cooked brown rice
1 lime, halved, one half cut into wedges
200g fresh white crabmeat
Handful of coriander leaves

A comforting bowl of rice and coconut topped with white crabmeat and a good squeeze of lime. The base can be made up to 2 days in advance, then reheated and finished with the toppings. Serve with sugar snap peas or long-stem broccoli.

1. Place the shallot, ginger and chilli, if using, in a mini food processor and blitz until it reaches a paste consistency. Alternatively, do this in a pestle and mortar.

2. Heat the oil in a saucepan over a medium heat. Add the shallot and ginger paste and cook for 7 minutes, stirring often and adding a splash of water, if the mixture starts to colour or looks dry.

3. Stir in the turmeric, lemongrass and lime leaves, if using. Pour in the coconut milk and soy sauce and bring to the boil. Reduce the heat and simmer for 20 minutes, stirring occasionally.

4. Add the frozen spinach and cook, stirring, until it defrosts and heats through.

5. Remove the lemongrass and lime leaves, if necessary, then add the rice and the juice of ½ lime. Stir and cook for a couple of minutes until the rice is thoroughly heated. Add a splash of water, if the stew is too thick. Check the seasoning.

6. Divide the stew between two shallow bowls. Top with the crabmeat and a few coriander leaves and serve with a wedge of lime for squeezing and some extra finely diced chilli, if you like.

NUT FREE | DAIRY FREE

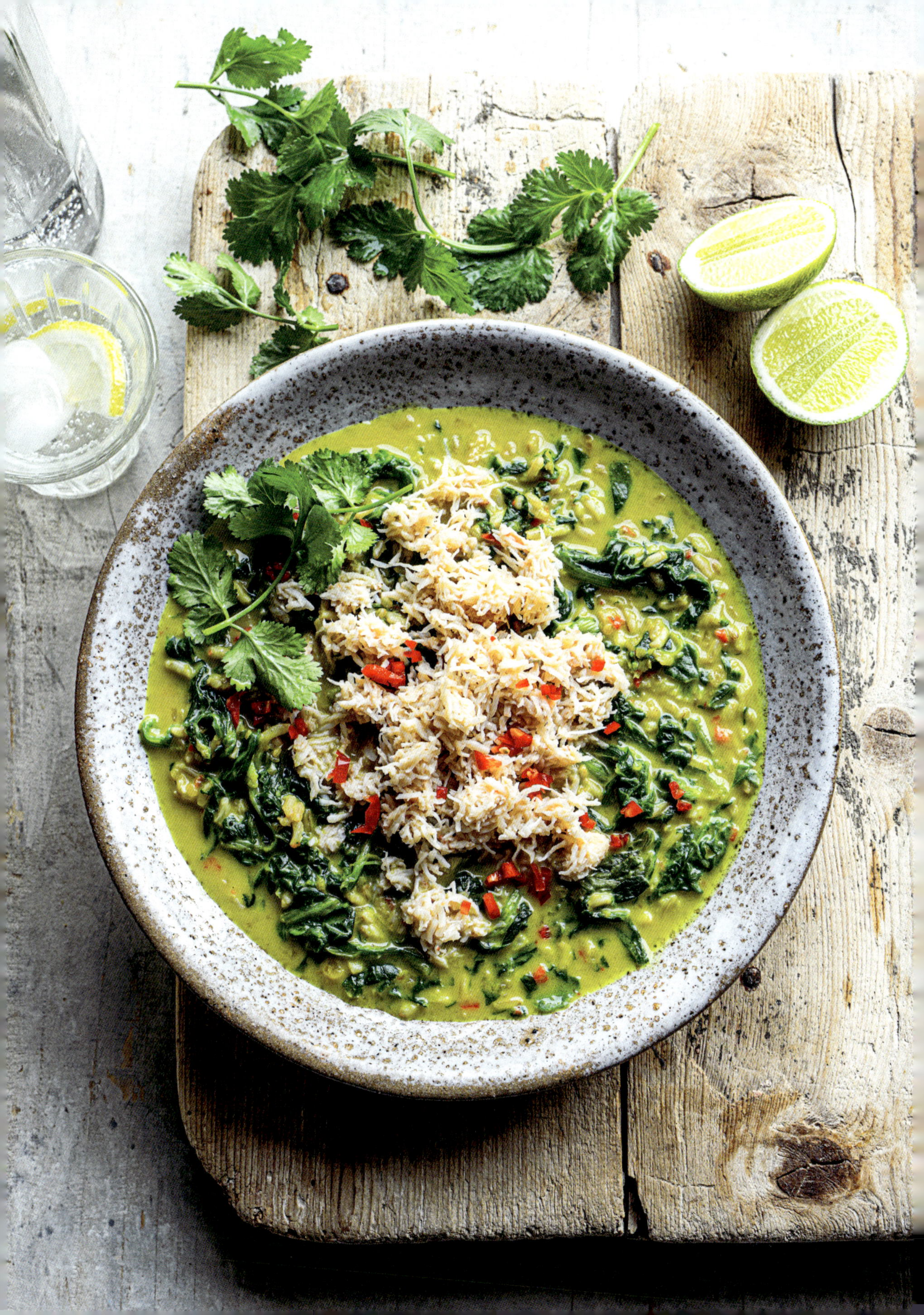

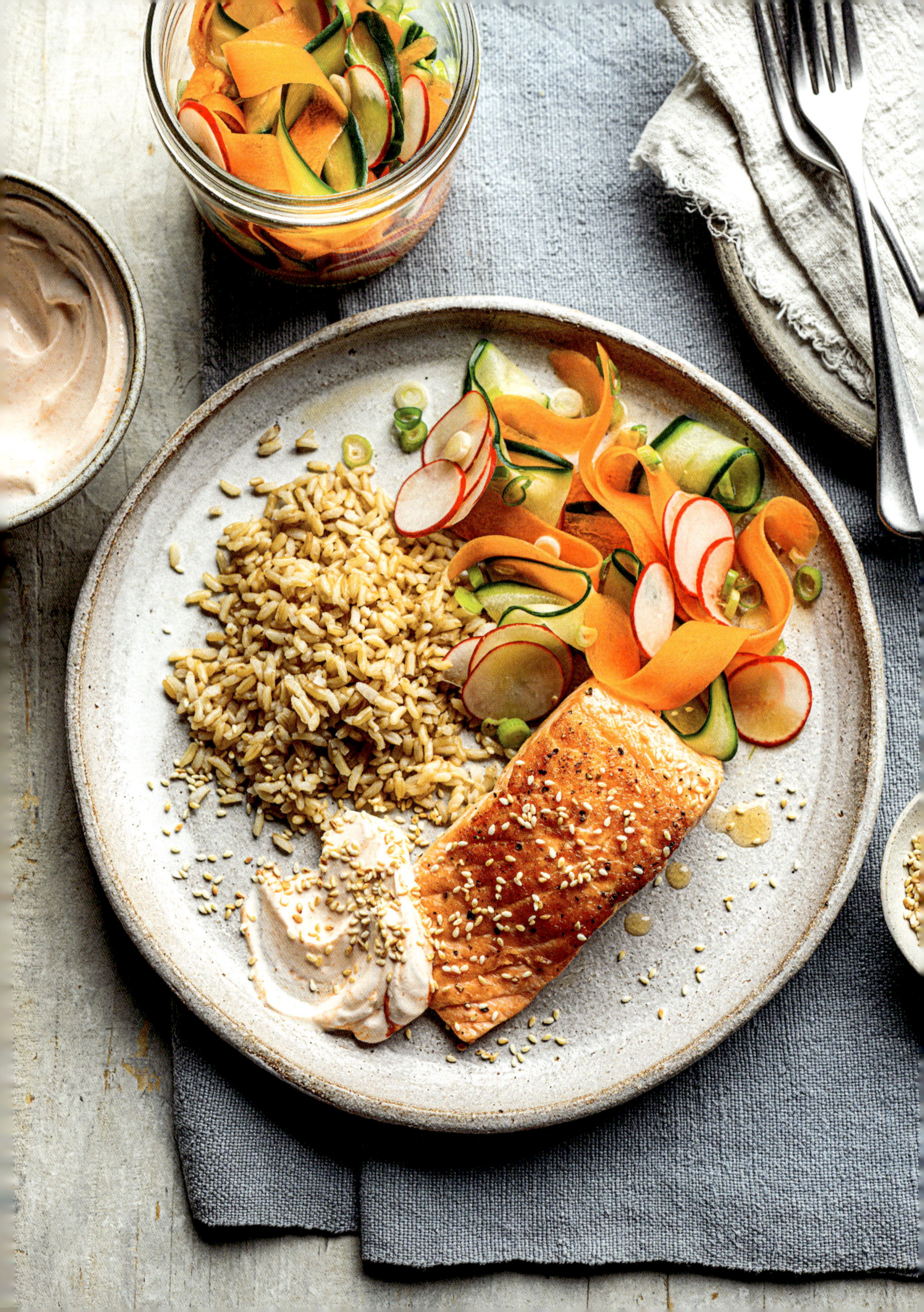

PER SERVING | **210cals** | PROTEIN **21.5g** | CARBS **5g** | FIBRE **1.5g**

UNDER 300 CALORIES

Pink Trout with Pickled Vegetables

SERVES **2** | PREP **30** mins | COOK **6** mins

2 pink trout fillets (about 100g each)
1 tbsp olive oil
1 tsp toasted sesame seeds
1 × quantity Creamy Hot Sauce (see page 242), to serve (optional)

For the pickled vegetables
2 tbsp rice vinegar or apple cider vinegar
Juice of 1 orange
6 radishes, thinly sliced
1 small carrot, pared into ribbons
1 snack cucumber, pared into ribbons
1 spring onion, finely sliced

The pickled vegetables can be made a day in advance, meaning this nutritious, light meal comes together in mere minutes. You can serve it with a portion of brown rice or noodles for a more substantial dish. I would fill half the plate with greens, such as spinach or kale (high in magnesium, iron and vitamins) and add a dash of butter or olive oil.

1. To make the pickled vegetables, mix together the vinegar and orange juice in a bowl. Season with salt, then add all the prepared vegetables and toss to coat. Leave for 15 minutes, or longer if liked (the pickles will keep for up to 1 day in the fridge).

2. To cook the fish, season the fillets and place them, skin-side down, in a frying pan with the olive oil over a medium heat. Cook for 4–5 minutes, until the skin is crisp, then turn and cook for another 30–60 seconds on the other side, until just cooked through.

3. Using a spatula, lift the fillets onto serving plates. Spoon over the pickled vegetables and finish with a sprinkling of sesame seeds. Serve with a spoonful of the creamy hot sauce, if you like.

AIR-FRYER TIP

Preheat the air fryer to 190°C, if needed. Prepare the pickle as Step 1. Cook the trout, skin-side up, for 4–5 minutes, until crisp. Turn the fillets over and cook for another 2 minutes, until just cooked through. Serve as above.

GLUTEN FREE · NUT FREE · DAIRY FREE

UNDER 300 CALORIES

PER SERVING | **226cals** | PROTEIN **26g** | CARBS **5g** | FIBRE **0.5g**

Gochujang Mussels

SERVES **2** | PREP **15** mins | COOK **10** mins

1kg mussels, cleaned and scrubbed
2 tsp neutral oil
1 large banana shallot, diced
3 garlic cloves, sliced
1 tbsp gochujang paste
1 tbsp light soy sauce
3 tbsp coconut cream
Handful of coriander leaves, chopped
½ lime, cut into wedges

The thick, sticky Korean spice paste, gochujang, adds flavour to the juicy steamed mussels. Michael loved mussels, especially as they are such a sustainable and high-quality source of protein. On a non-fast day, serve with crusty wholegrain sourdough.

1. Check the mussels and discard any with broken shells or that don't close when tapped lightly.

2. Heat the oil in a large saucepan or deep frying pan over a medium heat. Add the shallot and cook for 4 minutes. Stir in the garlic and cook for 1 minute, until softened and aromatic. Stir in the gochujang, soy sauce and 200ml water, then bring to the boil.

3. Tip the mussels into the pan, cover with a lid and cook for 4–5 minutes, shaking the pan occasionally, or until the mussels have opened.

4. Using a slotted spoon, transfer the mussels to two large shallow serving bowls, discarding any that haven't opened. Add the coconut cream to the broth in the pan and cook for 1–2 minutes, until slightly reduced and thickened. Check the seasoning.

5. Ladle the broth over the mussels, scatter over the coriander and serve with wedges of lime for squeezing.

NUT FREE
DAIRY FREE

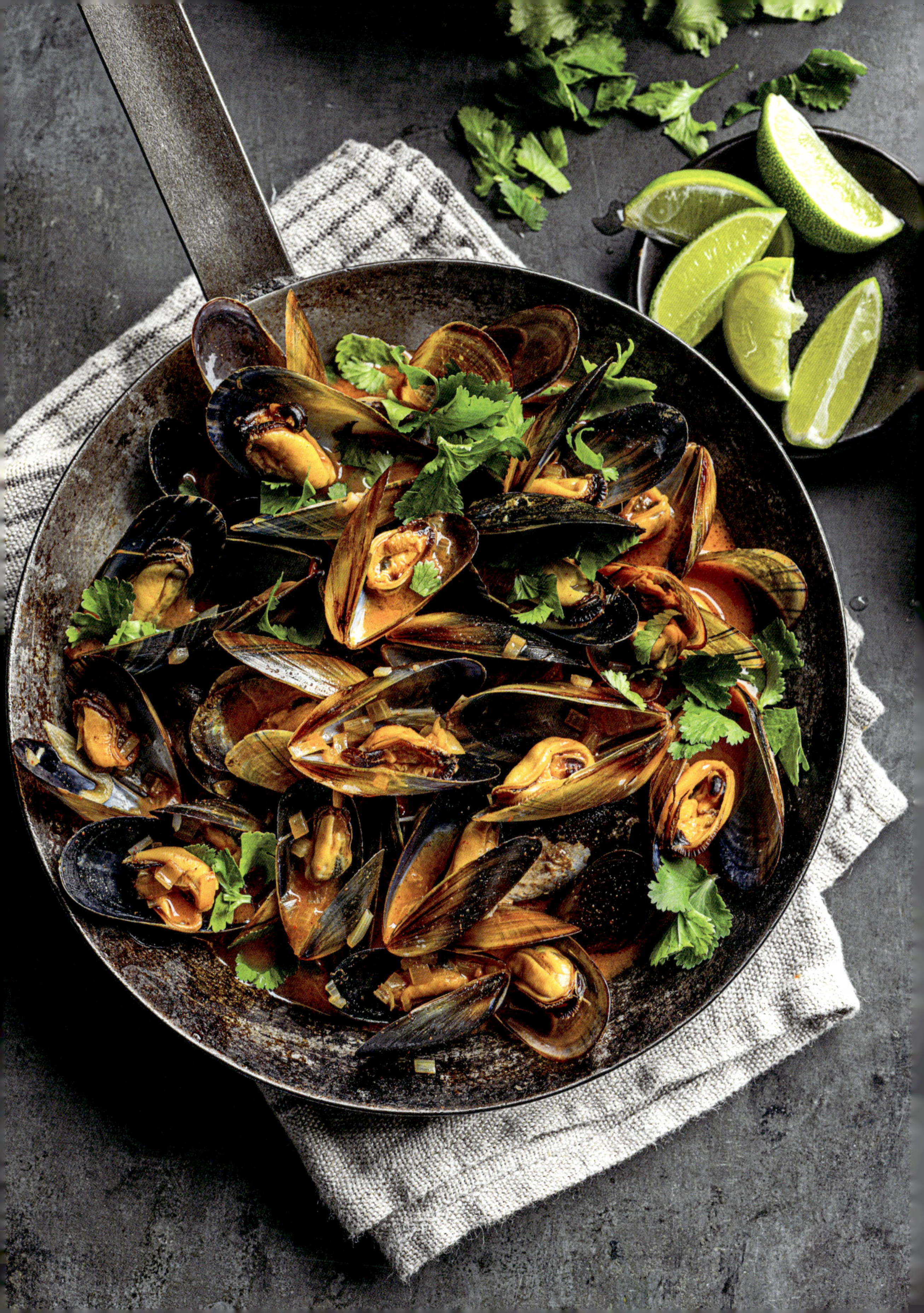

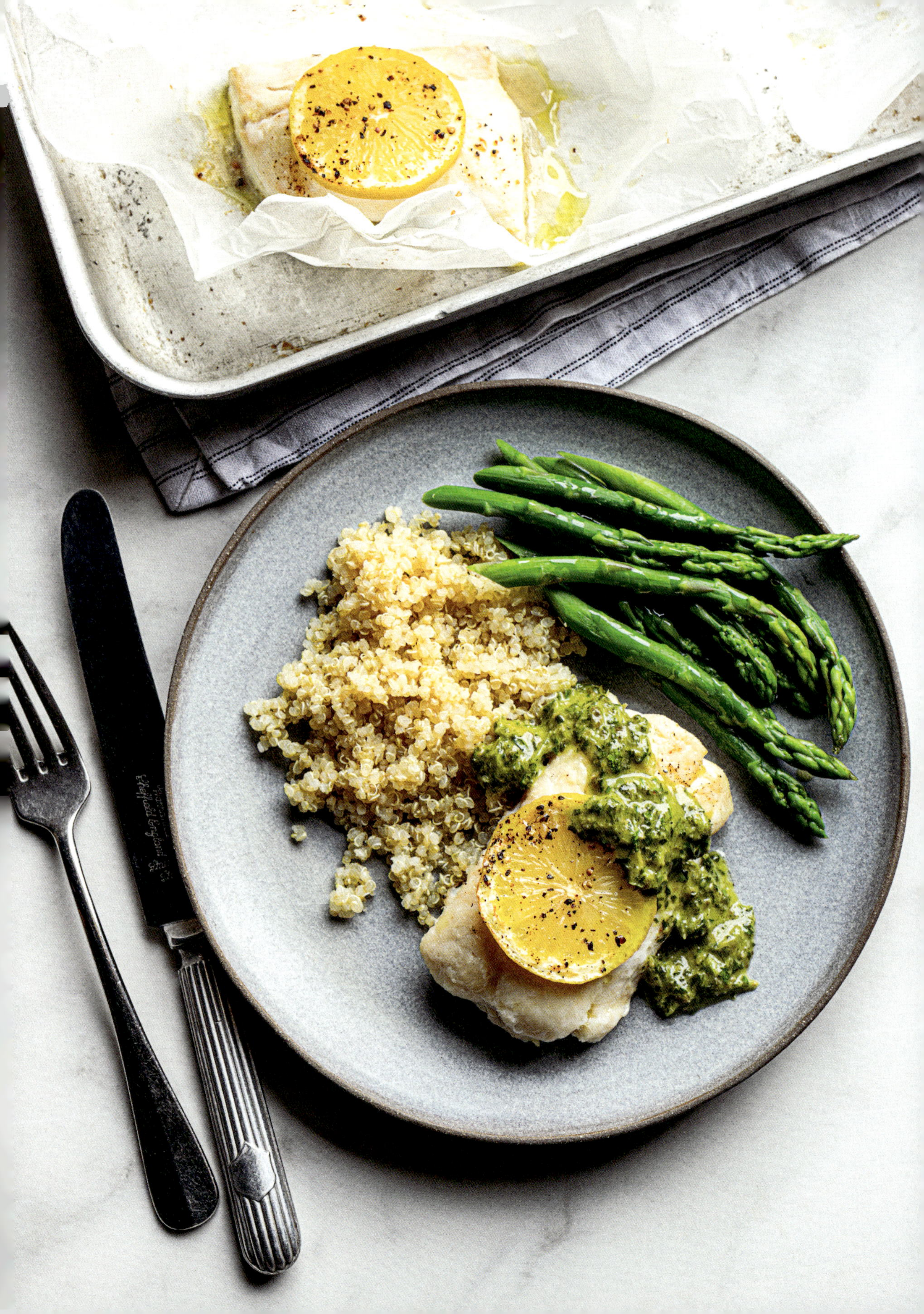

PER SERVING | **185cals** | PROTEIN **26.5g** | CARBS **0.5g** | FIBRE **0g**

UNDER 200 CALORIES

Baked White Fish with Salsa Verde

SERVES **2** | PREP **15** mins | COOK **15** mins

2 thick white fish fillets (such as cod, haddock or hake)
2½ tbsp extra-virgin olive oil
2 slices of lemon and the juice of ½ lemon
30g parsley, leaves and stalks
1 garlic clove, minced
1 tbsp small capers, drained
2 tsp Dijon mustard

The fish fillets are cooked in a parcel with slices of lemon to keep them moist – it's a simple, mess-free way to cook fish. The herby, lemony sauce adds a boost of flavour, colour and freshness. There is enough salsa verde here for 4 servings, so save half for another day. Serve it with quinoa and green veg on the side.

1. Preheat the oven to 200°C/Fan 180°C/Gas 6.

2. Place the fish on a sheet of non-stick baking paper, large enough to make a parcel. Season with salt and pepper, drizzle over 1 teaspoon of the olive oil and place a slice of lemon on top of each fillet. Fold over the edges of the paper to seal, then place the parcel on a baking tray. Bake the fish for 12–15 minutes, until opaque and the fish flakes easily.

3. Meanwhile, make the salsa verde. Put the remaining oil in a food processor with the parsley, garlic, capers, mustard and the juice of ½ lemon, and blitz to a coarse purée. Alternatively, finely chop the parsley, garlic and capers, and mix in a bowl with the mustard and lemon juice. Season to taste.

4. To serve, unwrap the fish parcels and place on serving plates with a spoonful of the salsa verde on top.

GLUTEN FREE | NUT FREE | DAIRY FREE

UNDER 400 CALORIES

PER SERVING | **385cals** | PROTEIN **36.5g** | CARBS **4g** | FIBRE **3g**

Baked Crispy White Fish

SERVES 2 | PREP 15 mins | COOK 15 mins

1 tbsp olive oil
2 thick white fish fillets (such as cod, hake or haddock)
40g ground almonds
Finely grated zest of 1 lemon
1 tsp garlic granules
2 tbsp mixed seeds
1 egg

There is something iconic about a plate of good fish and chips, especially by the sea, but so often they are greasy, starchy and likely to spike your sugars. With a few simple tweaks you can enjoy a satisfying healthy version. A combination of ground almonds, lemon zest and seeds makes the perfect crispy coating for white fish fillets, and they are baked rather than fried. Serve with Sweet Potato Chips and Smashed Minty Peas (see pages 238 and 232).

1. Preheat the oven to 220°C/Fan 200°C /Gas 7. Place a rack on a baking tray and oil it lightly.

2. Season the fish fillets on both sides with salt and pepper.

3. In a shallow bowl, combine the ground almonds, lemon zest, garlic granules and mixed seeds.

4. Beat the egg in a separate shallow bowl.

5. To coat the fish, first dunk the fillets in the egg, then transfer to the ground almond mixture, turning them once to coat both sides. Pat the coating to help it stick.

6. Place the fish on the oiled rack and, using a pastry brush, dab the remaining oil on top of the fish. Cook in the preheated oven for 12–15 minutes, depending on the thickness of the fillets, until the outside is crisp and the fish is cooked and flaky.

7. Serve the crispy fish with minty peas and fries on the side, if you like. Cut half the lemon into wedges for squeezing over.

GLUTEN FREE | DAIRY FREE

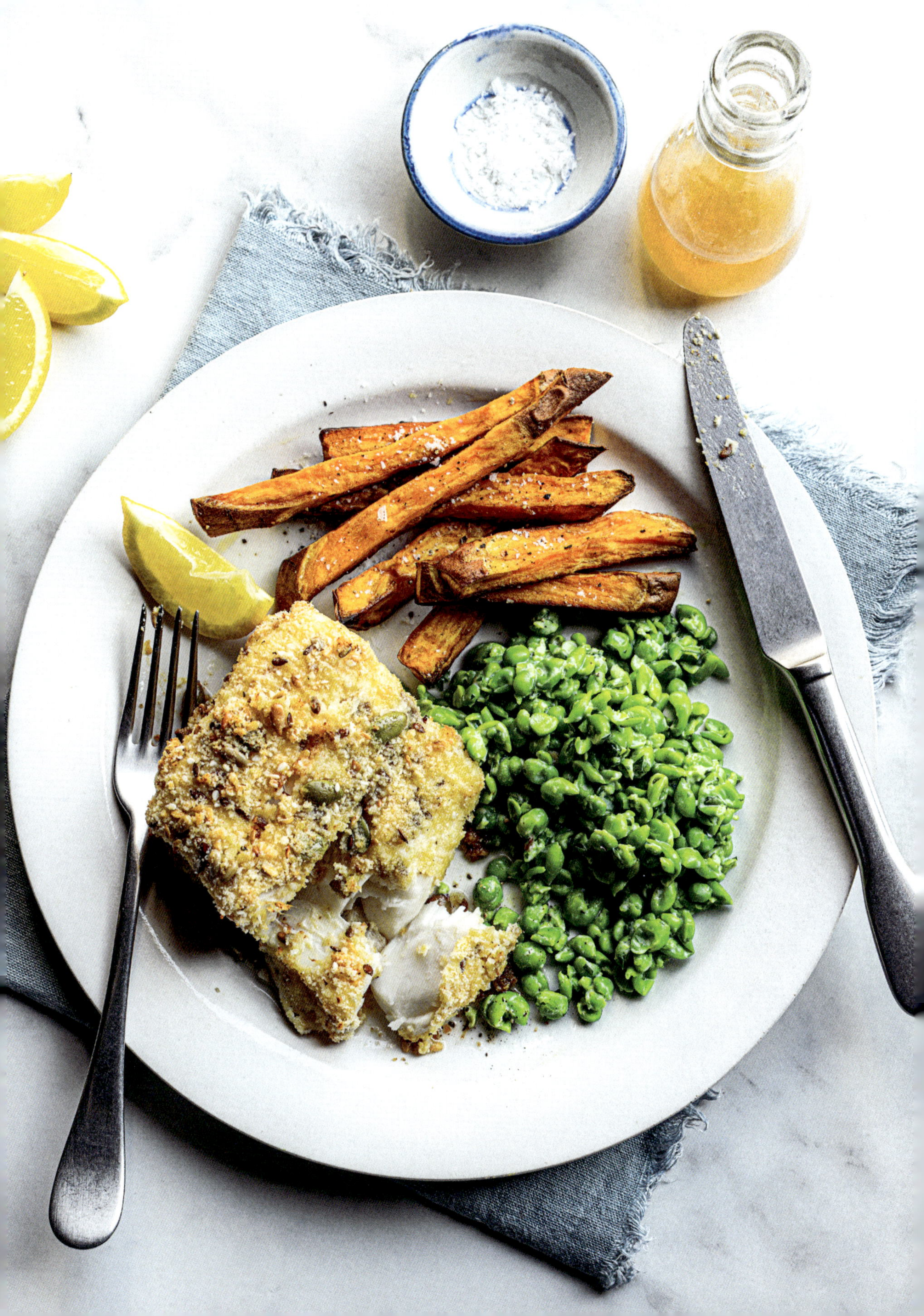

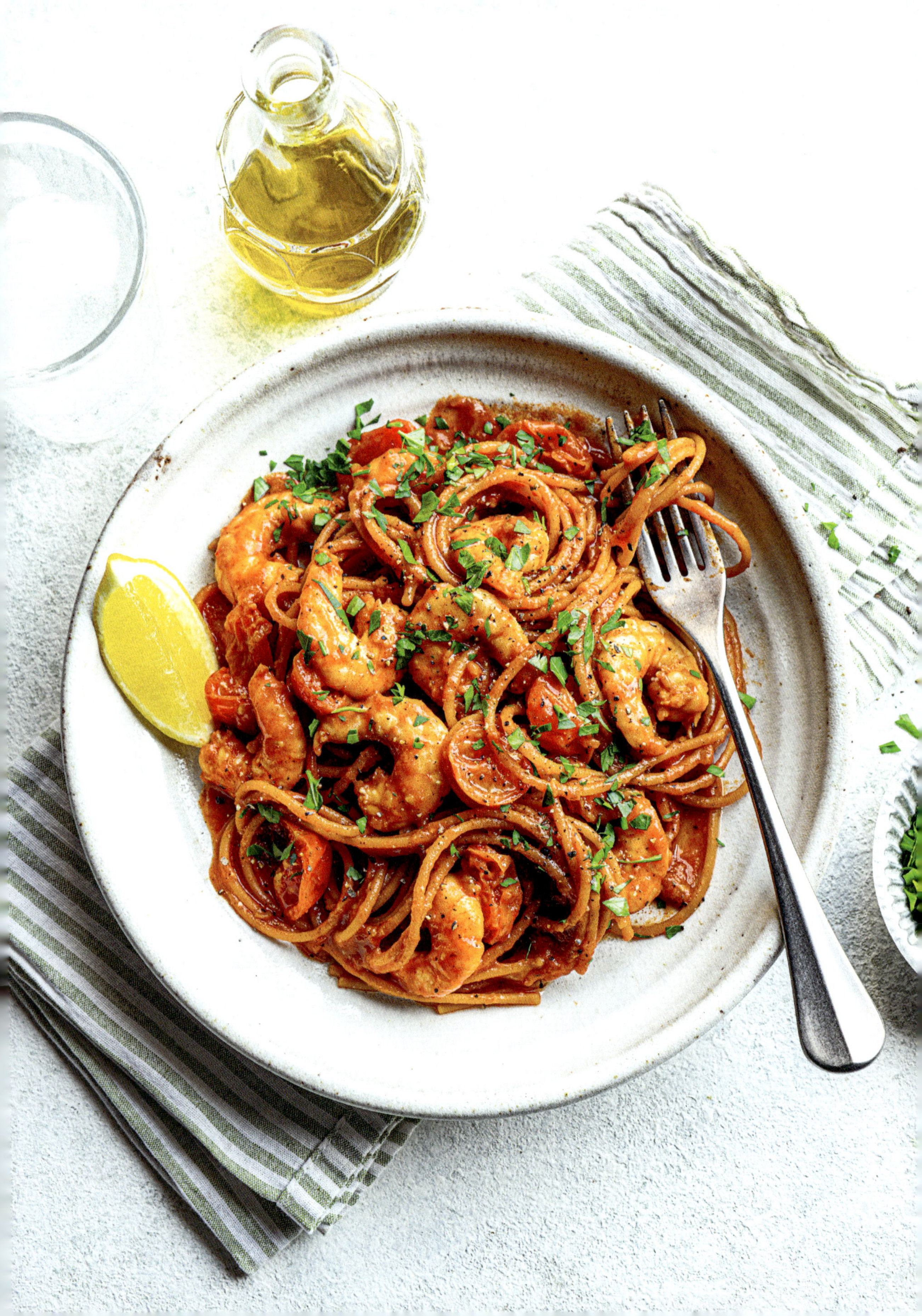

PER SERVING | **360cals** | PROTEIN **35g** | CARBS **33g** | FIBRE **8g**

UNDER 400 CALORIES

Sautéed Harissa Prawns

SERVES **2** | PREP **10** mins | COOK **10** mins

200g raw peeled king prawns
1 tbsp harissa paste
1 tbsp olive oil
2 tbsp tomato purée
2 garlic cloves, minced
10 cherry tomatoes, halved
120g high-protein pasta of choice
Squeeze of lemon
2 tbsp chopped parsley leaves

These harissa-coated prawns are served with pasta – look for a high-protein version, such as one made with lentils, black beans or chickpeas, as it is likely to contain up to four times more protein and fibre. Alternatively, swap the pasta for quinoa or brown rice.

1. In a bowl, mix the prawns with the harissa paste and 1 teaspoon of the olive oil. If you have time, leave them to marinate in the fridge for up to 1 hour; they can also be used straight away.

2. Cook the pasta in a pan of boiling salted water according to the packet instructions, until al dente. Drain the pasta, reserving 100ml of the cooking water. Return the pasta to the pan.

3. Meanwhile, heat the remaining olive oil in a saucepan with the tomato purée and cook, stirring, for 3 minutes. Add the garlic and tomatoes and cook for another 2 minutes. Tip in the prawns and any remaining harissa from the bowl, and cook for 3 minutes, until they turn pink and are cooked through. Add enough of the reserved cooking water (at least 50ml) to make a sauce. Season with salt and pepper, to taste.

4. Tip the tomato harissa prawn sauce into the pasta and toss until combined, adding a splash more water if needed, then heat through briefly. Add a squeeze of lemon and serve sprinkled with parsley.

NUT FREE | DAIRY FREE

UNDER **500** CALORIES

PER SERVING | **433cals** | PROTEIN **21g** | CARBS **17g** | FIBRE **3g**

Mackerel with Orange, Olive and Quinoa Salad

SERVES **2** | PREP **15** mins | COOK **5** mins

2 fresh mackerel fillets (about 90g each)
1 tbsp extra-virgin olive oil
80g cooked quinoa (from a pouch)
1 small shallot, diced
1 orange, peeled and segmented
50g pitted black olives, halved
60g watercress
1 lemon, cut into wedges, to serve

In this easy light meal, the fresh, fruity salad partners beautifully with the richness of the mackerel. Mackerel, being high in omega 3, provides anti-inflammatory benefits, but you could swap it for salmon, pink trout or prawns, if you prefer. Serve it at room temperature for the best flavour and add some steamed greens, too, if you like.

1. Brush both sides of the mackerel fillets with some of the olive oil and season with salt and pepper. Set aside.

2. Tip the quinoa into a shallow serving bowl. Add the shallot, orange, olives, watercress, the remaining oil and the juice of ½ lemon, then season and toss until combined.

3. Place a frying pan over a medium heat. When hot, add the mackerel fillets, skin-side down, and cook without moving for 3–4 minutes until the skin crisps. Turn them over and cook for another minute, or until just cooked through.

4. Place the mackerel on plates and serve with the salad on the side and some lemon wedges for squeezing.

AIR-FRYER TIP

Preheat the air fryer to 190°C, if needed. Prepare the mackerel and salad as steps 1–2. Cook the mackerel, skin-side up, for 4–5 minutes, until crisp. Turn the fillets over and cook for another 2–3 minutes, until just cooked through. Serve as above.

GLUTEN FREE | NUT FREE | DAIRY FREE

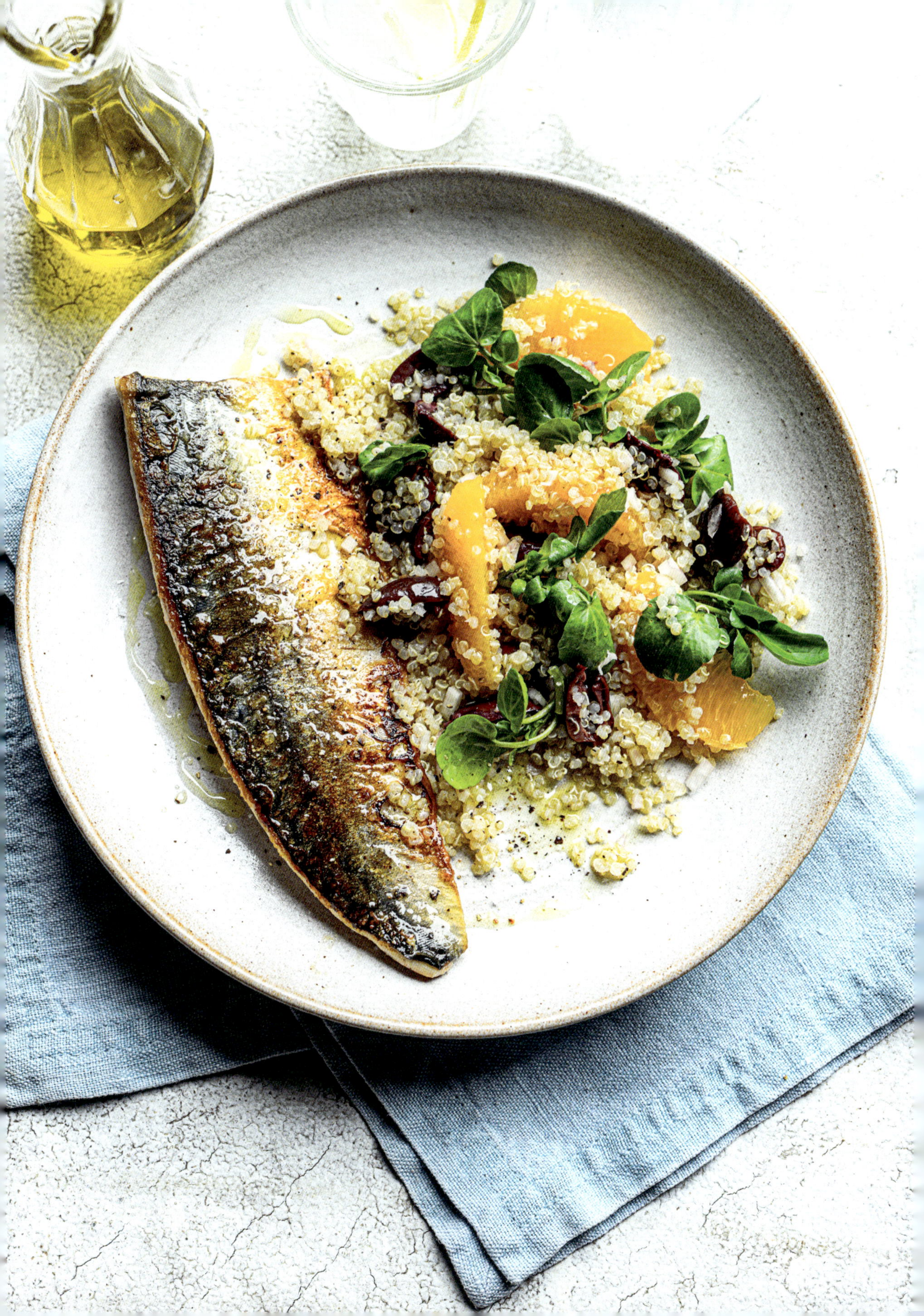

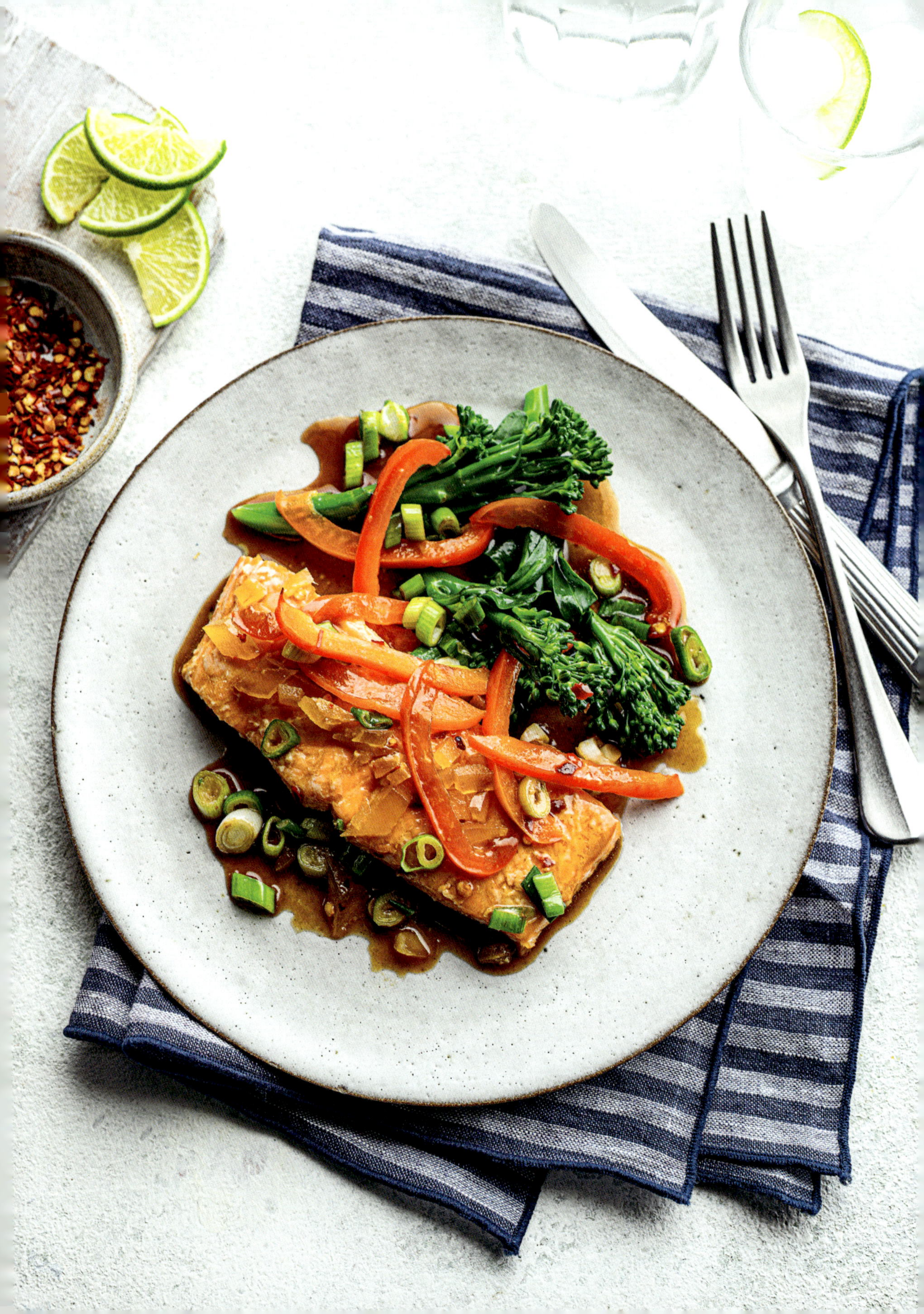

PER SERVING | **491cals** | PROTEIN **41g** | CARBS **18g** | FIBRE **6g**

UNDER 500 CALORIES

Poached Ginger Salmon with Broccoli

SERVES 2 | PREP 10 mins | COOK 30 mins

2 salmon fillets (about 180g each)
2 tbsp light soy sauce or fish sauce
1 ball stem ginger in syrup, drained and diced
½ red pepper, deseeded and finely sliced
Juice of 1 small orange
Dried chilli flakes (optional)
200g tenderstem broccoli, any thick stems sliced lengthways
3 spring onions, roughly chopped

A soothing dish with a delicate ginger flavour, it is easy to prepare, too. You can also use a normal head of broccoli – just break it into small florets.

1. Preheat the oven to 190°C/Fan 170°C/Gas 5 and place a baking tray in the oven to heat up.

2. Place the salmon on a sheet of foil, large enough to make a parcel. Sprinkle over the soy sauce, ginger, pepper, orange juice and chilli flakes, if using. Wrap the foil over the salmon to make a parcel.

3. Place the foil parcel on the hot baking tray in the oven and cook for 15 minutes.

4. Remove the salmon from the oven, open the parcel and add the broccoli and spring onions. Season with black pepper, then rewrap and return to the oven for a final 15 minutes.

5. Serve the salmon with the broccoli and pepper alongside and any cooking juices drizzled over the top.

NUT FREE | DAIRY FREE

UNDER 500 CALORIES | PER SERVING | 480cals | PROTEIN 36g | CARBS 13g | FIBRE 8g | DAIRY FREE

Quick Tuna Stir-fry

SERVES 2 | PREP 15 mins | COOK 5 mins

1 × 200g tin tuna in olive oil, drained, reserving 1 tbsp of the oil (150g drained weight)
1 × 300g pack of stir-fry veg
1 tsp finely chopped or grated fresh root ginger
2 eggs, beaten
2 tbsp light soy sauce or fish sauce
2 tbsp chia seeds
2 handfuls of cashew nuts

Full of aromatic flavour, protein and fibre, this is super easy to make and is one of my go-to recipes when the fridge looks bleak. A pack of stir-fry veg makes it easier, but you can use diced cabbage or pak choi instead.

1. Place a large frying pan or wok over a high heat until just smoking. Add 1 tablespoon of the oil from the tin of tuna, followed by the veg and ginger. Stir fry for 4–5 minutes.

2. Add the tuna to the pan and, when it is hot, stir in the eggs. Fry for a couple of minutes, then add the soy sauce, chia seeds and 2–3 tablespoons of water, to loosen, and mix well.

3. Remove from the heat and divide between two plates. Scatter with the cashews to serve.

UNDER 400 CALORIES | PER SERVING | 311cals | PROTEIN 30g | CARBS 2.5g | FIBRE 3g | GLUTEN FREE | NUT FREE

White Fish with Lemon and Asparagus

SERVES 2 | PREP 15 mins | COOK 5 mins

150g white fish (such as cod, haddock or hake)
½ tbsp olive oil
1 tbsp butter
1 bunch of asparagus or 100g tenderstem broccoli, any thick stems sliced lengthways
Juice of ½ small lemon and 1 tsp finely grated lemon zest

This is highly nutritious and promotes digestive health.

1. Season the fish with salt and ground black pepper, and place a frying pan over a medium heat. Add the olive oil, butter, asparagus and lemon juice and zest to the pan, then add the fish, skin-side down, and cook for 2–3 minutes. Turn and cook for another 2–3 minutes, until the fish is opaque and flakes easily. Be careful not to overcook.

2. Turn the asparagus to coat in the sauce, then place on a warm plate. Arrange the fish on top, and drizzle any cooking juices over to serve.

PER SERVING | **370cals** | PROTEIN **31g** | CARBS **14g** | FIBRE **8g**

UNDER 400 CALORIES

Sea Bass, Fennel and Jerusalem Artichokes

SERVES 2 | PREP 8 mins | COOK 30 mins

1 tbsp olive oil
1 small fennel bulb, core removed, finely sliced
250g Jerusalem artichokes, washed and finely sliced
2 sea bass fillets
1 tbsp apple cider vinegar
Handful of chopped parsley, to garnish

One of my favourite recipes, light and with a delicate flavour, the fennel is sautéed with gut-friendly Jerusalem artichokes. They look like small knobbly potatoes and have a nutty flavour. You could also serve this with 2–3 tablespoons of quinoa or brown rice.

1. Place a frying pan over a medium–high heat. Add the oil, fennel and artichokes and cook for 20 minutes, stirring occasionally, until soft but crisping at the edges.

2. Season with salt and pepper, then push the veg to one side of the pan. Add the fish, skin-side down, and fry for 3–4 minutes, then turn over and cook for a few minutes on the other side, until cooked through.

3. Divide the veg between two plates, drizzle with apple cider vinegar, then top with the sea bass fillets. Scatter over the chopped parsley to serve.

GLUTEN FREE | NUT FREE | DAIRY FREE

UNDER 600 CALORIES

PER SERVING | **561cals** | PROTEIN **38g** | CARBS **23g** | FIBRE **6g**

Thai-style Fish Cakes

SERVES 2 | PREP 20 mins | COOK 20 mins

1 snack cucumber, seeds removed, finely sliced
2 tbsp apple cider vinegar
300g cooked skinless salmon (fresh or tinned), flaked
200g cooked sweet potato, mashed and left to cool
1 large egg, beaten
1 tbsp chia seeds
1 tbsp red Thai curry paste
Large handful of coriander leaves, finely chopped
1 tbsp olive oil, to drizzle

Colourful, mildly spiced and with a pleasing sweetness, these fish cakes are delicious and improved by the addition of quick pickled cucumber. Serve the fish cakes with cauliflower rice and 1–2 tablespoons of cooked edamame beans to top up the protein.

1. Preheat the oven to 200°C/Fan 180°C/Gas 6.

2. Place the cucumber in a bowl and drizzle over the apple cider vinegar. Season with a pinch of salt and pepper, and set aside.

3. Combine the salmon, sweet potato, egg, chia seeds, Thai paste, and half the coriander in a large bowl. Season with salt and pepper and mix well. Form into 8 small patties, then set aside in the fridge for 15 minutes to firm up.

4. Arrange the patties on a baking tray, lined with baking paper, and drizzle with a little oil. Cook in the oven for 20 minutes, carefully turning halfway.

5. Divide the patties between two plates, garnish with the remaining coriander and serve with the pickled cucumber alongside.

AIR-FRYER TIP

Preheat the air fryer to 180°C, if needed. Prepare the cucumber pickle and patties as steps 2–3. Spray the patties with oil and cook for 15 minutes, turning halfway, until cooked through. Serve as above.

NUT FREE · DAIRY FREE

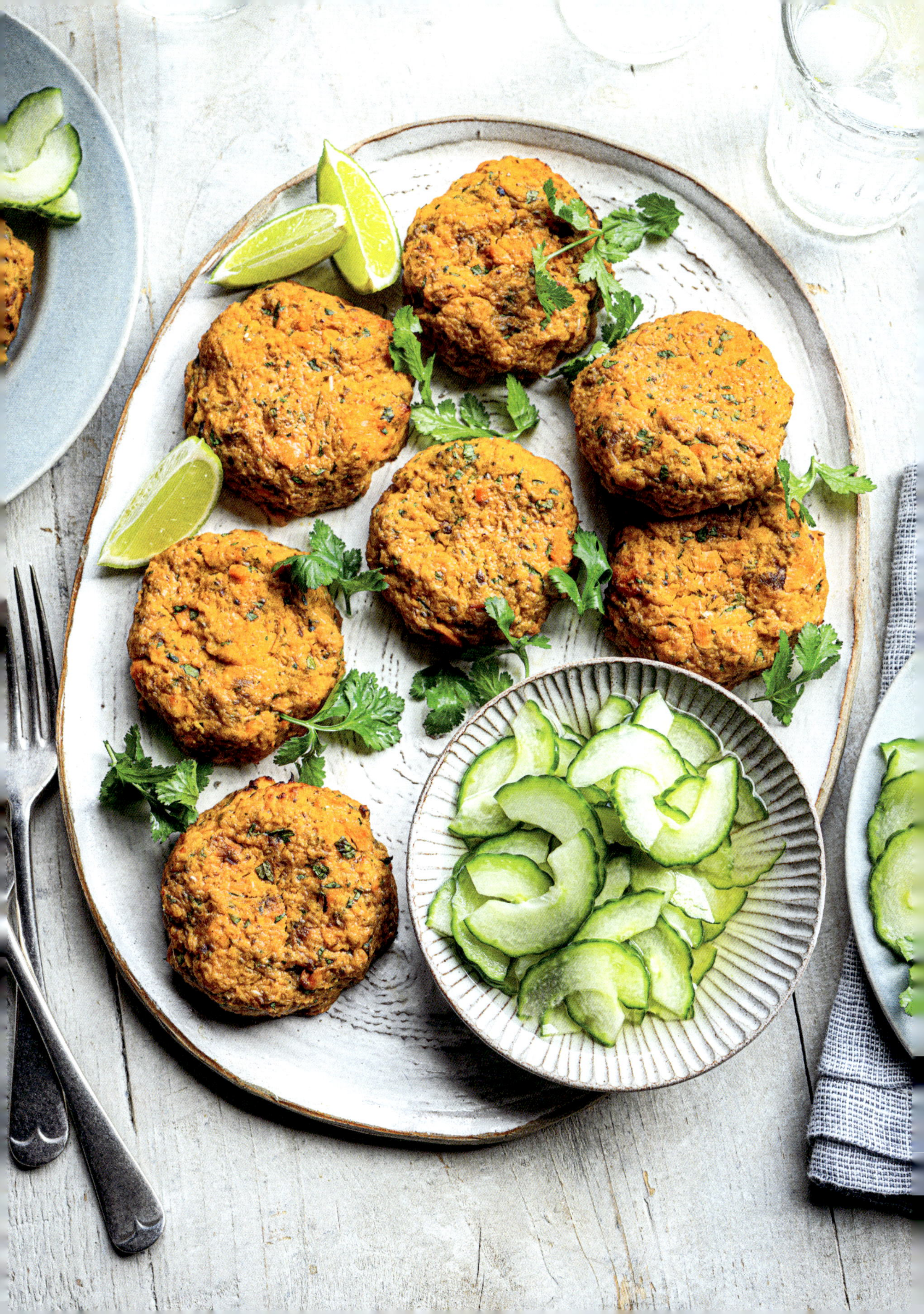

UNDER 400 CALORIES

PER SERVING | **310cals** | PROTEIN **32g** | CARBS **24g** | FIBRE **6g**

Caribbean-style Fish Traybake

SERVES 2 | PREP 15 mins | COOK 15 mins

2 thick haddock fillets, or your choice of white fish
¾ tsp jerk spice mix
1 lime, halved
2 tsp olive oil
100g drained tinned pinto or black beans, rinsed
65g cooked brown, red and black rice mixture (or just use brown)
2 tbsp coconut cream
1 orange, segmented
1 small red pepper, deseeded and diced
¼ small red onion, diced
1 tbsp chopped coriander leaves

The fish is flavoured with jerk spices and lime juice, then baked with rice and beans. An orange and lime salsa adds colour and freshness to the dish.

1. Preheat the oven to 200°C/180°C fan/Gas 6. Pat the fish fillets dry with kitchen paper.

2. Mix together the jerk spices, 1 teaspoon of the lime juice and half of the olive oil. Season with salt and pepper.

3. Mix together the remaining oil, the beans, cooked rice, 1 teaspoon of lime juice and the coconut cream in a medium roasting tin. Place the fish fillets on top and spoon over the jerk spice marinade. Cook in the oven for 12–15 minutes, until opaque and the fish flakes easily.

4. While the fish is cooking, mix the orange, red pepper, onion and coriander together in a bowl with the remaining lime juice (there should be ½ a lime left).

5. Serve the fish on top of the coconut rice and beans with the orange salsa spooned on top.

GLUTEN FREE · NUT FREE · DAIRY FREE

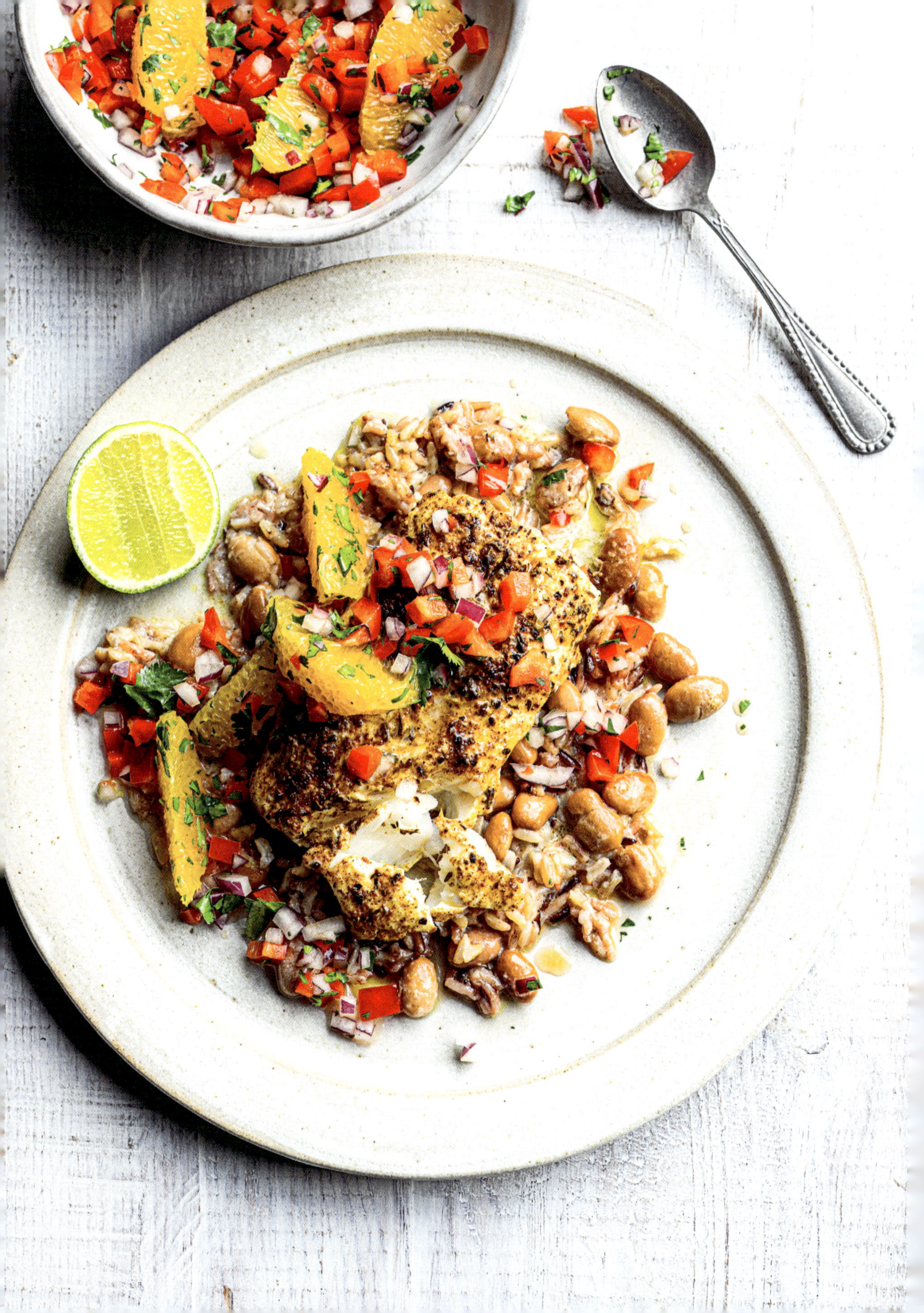

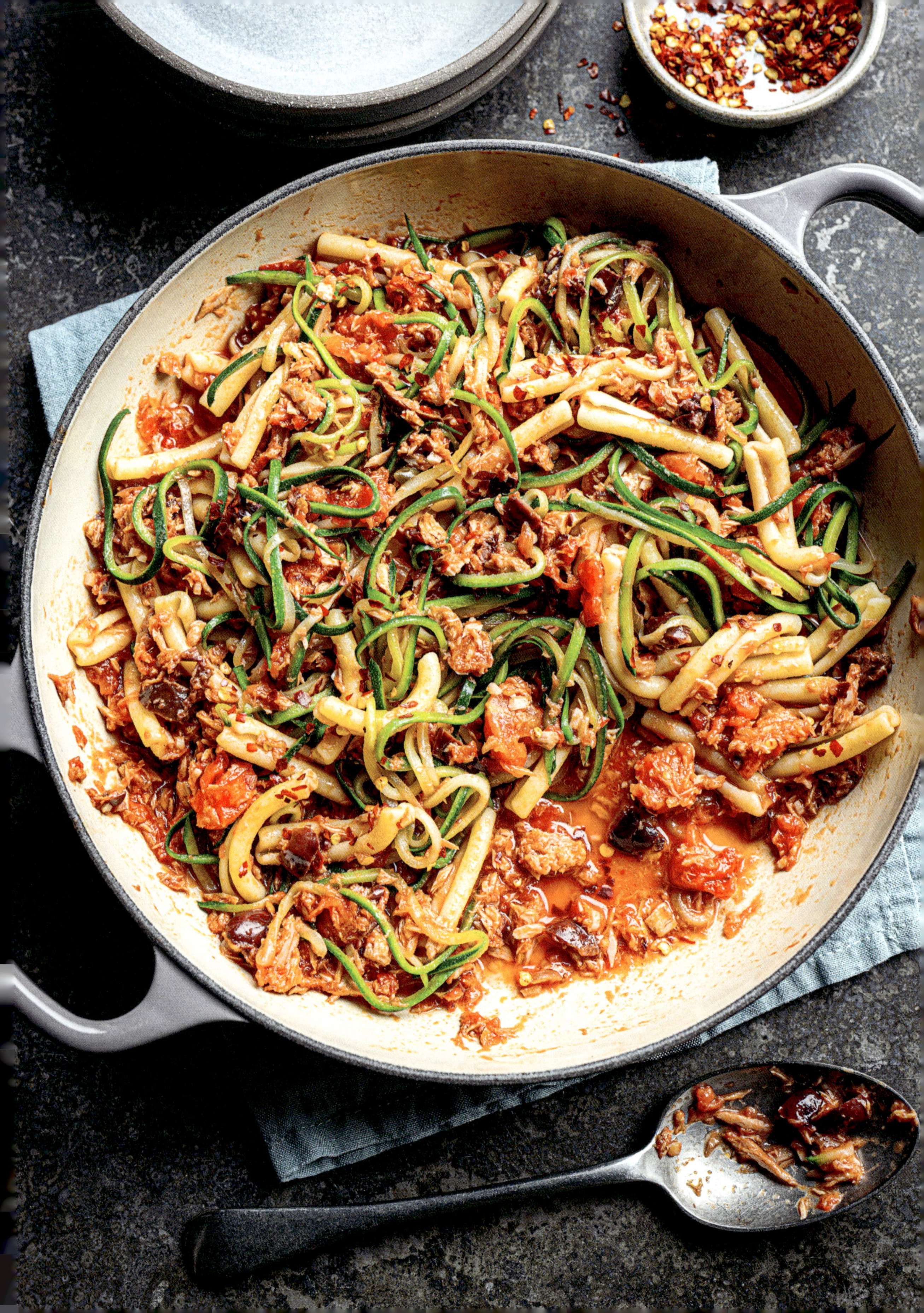

PER SERVING | **416cals** | PROTEIN **25g** | CARBS **31g** | FIBRE **6g**

UNDER **500** CALORIES

Tuna Pasta in Puttanesca Sauce

SERVES **2** | PREP **10** mins | COOK **10** mins

1 × 150g tin tuna in olive oil, drained, reserving 1 tbsp of the oil
1 × 400g tin chopped tomatoes
55g pitted black olives (about 12)
1 tbsp capers
4 small anchovies, diced
2 garlic cloves, diced
Finely grated zest and juice of ½ lemon
60g dried pasta
2 medium courgettes, trimmed and spiralised (also available in a pack already spiralised)
Dried chilli flakes (optional)

A lovely supper made with some store-cupboard staples. If you don't have a spiraliser, just grate or finely slice the courgettes. I try and keep a couple of tins of tuna in the cupboard for an emergency dinner, such as this. It's a valuable source of protein, omega 3, vitamins and minerals, including vitamin D and B12.

1. Place a large frying pan or flameproof casserole over a medium heat and add 1 tablespoon of the oil from the tuna tin. Add the tuna, chopped tomatoes, olives, capers, anchovies, garlic, lemon zest and juice, and cook for a few minutes, until heated through, stirring occasionally.

2. Meanwhile, cook the pasta according to the packet instructions. Just before you drain it, add the spiralised courgette to the pan to warm through and soften. Drain everything well and add to the pan with the sauce.

3. Add dried chilli flakes, to taste, and mix well to coat the pasta and courgette in the sauce.

4. Divide between two plates and serve immediately.

NUT FREE | DAIRY FREE

UNDER 600 CALORIES

PER SERVING | **583cals** | PROTEIN **41g** | CARBS **20.5g** | FIBRE **13g**

Green Thai-style Coconut Prawns

SERVES **2** | PREP **5** mins | COOK **10** mins

1 tbsp coconut oil
1 small onion, diced
4 pak choi, sliced lengthways
155g frozen edamame beans
½ × 190g jar green Thai curry paste
1 × 400ml tin reduced-fat coconut milk
300g cooked jumbo prawns

So easy to throw together, you might like to have this with cauliflower rice on a fast day, or with 2–3 tablespoons of brown rice (which has 3 times the amount of fibre as white rice) on a non-fast day. Serve the prawns with some steamed green vegetables on the side, if you like. You could use raw instead of cooked prawns – just add them to the simmering sauce and cook until pink.

1. Place a medium saucepan over a gentle heat. Add the oil and onion and cook gently for 5 minutes, stirring occasionally.

2. Tip in the pak choi and edamame and stir-fry for 2 minutes.

3. Stir in the Thai paste to coat the veg, then pour in the coconut milk. Bring up to a simmer.

4. Add the prawns to the pan and cook in the sauce for a couple of minutes, until heated through. Serve straight away.

GLUTEN FREE NUT FREE DAIRY FREE

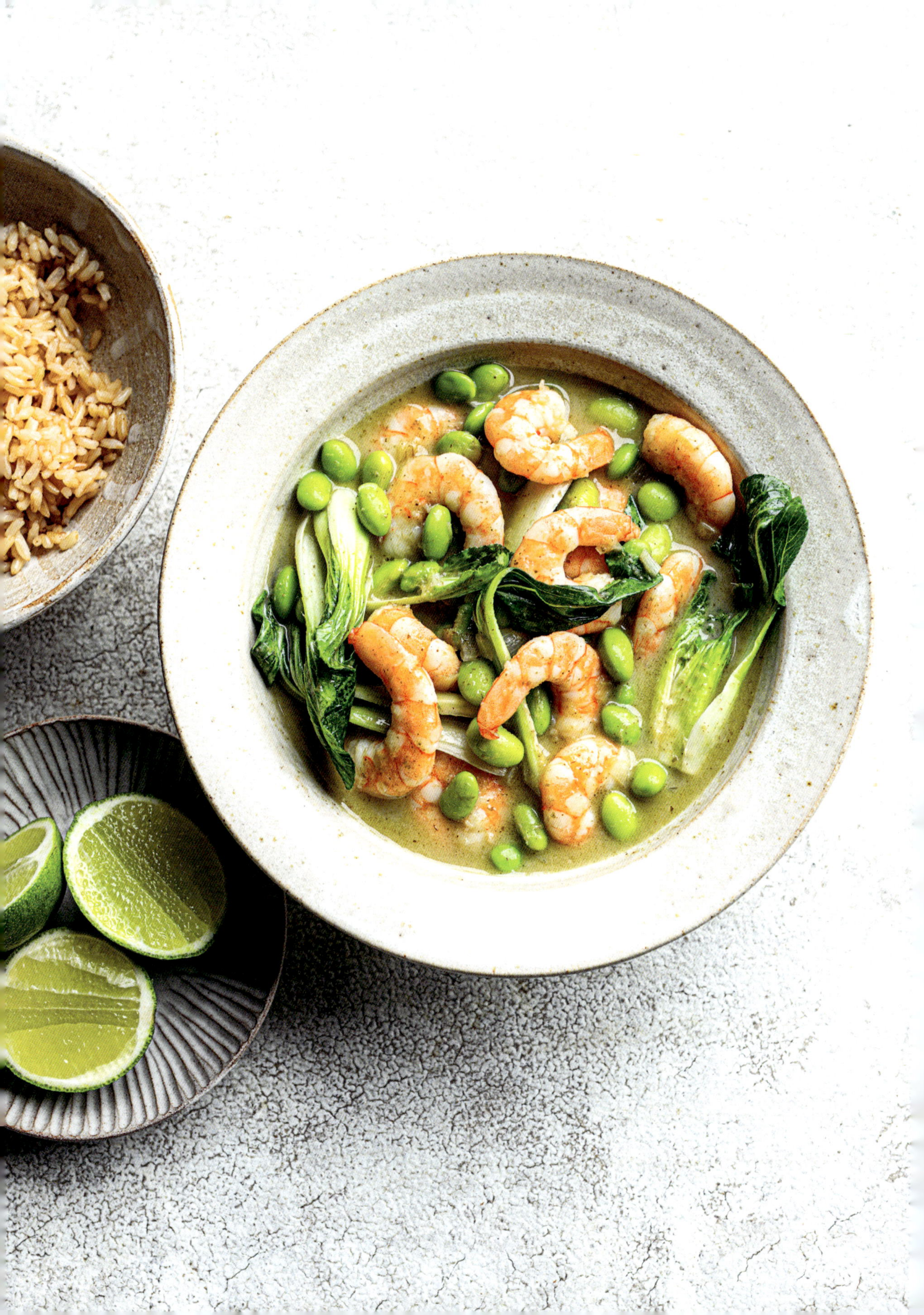

UNDER 500 CALORIES

PER SERVING | **420cals** | PROTEIN **38g** | CARBS **2g** | FIBRE **5.5g**

Salmon Ceviche

SERVES 2 | PREP 45 mins

2 good-quality and very fresh salmon fillets, skinned (about 180g each)
½ spring onion, finely chopped
Handful of coriander leaves, roughly chopped
1 small garlic clove, finely chopped
½ celeriac, peeled and finely sliced (about 200g prepared weight)
Juice of ½ lemon
1 tbsp apple cider vinegar
Pinch of dried chilli flakes (optional)

Light, zesty and with a hint of garlic, if you can find very fresh and good-quality fish, this is a lovely way to serve it. You could serve this with a small slice of sourdough.

1. Place all the ingredients in a bowl and toss to coat the fish and vegetables in the lemon juice and vinegar. Leave to marinate in the fridge for 30 minutes.

2. Remove the fillets from the bowl and cut into small, bite-sized pieces. Return the fish to bowl, sprinkle with dried chilli flakes, if you like, and toss a final time before serving.

GLUTEN FREE | NUT FREE | DAIRY FREE

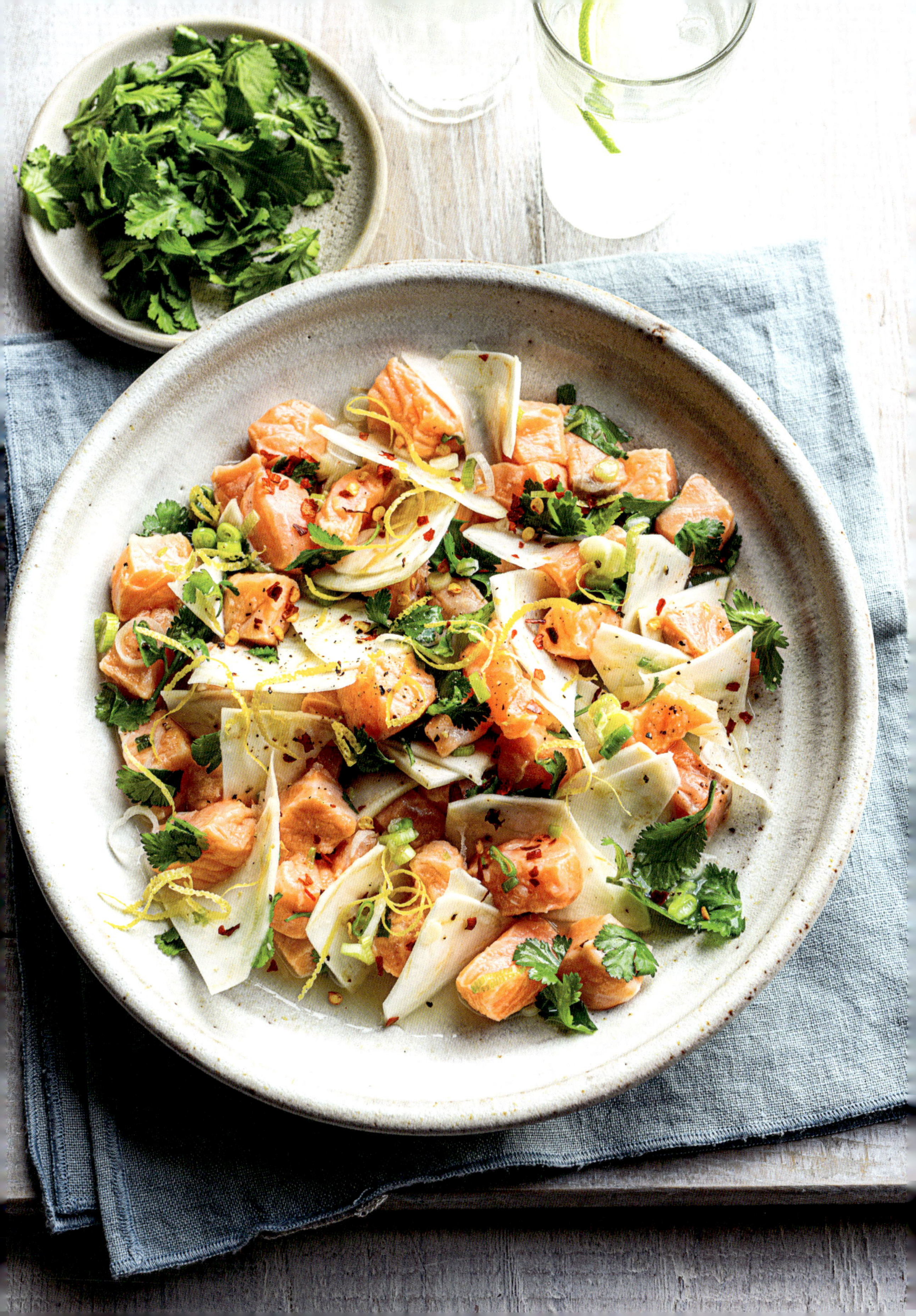

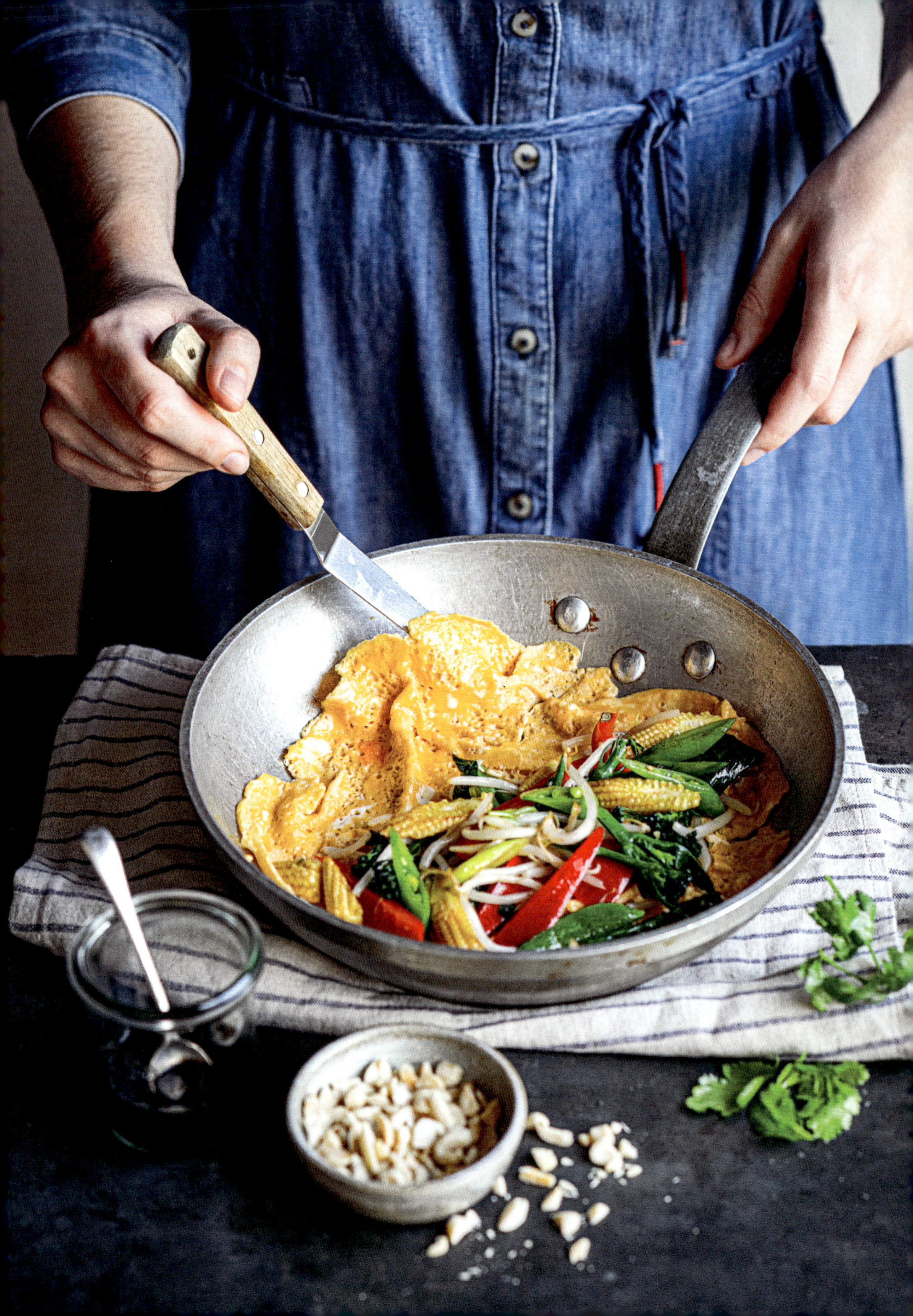

Meat-free

UNDER 400 CALORIES

PER SERVING | **335cals** | PROTEIN **20g** | CARBS **10g** | FIBRE **5g**

Omelette Spring Roll

SERVES **1** | PREP **5** mins | COOK **8** mins

Filled with a generous amount of stir-fried vegetables, this 'spring roll' uses an omelette as the wrapper, instead of the usual white flour pastry.

2 eggs
1 tsp light soy sauce
1 tbsp olive oil
200g mixed stir-fry veg
1cm piece of fresh root ginger, peeled and finely grated
1 tbsp chopped unsalted roasted peanuts (optional)
Small handful of coriander leaves (optional)

1. Lightly beat the eggs with the soy sauce. Season with pepper and set aside.

2. Heat 2 teaspoons of the oil in a frying pan or wok over a medium–high heat. Add the vegetables and ginger, and stir-fry for 3–5 minutes, until softened but still with some crunch. Season with salt and pepper, then tip the vegetables onto a plate and set aside.

3. Wipe the pan clean and set over a medium–low heat. Heat the remaining oil, then pour in the egg mixture. Tilt the pan to cover the base in an even layer, then cook the omelette, drawing the cooked egg at the edges towards the middle of the pan and tilting the pan to allow any uncooked egg to fill the gaps.

4. When the base of the omelette is set and the top is still slightly runny, spoon the vegetables down one side. Fold the omelette over the vegetables to form a roll, heat through briefly, then slide it onto a serving plate. Scatter the peanuts and coriander leaves over the top to serve, if using.

VEGGIE DAIRY FREE

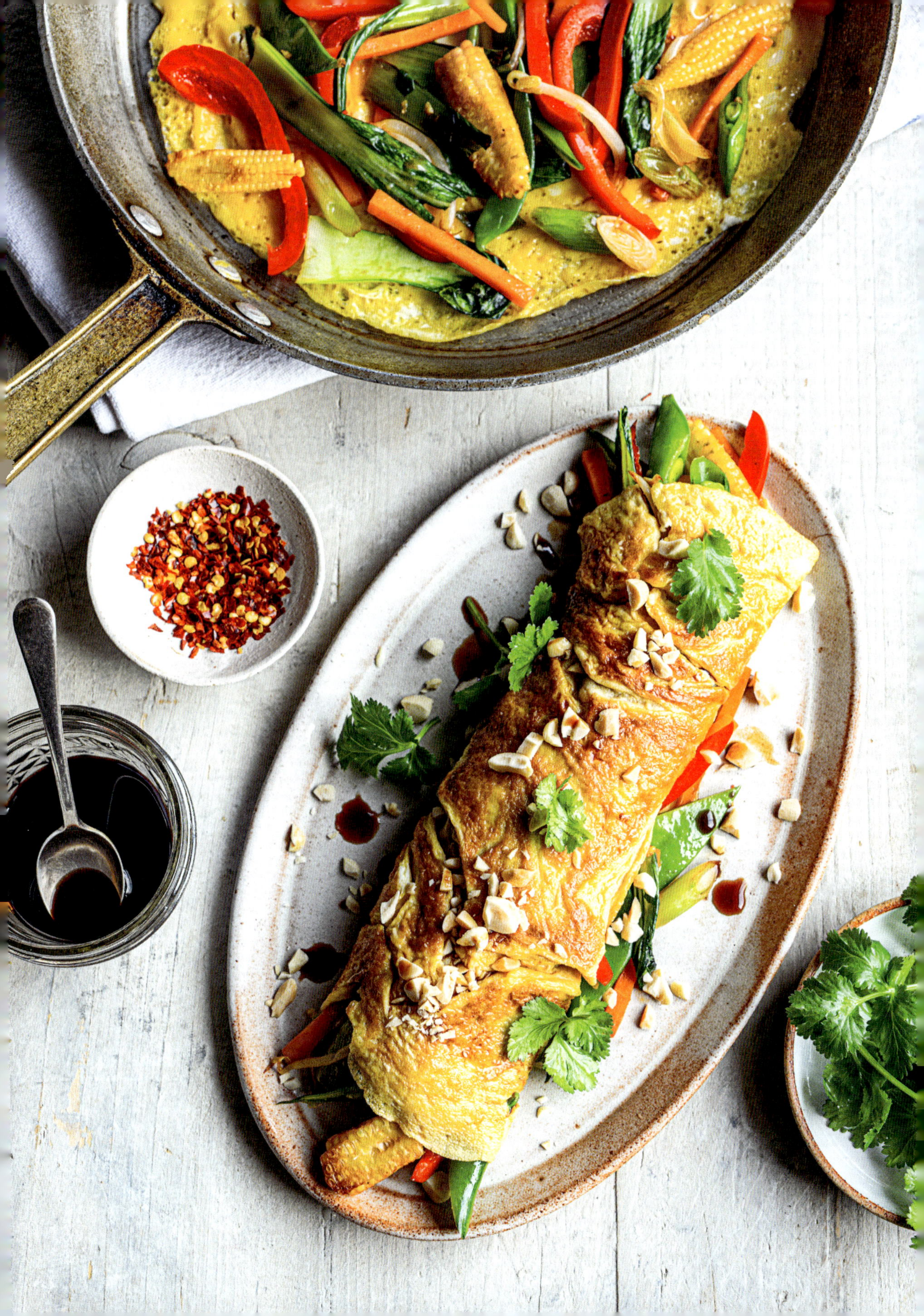

UNDER 500 CALORIES

PER SERVING | **453cals** | PROTEIN **29g** | CARBS **34g** | FIBRE **12g**

Broccoli and Almond Pesto Pasta

SERVES **2** | PREP **15** mins | COOK **10** mins

This recipe uses lentil pasta, which is higher in protein than regular wheat pasta, but you can opt for high-protein pasta or wholemeal options, if easier.

120g lentil pasta
200g broccoli florets
2 tbsp toasted flaked almonds
1 garlic clove, minced
Finely grated zest of 1 lemon and juice of ½
1 tbsp extra-virgin olive oil
2 tbsp finely grated Parmesan, plus extra to serve (optional)
Handful of basil leaves

1. Cook the pasta in a saucepan of boiling salted water according to the packet instructions. Drain, reserving 100ml cooking water, then return the cooked pasta to the pan.

2. Meanwhile, steam the broccoli for 4–5 minutes, until just tender, then refresh under cold running water until cool.

3. Put 80g of the cooked broccoli in a blender with 1 tablespoon of the flaked almonds, the garlic, lemon zest and juice, olive oil, Parmesan and 2 tablespoons of water. Blend until the consistency of pesto. Taste and season with salt and pepper, if needed.

4. Add the broccoli pesto to the pasta and pour in enough of the reserved cooking water to make a light sauce. Add the reserved whole broccoli florets and warm through.

5. Serve the pasta, sprinkled with the remaining almonds and extra Parmesan, if you like. Finish with a scattering of basil leaves.

GLUTEN FREE

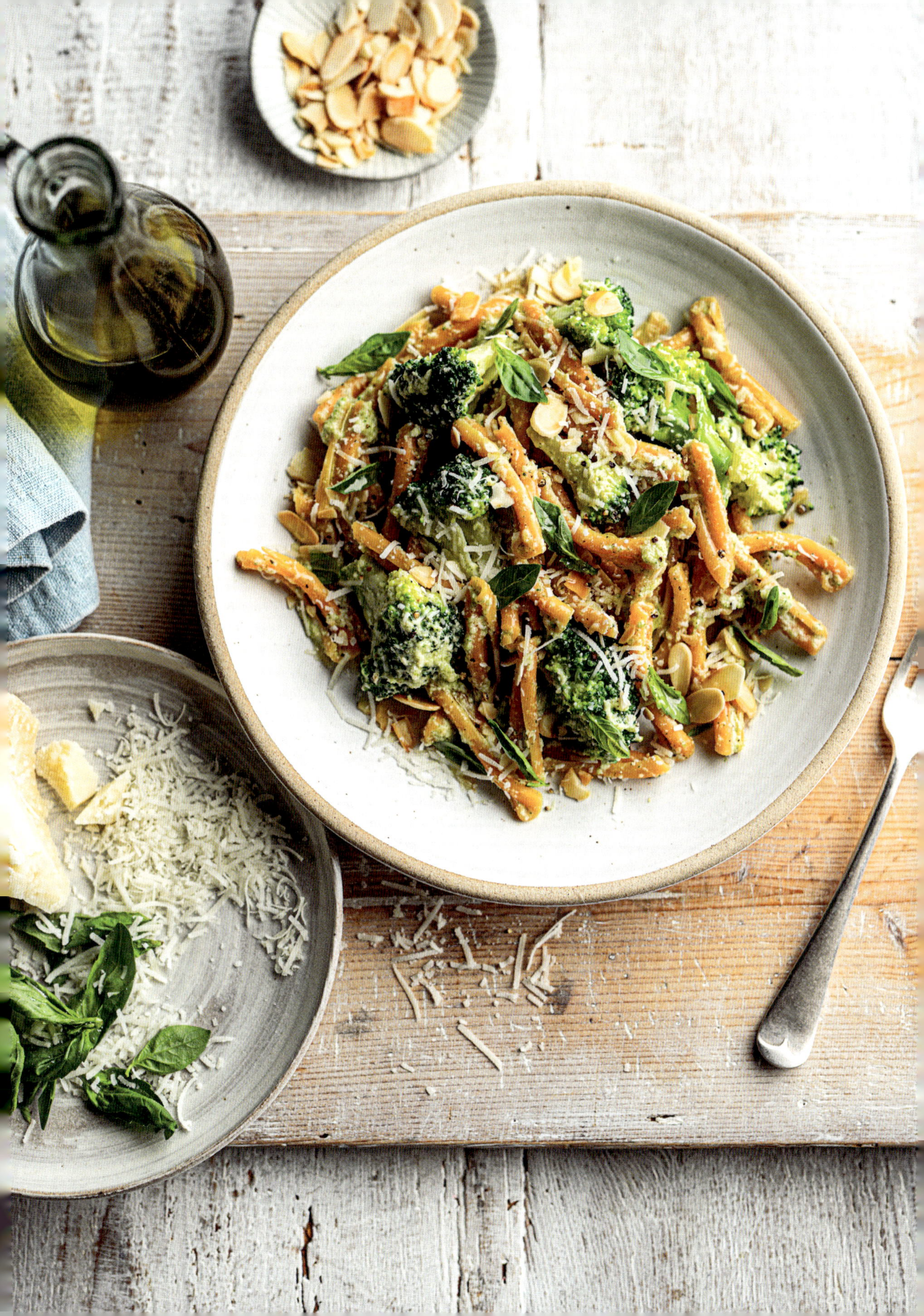

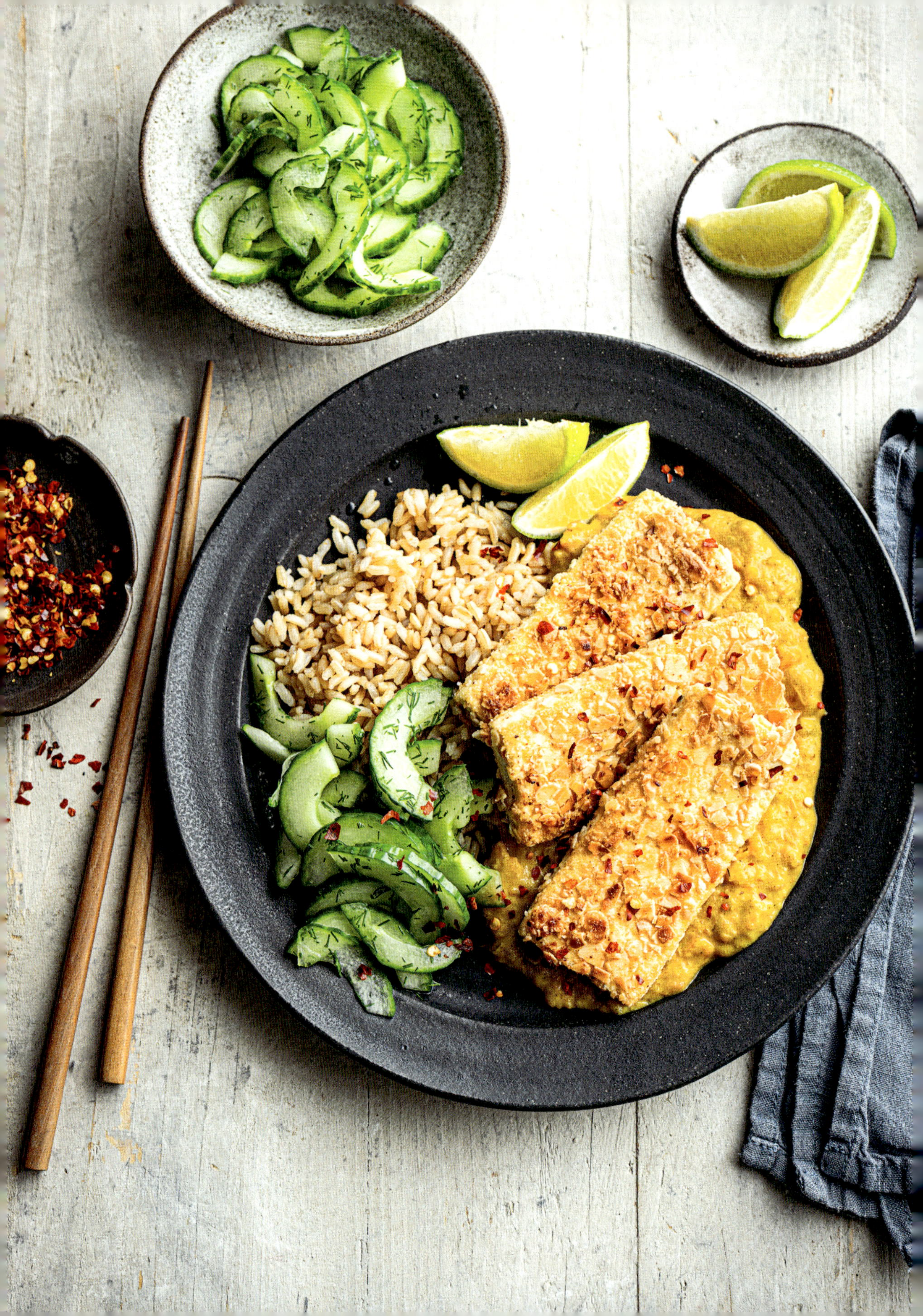

PER SERVING | **538cals** | PROTEIN **29g** | CARBS **13.5g** | FIBRE **9g**

UNDER 600 CALORIES

Crispy Katsu Tofu Steaks

SERVES **2** | PREP **15** mins | COOK **25** mins

2 tbsp olive oil
1 onion, diced
1 large carrot, thinly sliced
2.5cm piece of fresh root ginger, peeled and grated
1 large garlic clove, finely chopped
2 tsp mild curry powder
½ tsp turmeric powder (optional)
175ml vegetable stock
1 tbsp coconut cream
50g toasted flaked almonds or ground almonds
1 egg
225g firm tofu, drained, patted dry and cut into 6 × 1cm thick slices
Quick Pickled Cucumber **(see page 222)****, to serve (optional)**
½ lime, cut into wedges (optional)

The tofu is in a crisp, protein-rich, almond coating, and is served with a lightly spiced carrot sauce. You could have some cauli rice alongside, or 2–3 tablespoons of brown rice. Serve with steamed green veg.

1. To make the katsu sauce, heat ½ tablespoon of the oil in a saucepan over a medium–low heat, add the onion and carrot and cook for 6 minutes, until softened, adding a splash of water if the pan becomes dry. Stir in the ginger and garlic and cook for 1 minute. Stir in the curry powder and turmeric, if using, and cook another minute, then add the stock and coconut cream. Bring to a simmer and cook for 10 minutes, until reduced. Use a stick blender to blend until smooth. Return the sauce to the pan, then set aside.

2. Blitz the toasted almonds in a mini food processor or blender until fine crumbs, then tip into a shallow bowl, or simply add the ground almonds to the bowl. Season with salt and pepper. Beat the egg in a separate shallow bowl.

3. Take the tofu and dip the pieces, one at a time, into the egg, then into the almond crumbs until coated.

4. Heat the remaining oil in a large pan over a medium heat, add the tofu and cook for 3–4 minutes on each side, until golden. Remove to kitchen paper to absorb the excess oil.

5. Meanwhile, reheat the sauce. Spoon the sauce onto plates and top with the crispy tofu. Serve with rice, pickled cucumber and wedges of lime for squeezing over, if you like.

AIR-FRYER TIP

Preheat the air fryer to 190°C, if needed. Prepare the sauce and tofu as in Steps 1–3. Brush oil onto both sides of the coated tofu, then air fry for 5 minutes on each side until crisp and golden. Serve as above.

VEGGIE | GLUTEN FREE | DAIRY FREE

UNDER 500 CALORIES

PER SERVING | 470cals | PROTEIN 27.5g | CARBS 2.5g | FIBRE 0g

Pizza Omelette

SERVES 2 | PREP 10 mins | COOK 10 mins

4 eggs
½ tsp dried oregano
10g butter or 1 tbsp olive oil
2 tbsp sun-dried tomato pesto
1 × 125g ball of mozzarella, drained
40g pitted black olives, halved
Good pinch of dried chilli flakes (optional)
Basil leaves, to serve

A herby omelette replaces the more usual carb-heavy base in this super easy pizza. Feel free to experiment with your favourite toppings, such as mushrooms, peppers, artichokes, tuna, prawns, or cooked chicken. Serve with a leafy salad.

1. Preheat the grill to high.

2. Using a fork, beat together the eggs and oregano in a bowl, then season with salt and pepper.

3. Melt the butter or oil in a small, non-stick ovenproof frying pan over a medium–low heat. Pour in the beaten egg and cook, drawing the cooked set edges in with a spatula and tilting the pan to tip any uncooked egg to replace it. Cook until the base is set and light golden in places, and the top of the omelette has only small patches of uncooked egg. Remove the pan from the heat.

4. Place small dollops of pesto all over the top of the omelette, then tear the mozzarella into chunks and add that, too. Sprinkle with the olives and chilli flakes, if using, then place the pan under the grill for about 3–5 minutes until the cheese has melted.

5. Scatter over the basil leaves to serve.

VEGGIE · GLUTEN FREE · NUT FREE

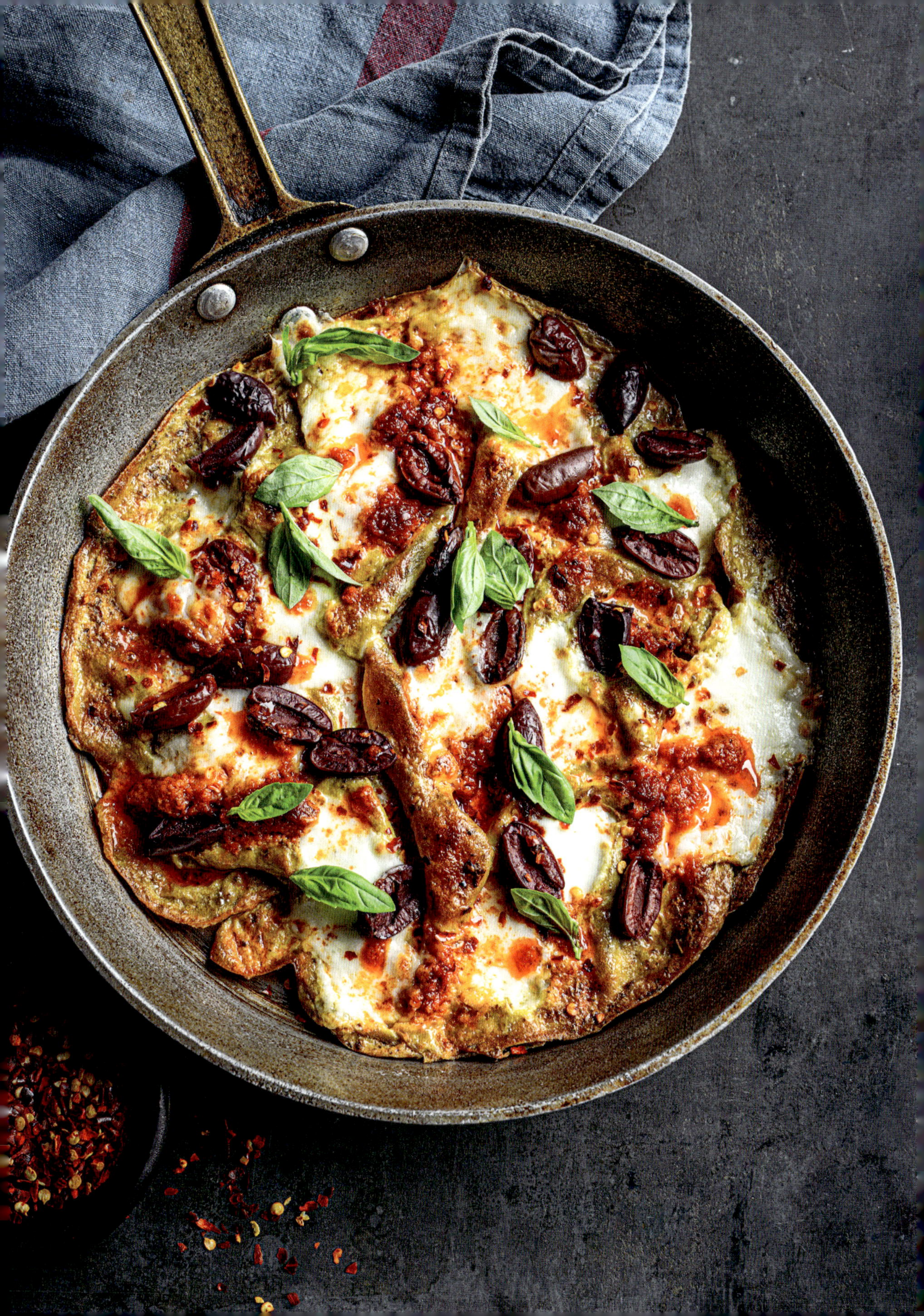

UNDER 500 CALORIES

PER SERVING | **414cals** | PROTEIN **16g** | CARBS **32g** | FIBRE **15g**

Falafel Burgers with Pitta Pockets

SERVES **2** | PREP **45** mins | COOK **6** mins

1 × 400g tin chickpeas, drained
1 tsp chia seeds
2 garlic cloves, minced
1 tbsp ras el hanout
2 tbsp olive oil
1 wholemeal pitta bread
4 Little Gem lettuce leaves
4 tbsp hummus
4 tsp Quick Pickled Pink Onions (see page 222), sliced jalapeños or sriracha, to serve

Lightly spiced, these chickpea burgers are delicious stuffed into a warm pitta with lettuce, hummus and pickles. On a non-fast day use half a pitta for each burger, rather than sharing 1 pitta between 2 people. Serve them with a green salad on the side.

1. Tip the chickpeas into a food processor with the chia seeds, garlic and ras el hanout. Season with salt and pepper. Blend to a coarse paste, then shape the chickpea mixture into 4 burgers. Place in the fridge to chill for 30 minutes.

2. Heat the olive oil in a large frying pan over a medium heat and fry the burgers for 3 minutes on each side, until golden and crisp. Take care turning the burgers as they will be slightly crumbly.

3. Meanwhile, warm the pitta bread, then cut it in half and open out to make a pocket. Divide the lettuce leaves, hummus, pickled onions, jalapeños or sriracha between each pitta pocket, then add the burgers. Serve straight away.

VEGAN | NUT FREE | DAIRY FREE

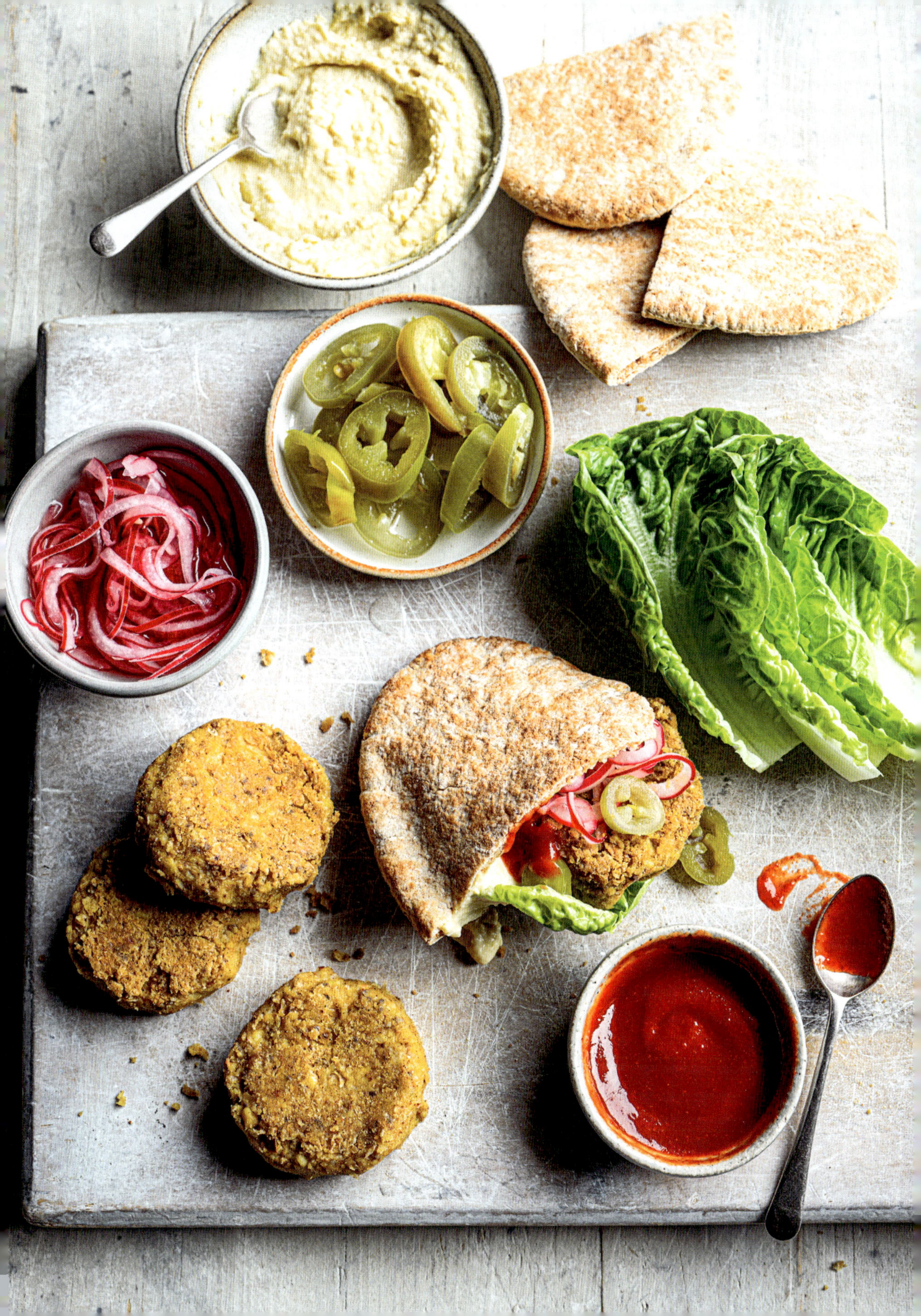

UNDER 500 CALORIES

PER SERVING | **412cals** | PROTEIN **22g** | CARBS **14g** | FIBRE **6g**

Fridge-raid Supper

SERVES **1** | PREP **5** mins | COOK **5** mins

This lunch or supper dish is great for using up whatever leftovers you have in the fridge. This recipe is a template that you can adapt to suit your tastes and according to what you need to use up. It comes topped with 2 poached eggs, but it is equally good with a spoonful of hummus, a few chunks of cheese, or cooked prawns or chicken.

2 medium eggs
Splash of apple cider vinegar
1 tbsp olive oil
50g kale, tough stalks removed and leaves torn into small pieces
6 cherry tomatoes, halved
60g drained tinned beans, such as cannellini, butter beans or chickpeas, rinsed
30g pitted black olives
1 garlic clove, finely chopped
½ tsp Dijon or English mustard
Juice of ½ lemon

1. To poach the eggs, crack them into 2 small bowls and bring a small, deep saucepan of water to the boil. Once boiling, add the vinegar and turn the heat down so the water is barely simmering. Stir the water, then slide the eggs into the pan one at a time. Simmer for 3–4 minutes until the white is set, and the yolk remains runny.

2. Meanwhile, heat the oil in a frying pan over a medium heat. Add the kale, tomatoes, tinned beans and olives and fry, turning frequently, for 2 minutes, until softened. Add the garlic and cook for another minute, then stir in the mustard and lemon juice. Season with salt and pepper.

3. Spoon the kale and bean mixture onto a serving plate, then scoop out the poached eggs with a slotted spoon, drain briefly on kitchen paper, and place on top of the veg. Season to taste and serve.

VEGGIE · GLUTEN FREE · NUT FREE · DAIRY FREE

PER SERVING | **353cals** | PROTEIN **23g** | CARBS **28g** | FIBRE **7.5g**

UNDER 400 CALORIES

One-pot Kimchi Tofu

SERVES 2 | PREP 10 mins | COOK 27 mins

1 tbsp neutral oil
1 onion, finely sliced
2 large garlic cloves, finely chopped
1 tbsp gochujang paste
1 × 400g tin chopped tomatoes
75g kimchi (shop-bought or homemade, see page 225)
225g firm tofu, drained and cut into 1cm-thick slices
1 lime, cut into wedges

This recipe is super easy and doesn't require long preparation or marinating, relying instead on the kimchi and the Korean-spice paste gochujang to add flavour. Serve it with 2–3 tablespoons of cooked brown rice, quinoa or brown noodles.

1. Heat the oil in a saucepan over a medium heat. Add the onion and cook for 7 minutes, until tender. Add the garlic and cook for another minute.

2. Stir in the gochujang paste, then the tinned tomatoes, kimchi and 150ml water. Bring to the boil, then reduce the heat and simmer for 10 minutes.

3. Add the tofu to the pan, spooning the sauce over the top and taking care not to break it up, and cook for another 10 minutes, until the sauce has reduced and thickened and the tofu has taken on the flavours of the sauce. Season with salt and pepper to taste.

4. Serve in bowls with green veg and rice, quinoa or brown noodles and with lime wedges on the side for squeezing over.

VEGAN | NUT FREE | DAIRY FREE

UNDER **500** CALORIES

PER SERVING | **452cals** | PROTEIN **24.5g** | CARBS **28g** | FIBRE **10g**

Roasted Cauliflower, Chickpea and Halloumi Salad

SERVES **2** | PREP **10** mins | COOK **25** mins

1 tbsp olive oil
1 tsp smoked paprika
1 tsp turmeric powder (optional)
1 tsp ground cumin
120g drained tinned chickpeas, rinsed
1 small cauliflower, cut into small florets
75g halloumi, cut into large bite-sized chunks
50g rocket leaves
2 tbsp toasted pumpkin seeds
2 tbsp Herby Tahini Dressing (see page 241) (optional)

This salad is substantial enough to make a meal in itself, and comes with a healthy quota of protein and fibre from the vegetables, beans and seeds, as well as a lovely herby tahini dressing.

1. Preheat the oven to 200°C/180°C fan/Gas 6.

2. Mix the oil and spices with 1 tablespoon of water in a bowl, then season with salt and pepper.

3. Tip the drained chickpeas into the bowl. Add the cauliflower and halloumi, then turn until everything is combined and coated in the spicy oil.

4. Tip into a roasting tin and spread out evenly. Roast in the oven for 20–25 minutes, turning once, until everything is golden and cooked through.

5. Divide the rocket leaves between two serving plates and spoon the cauliflower mixture alongside, then finish with the pumpkin seeds and a spoonful of the dressing, if using.

AIR-FRYER TIP

Preheat the air fryer to 180°C. Prepare the cauliflower, chickpeas and halloumi as Steps 2–3, then cook in the air fryer (you may need to do this in batches) for 15–20 minutes, turning once or twice. Serve as above.

VEGGIE | GLUTEN FREE | NUT FREE

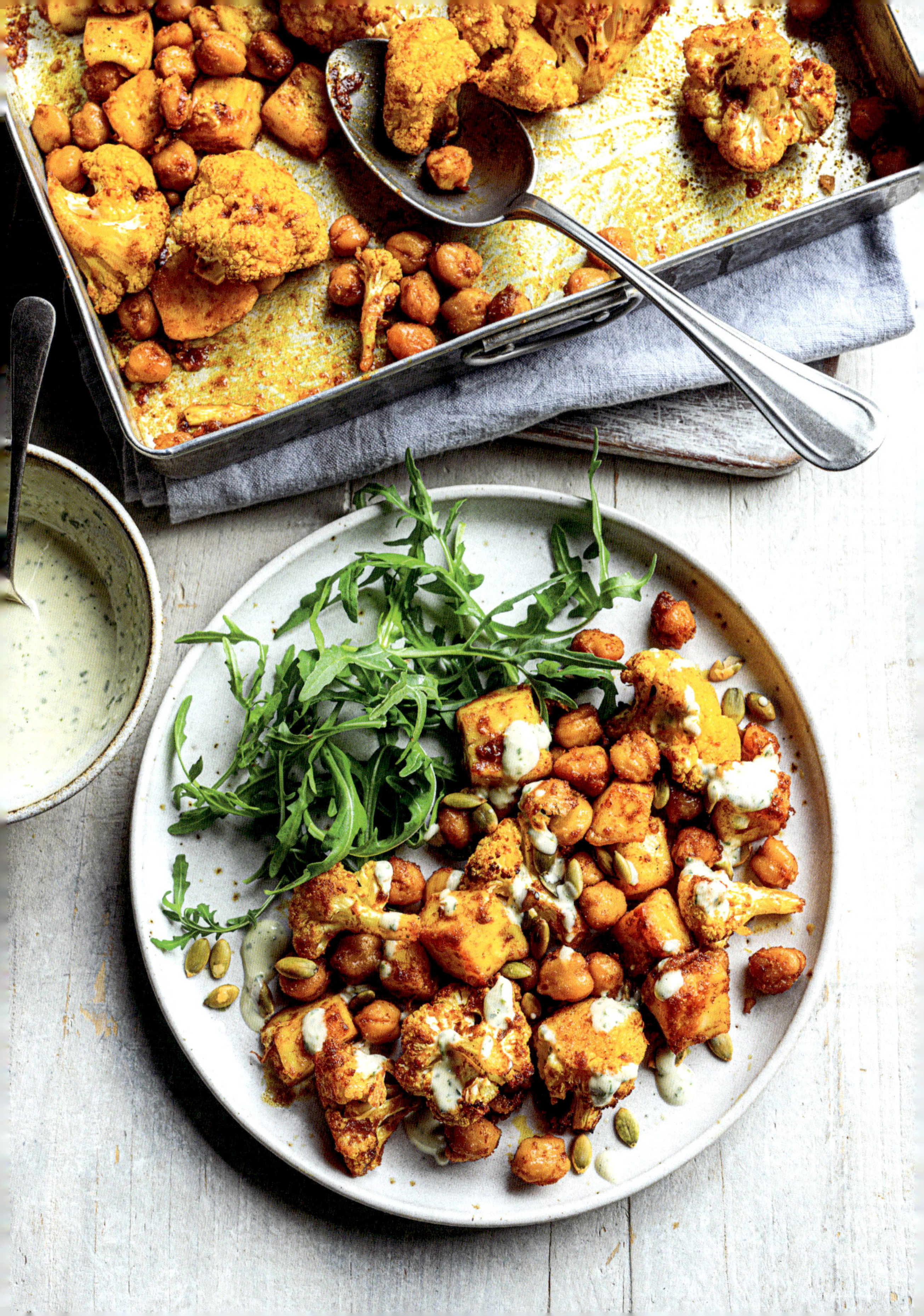

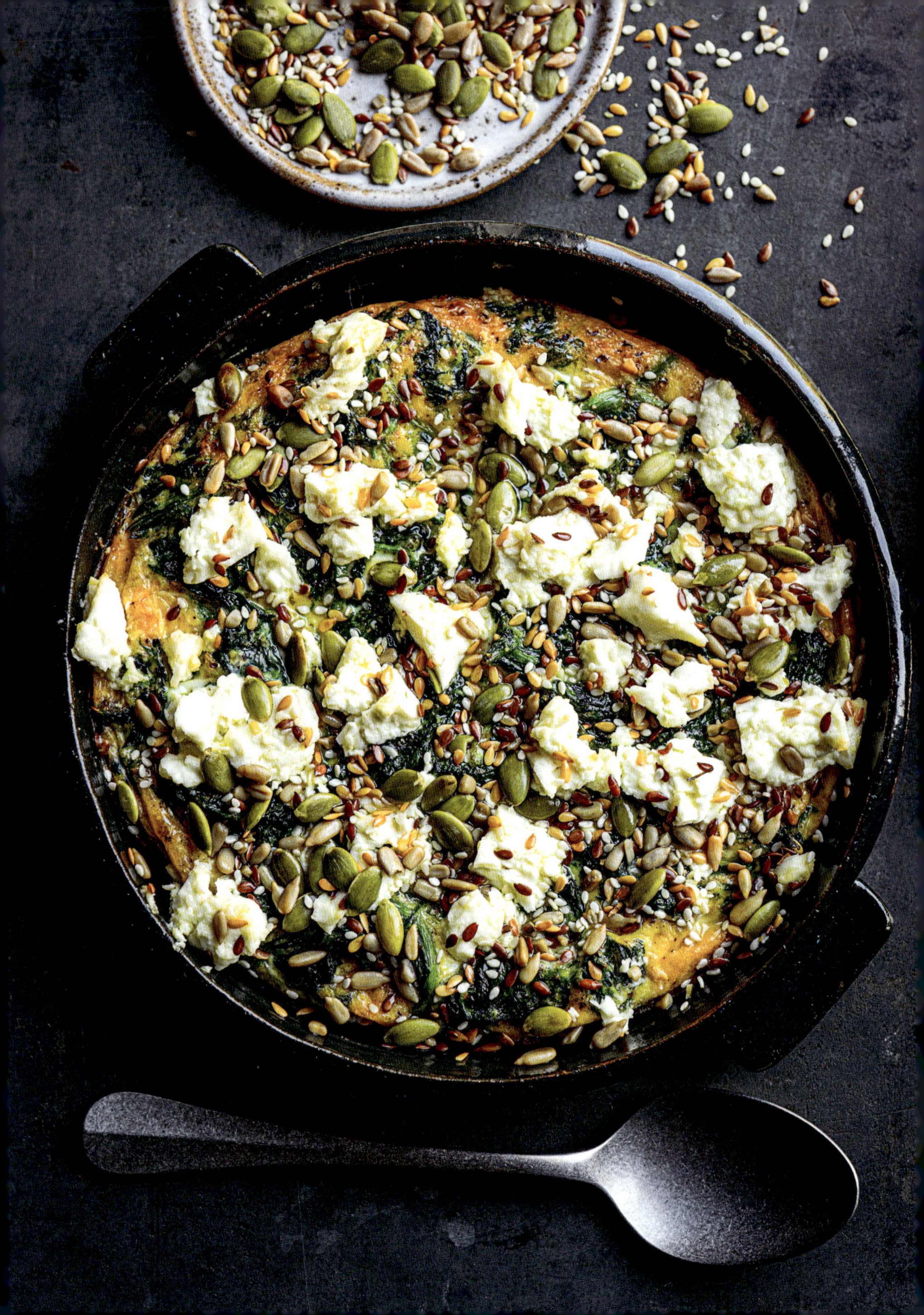

PER SERVING | **370cals** | PROTEIN **26.5g** | CARBS **3.5g** | FIBRE **1.5g**

UNDER 400 CALORIES

Baked Eggs with Spinach, Feta and Toasted Seeds

SERVES 2 | PREP 5 mins | COOK 20 mins

½ tbsp olive oil, for greasing
4 frozen spinach balls, defrosted and drained well
½ tsp ground nutmeg
4 eggs, beaten
100g feta
2 tbsp mixed seeds

Tasty, quick, versatile and easy to assemble, this makes a lovely nutritious brunch or lunch box.

1. Preheat the oven to 190°C/Fan 170°C/Gas 5 and grease a 20cm oven dish with olive oil.

2. Combine the spinach, nutmeg and eggs in the dish, and season with salt and plenty of black pepper.

3. Cook in the oven for 10–20 minutes, until golden brown in places and cooked through.

4. Crumble the feta over the top and sprinkle with the seeds. Return to the oven for 5 minutes, until golden, then serve.

AIR-FRYER TIP

Preheat the air fryer to 170°C, if needed. Prepare the spinach and eggs as above. Pour the egg mixture into the prepared dish and cook for 8–10 minutes, until golden and cooked through. Crumble the feta over the top and sprinkle with the seeds. Return to the air fryer for another 3–4 minutes, until slightly golden, then serve.

VEGGIE | GLUTEN FREE | NUT FREE

UNDER 500 CALORIES

PER SERVING | **472cals** | PROTEIN **18g** | CARBS **24g** | FIBRE **12g**

Homemade Nacho Platter

SERVES 2 | PREP 15 mins | COOK 30 mins

1 small wholemeal tortilla, halved and each half cut into triangles
150g cauliflower, broken into small florets
1 tbsp olive oil
2 tsp fajita spice mix
10 cherry tomatoes, quartered
100g drained tinned pinto or black beans, rinsed
½ small red onion, diced
1 small ripe avocado, peeled, destoned, and cut into bite-sized chunks
1 tbsp chopped jalapeños (optional)
1 lime, halved
60g mature Cheddar, coarsely grated
4 tbsp full-fat Greek yoghurt or soured cream

This makes a great informal, picky meal when you're looking for something light, easy and tasty. The homemade tortilla chips are a great alternative to the overly salty, high-fat ones.

1. Preheat the oven to 200°C/Fan 180°C /Gas 6.

2. Place the tortilla triangles on a baking tray and cook in the oven for 5 minutes, turning halfway, until golden and crisp. Remove from the oven and leave to cool and crisp up further. Set aside.

3. Meanwhile, place the cauliflower in a roasting tin and toss in the olive oil, spice mix and 1 tablespoon of water until combined. Season with salt and pepper, then roast for 20–25 minutes, turning halfway, until golden and tender.

4. Combine the tomatoes, tinned beans, red onion, avocado and jalapeños, if using, in a bowl. Season and squeeze over the juice of ½ lime. Cut the remaining lime half into wedges.

5. Remove the cauliflower from the oven and spoon the tomato mixture on top, then scatter over the cheese. Return to the oven for another 5 minutes, until the cheese is melted.

6. Spoon the cauliflower mixture onto a serving plate and top with small dollops of Greek yoghurt. Serve with wedges of lime for squeezing over and the crispy tortillas.

AIR-FRYER TIP

Preheat the air fryer to 180°C, if needed. Prepare the tortilla and air-fry for 3–4 minutes, turning once; keep an eye on it as it can easily burn. Leave to cool while you prepare and cook the cauliflower for 15–20 minutes, turning once. Top with the tomato mixture and the cheese and cook for another 3–4 minutes. Serve as above.

VEGGIE | NUT FREE

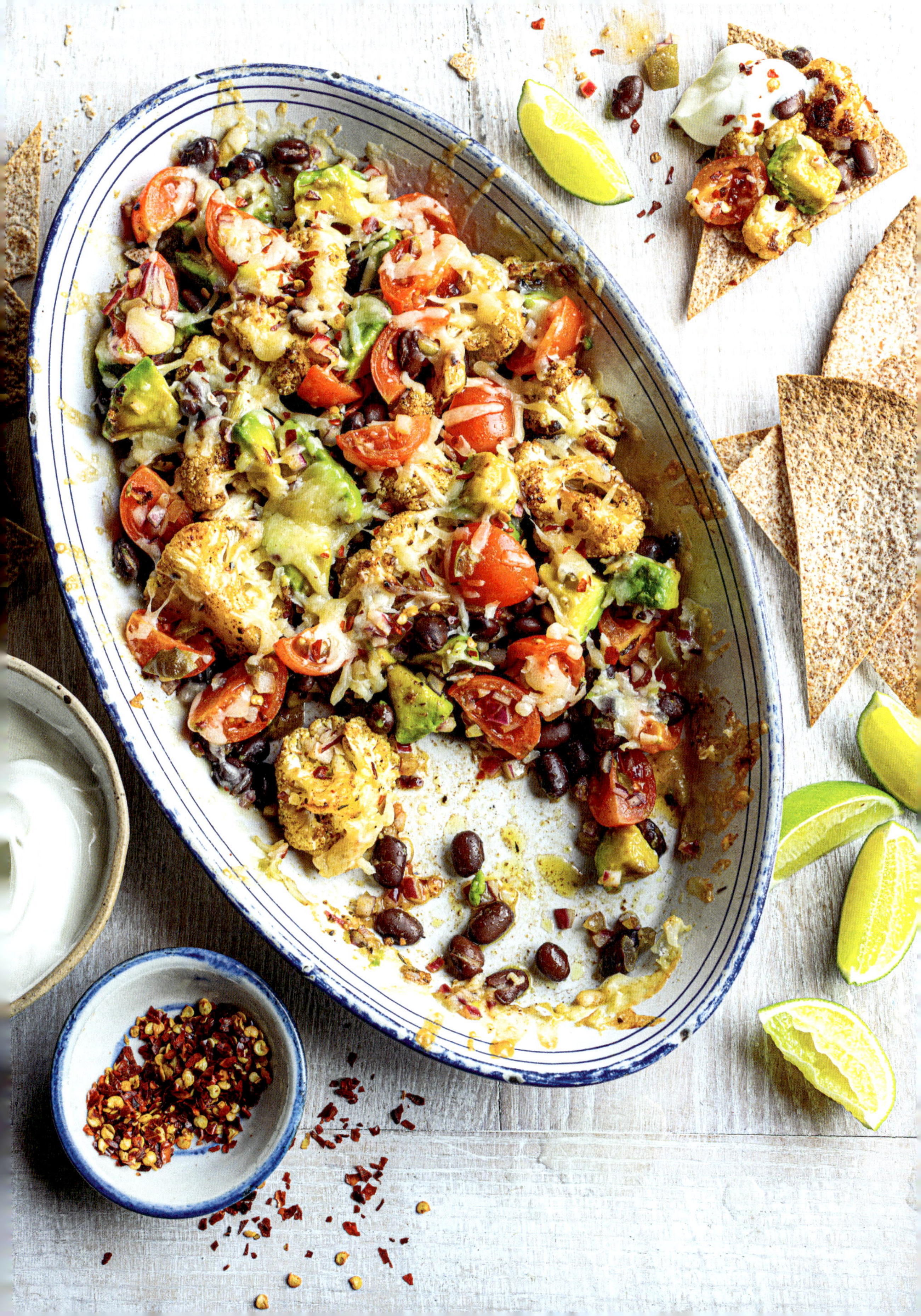

UNDER 300 CALORIES

PER SERVING | **284cals** | PROTEIN **18g** | CARBS **20g** | FIBRE **8.5g**

Meat-free Ragu

SERVES 4 | PREP 15 mins | COOK 40 mins

2 tbsp olive oil
1 onion, finely chopped
1 carrot, coarsely grated
1 celery stick, finely chopped
2 large garlic cloves, finely chopped
2 tsp dried mixed herbs
250g mushrooms, coarsely grated
200g tempeh, coarsely grated
150ml red wine or vegetable stock
2 tbsp tomato purée
1 × 400g tin chopped tomatoes
150g cooked Puy or green lentils (from a pouch or tin)

Tempeh is packed with protein and makes an excellent alternative to minced meat when coarsely grated. This makes a hearty vegan meal to serve with spiralised courgetti, adding lots of fibre and skipping the starchy alternatives. If you do crave pasta, use a small amount of wholemeal pasta (20–40g dried per person). Cook the pasta as usual and add the courgetti for the last 30 seconds to heat up but don't overcook it, or it will go soggy. You could serve the ragu with a sprinkling of grated Parmesan to boost the protein levels.

1. Heat the olive oil in a large saucepan over a medium heat. Add the onion, carrot and celery and cook, stirring, for 5 minutes, until softened. Stir in the garlic, herbs, mushrooms and tempeh and cook for 5 minutes, until the mushrooms soften and any liquid evaporates.

2. Pour in the wine or stock and cook over a medium–high heat until there is almost no liquid in the pan. Stir in the tomato purée, then tip in the tinned tomatoes. Fill the empty tin with water and add this to the pan. Stir until combined. Bring up to a boil, then turn the heat down, add the lentils and simmer for 30 minutes, until reduced and thickened.

3. Season with salt and pepper to taste before serving.

VEGAN · GLUTEN FREE · NUT FREE · DAIRY FREE

PER SERVING | **447cals** | PROTEIN **33g** | CARBS **25g** | FIBRE **10g**

UNDER 500 CALORIES

10-minute Smoked Tofu and Quinoa Bowl

SERVES **1** | PREP **10** mins

50g cooked quinoa (from a pouch)
1 tsp chia seeds
½ avocado, sliced
100g smoked tofu, cut into small bite-sized cubes
60g cooked edamame beans (podded weight)
1 snack cucumber, cut into ribbons
1 tbsp Quick Pickled Pink Onions (see page 222) or 1 spring onion, sliced diagonally
2 tbsp Mint Yoghurt Sauce (see page 242) (optional)
1 tsp Soy Seed Sprinkles (see page 39)

No cooking is needed to prepare this healthy salad bowl, packed full of fresh and nutritious ingredients, including protein and fibre. You can vary the ingredients, depending on your likes and what you have in the fridge. Hard-boiled eggs, prawns or cooked chicken are also good protein alternatives, if you're not a fan of tofu.

1. Measure the quinoa into a shallow serving bowl, then stir in the chia seeds.

2. Arrange the avocado, tofu, edamame, cucumber and pickled onion on top in individual piles.

3. Spoon the sauce over the fresh ingredients, if using, then sprinkle with the seeds to serve.

VEGGIE · NUT FREE · DAIRY FREE

UNDER 600 CALORIES

PER SERVING | **567cals** | PROTEIN **16g** | CARBS **34g** | FIBRE **10g**

Roasted Sweet Potatoes and Goats' Cheese

SERVES **2** | PREP **5** mins | COOK **30** mins

Sweet potatoes and carrots develop a caramelised flavour when roasted, which goes particularly well with the goats' cheese.

2 tbsp extra-virgin olive oil
1 medium sweet potato, peeled and cut into 2–3cm cubes
1 small onion, diced
2 carrots, cut into 2cm rounds
8 cherry tomatoes, halved
½ tsp dried thyme
100g soft goats' cheese, broken into pieces
40g walnut pieces
Handful of rocket, to serve

1. Preheat the oven to 190°C/Fan 170°C/Gas 5.

2. Place the olive oil, sweet potato, onion, carrots and tomatoes in a bowl. Season with salt and a generous amount of ground black pepper, and sprinkle over the dried thyme. Turn to coat the veg in the oil. Tip into a roasting tin, spreading everything out, and cook in the oven for 20 minutes, stirring once or twice.

3. Remove the tin from the oven and add the goats' cheese and the walnuts, then cook for another 5–10 minutes.

4. Divide between two plates and serve with the rocket.

AIR-FRYER TIP

Preheat the air fryer to 180°C, if needed. Prepare the vegetables as above and cook for 12–15 minutes, turning halfway. Scatter over the goats' cheese and walnuts and cook for a further 5 minutes. Serve as above.

VEGGIE | GLUTEN FREE

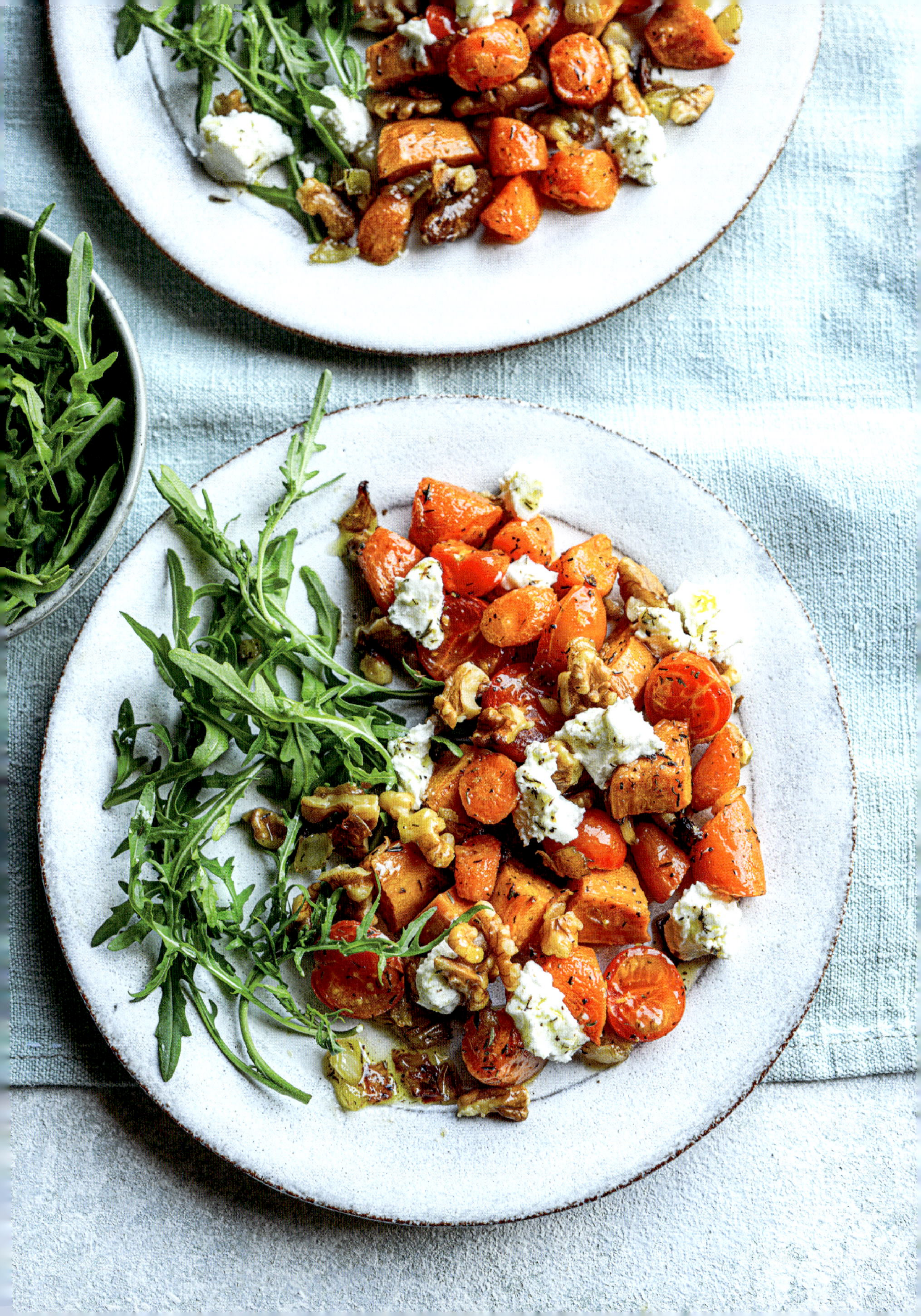

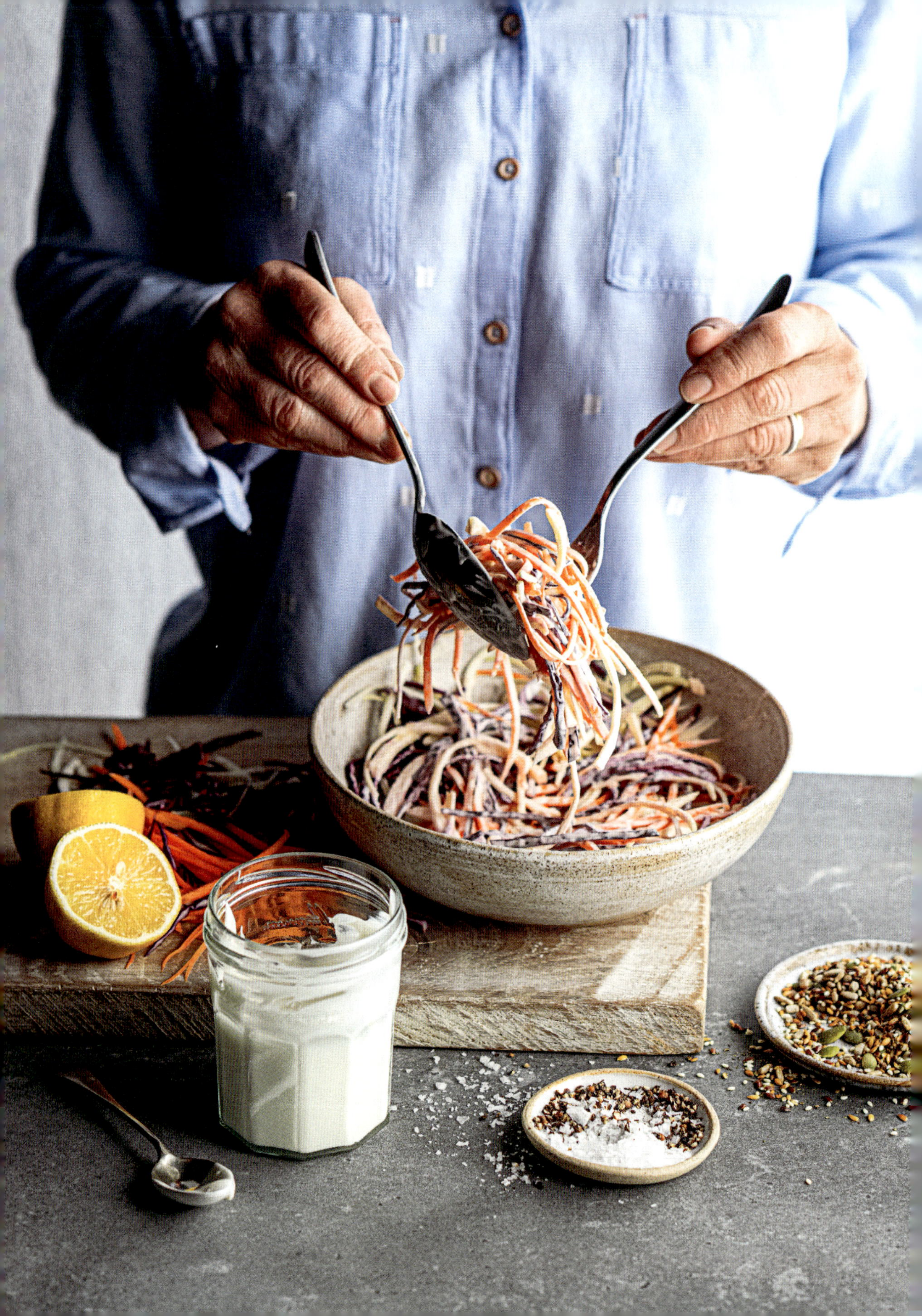

Vegetable Sides and Snacks

UNDER 100 CALORIES

PER PINK ONION SERVING	PER FENNEL SERVING	PER CUCUMBER SERVING
10cals	**6cals**	**8cals**
PROTEIN **0g**	PROTEIN **0.5g**	PROTEIN **0.5g**
CARBS **2g**	CARBS **0.5g**	CARBS **0.5g**
FIBRE **0.4g**	FIBRE **1g**	FIBRE **0.5g**

PICKLES 3 WAYS

SERVES 6 | PREP 20 mins

QUICK PICKLED PINK ONIONS
1 medium red onion, thinly sliced into rings
2 tbsp apple cider vinegar

QUICK PICKLED FENNEL
1 fennel bulb, trimmed and finely sliced
2 tbsp apple cider vinegar

QUICK PICKLED CUCUMBER
1 medium cucumber, cut lengthways, seeds removed and finely sliced
2 tbsp apple cider vinegar
1 tbsp chopped fresh dill

A spoonful of pickle adds flavour, zing and crunch to fish, meat, chicken and vegetarian dishes and stir-fries, as well as bean and grain dishes. Store in a jar in the fridge for up to 1 week.

1. Mix the ingredients together in a small dish, add a good pinch of salt, then leave to pickle for 15 minutes.

VEGAN · GLUTEN FREE · NUT FREE · DAIRY FREE

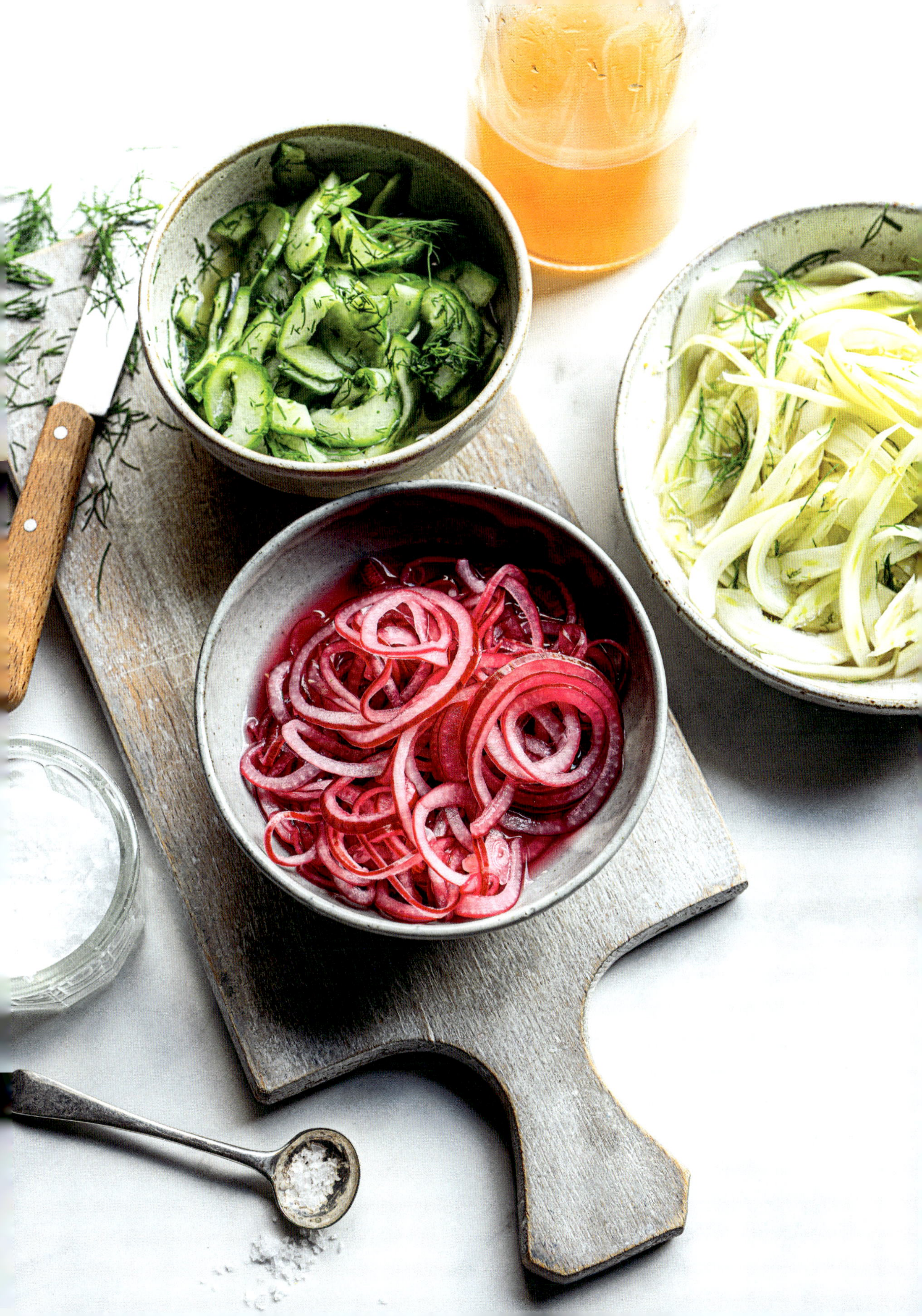

UNDER 200 CALORIES

PER SERVING | 192cals | PROTEIN 4g | CARBS 25g | FIBRE 12g

Sautéed Jerusalem Artichokes

SERVES 2 | PREP 5 mins | COOK 20 mins

1 tbsp olive oil
500g Jerusalem artichokes, washed and thinly sliced
Squeeze of lemon

These small gnarled tubers are high in soluble fibre and great for a healthy gut microbiome. They can be boiled, fried and made into soup and have a nutty, buttery taste.

1. Place the olive oil in a large frying pan over a medium heat. Add the artichokes and fry for 20 minutes, stirring occasionally, until the edges are browning and slightly crisp.

2. Tip them into a serving dish, squeeze over some lemon juice and sprinkle with a pinch of salt to serve.

VEGAN · GLUTEN FREE · NUT FREE · DAIRY FREE

PER 50G SERVING | **30cals** | PROTEIN **1.5g** | CARBS **4.5g** | FIBRE **3g**

UNDER 100 CALORIES

Kimchi

MAKES **1** litre | PREP **10** days

1 medium–large white cabbage, cored, quartered and sliced into 1.5–2cm ribbons
4 medium white onions, peeled, halved and thinly sliced
2 large carrots, trimmed and grated
2 tsp coriander seeds
2 tbsp sweet smoked paprika (optional)
1½ tbsp fine sea salt (such as Maldon or Kosher salt)

You will need
1 × 1 litre jar or 2 × 500ml jars

This sweet, tangy cabbage dish will cheer up an omelette and add flavour to a salad, fish or stir-fry. It's also a fabulous source of fibre that your gut microbiome will love. The helpful microbes in kimchi are good for better immunity, reducing blood sugar, improving mood and so much more.

1. With clean hands, mix the cabbage, onion, carrot, coriander seeds and paprika, if using, in a large bowl, sprinkling the salt between the layers as you mix.

2. Massage the salt into the veg, then press it down firmly, with a wooden spoon or the end of a wooden rolling pin, and leave it for 1–2 hours, for the juices to appear.

3. Spoon the contents into the jar(s) and press the contents down as you go. It is an anaerobic process, so we need to remove as much air as possible from the mixture. The mixture needs to remain submerged for the fermenting process to work properly. When packing the mixture into the jar, leave 1.5–2cm space at the top. If there is not enough liquid to cover the mixture you can top with brine (made with 1 teaspoon of sea salt dissolved in 200ml filtered water as needed).

4. Use a stone or piece of ceramic to keep the veg submerged – or use the end of the cabbage as a plug. Seal the jar(s) and place on a plate to catch any overflow. Keep at room temperature, out of direct sunlight.

5. For the first few days, open the jars daily and press down the contents, to release the bubbles formed by the vegetables fermenting. The more active, the better! Then repeat this process every few days. After 5–10 days you can place it in the fridge to slow the fermentation. The longer it ferments, the stronger the flavour.

6. Store the jars in the fridge for up to 2–3 months. Discard the kimchi if it blackens or smells off.

VEGAN | GLUTEN FREE | NUT FREE | DAIRY FREE

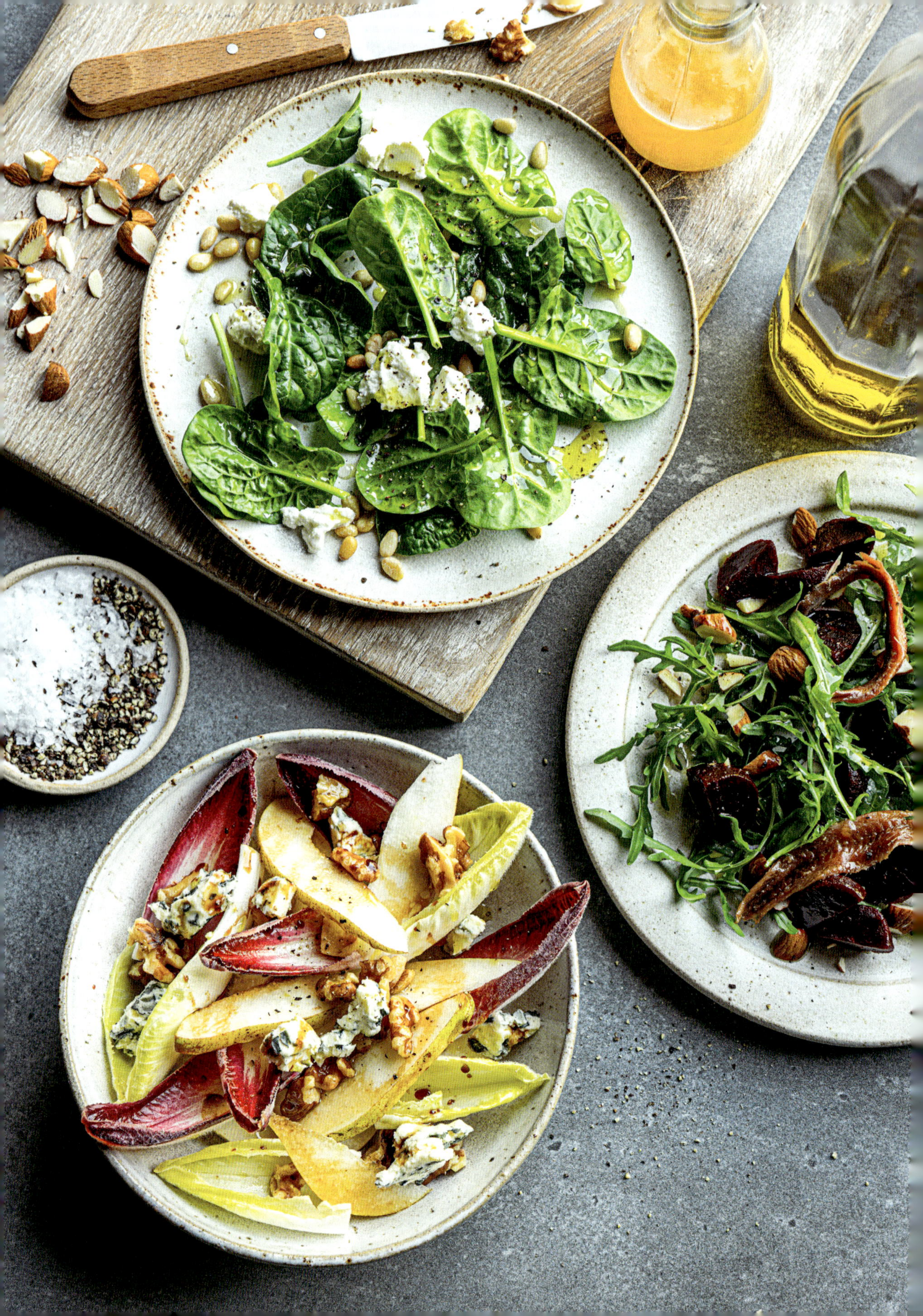

BITTER LEAVES FOR DIGESTION 3 WAYS

These foods are nutrient rich and high in antioxidants. Eating bitter salad leaves, such as rocket, radicchio and kale, has known health benefits, including stimulating digestive enzymes, improving liver function, and stimulating the taste buds to help increase saliva, break down food more easily and reduce bloating. Turn over to pages 228–9 to see the other bitter leaf recipes.

PER 50G SERVING | **235cals** | PROTEIN **6g** | CARBS **1g** | FIBRE **0.5g**

UNDER 300 CALORIES

Baby Spinach, Toasted Pine Nuts and Soft Goats' Cheese

SERVES **2** | PREP **2** mins

2 generous handfuls of baby spinach
30g soft goats' cheese, broken into pieces
2 tbsp toasted pine nuts
1½ tbsp extra-virgin olive oil
1 tbsp apple cider vinegar

1. Divide the spinach between two bowls. Season with ground black pepper and salt, then top with the goats' cheese and pine nuts.

2. Drizzle over the oil and vinegar to serve.

VEGGIE · GLUTEN FREE · NUT FREE

UNDER 200 CALORIES

PER SERVING | **185cals** | PROTEIN **6g** | CARBS **6g** | FIBRE **3g**

Beetroot Salad with Anchovies

SERVES **2** | PREP **4** mins

2 generous handfuls of rocket leaves
½ × 250g pack of cooked beetroot, diced
Handful of toasted almonds, chopped
4 anchovies
1½ tbsp extra-virgin olive oil
1 tbsp apple cider vinegar

1. Divide the rocket between two bowls. Season with ground black pepper and salt, then top with the beetroot, almonds and anchovies.

2. Drizzle over the oil and vinegar to serve. (See photo on page 226.)

GLUTEN FREE DAIRY FREE

PER SERVING | **361cals** | PROTEIN **8.5g** | CARBS **9g** | FIBRE **3.5g**

UNDER 400 CALORIES

Chicory, Walnut, Sliced Pear and Blue Cheese Salad

SERVES **2** | PREP **5** mins

2 heads of chicory, trimmed, leaves separated
½ pear, cored and thinly sliced
10 walnuts, crushed and toasted
30g blue cheese (St Agur or similar), broken into pieces
1½ tbsp extra-virgin olive oil
1 tbsp balsamic vinegar

1. Divide the chicory between two bowls. Season with ground black pepper and salt, then top with the pear, toasted walnuts and blue cheese.

2. Drizzle over the oil and vinegar to serve.
(See photo on page 226.)

VEGGIE GLUTEN FREE

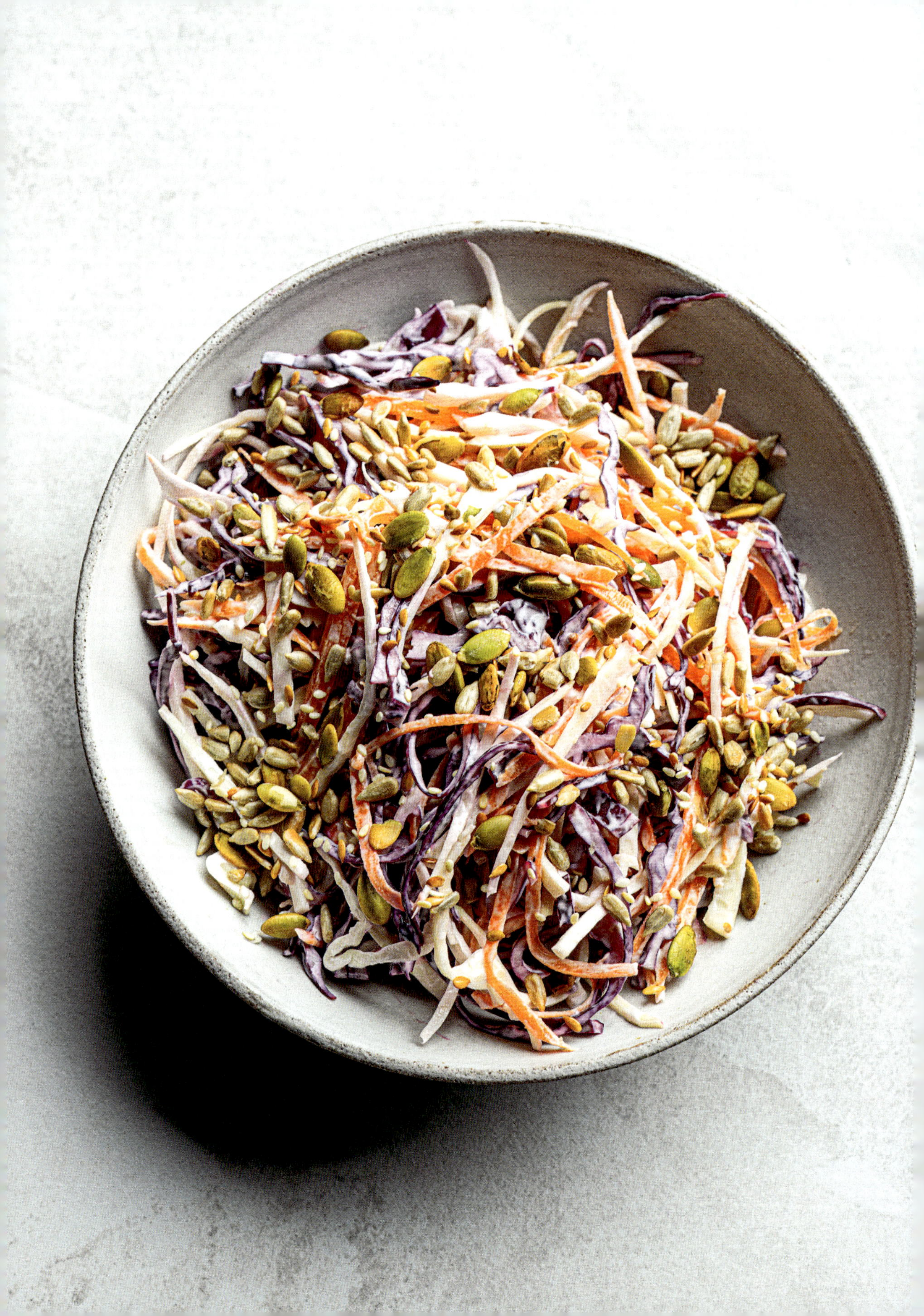

PER SERVING | **123cals** | PROTEIN **3g** | CARBS **6g** | FIBRE **2.5g**

UNDER 200 CALORIES

Seedy Slaw

SERVES 4 | PREP 10 mins

1 carrot, coarsely grated
100g red cabbage, finely shredded
80g white cabbage, finely shredded
100g full-fat Greek yoghurt
2 tbsp mayonnaise
Juice of ½ lemon
1 tsp Dijon or wholegrain mustard
1 tbsp Seedy Sprinkles (see page 39)

Packed with colourful veg, serve this coleslaw with the Cheat's Pulled Pork (see page 115).

1. Mix the prepared vegetables together in a large bowl.

2. In a small bowl, mix the yoghurt, mayonnaise, lemon juice and mustard, then season with salt and pepper. Add a splash of water if the dressing is too thick.

3. Spoon the dressing over the vegetables and turn to coat. Scatter over the seed mix just before serving.

VEGGIE · GLUTEN FREE · NUT FREE

UNDER 200 CALORIES

PER SERVING | **100cals** | PROTEIN **5.5g** | CARBS **8g** | FIBRE **4g**

Smashed Minty Peas

SERVES **2** | PREP **5** mins | COOK **5** mins

These go well as a side dish with the baked fish on page 176 or would be good spread on some sourdough as an open sandwich.

150g frozen peas
1 tbsp crème fraîche
1 tsp apple cider vinegar
1 tbsp chopped fresh mint

1. Cook the peas in a pan of boiling water for 2–3 minutes. Drain and return the peas to the pan, then lightly crush them with the back of a fork.

2. Stir in the crème fraîche, vinegar and mint, then season with salt and pepper to serve.

VEGGIE GLUTEN FREE NUT FREE

PER SERVING | **320cals** | PROTEIN **10.5g** | CARBS **14g** | FIBRE **13g**

UNDER 400 CALORIES

Charred Miso Cabbage

SERVES 2 | PREP 5 mins | COOK 35 mins

A combination of sweet, sour and umami flavours, combined with a bit of char – you could never imagine that simple cabbage can taste so good.

1 pointed/sweetheart cabbage, trimmed and halved lengthways
2 tbsp olive oil
1 tbsp miso paste
Juice of ½ lemon
Generous pinch of flaked sea salt (ideally a smoked version)
30g hazelnuts, toasted and chopped

1. Preheat the oven to 200°C/Fan 180°C/Gas 6.

2. Rub the cut side of the cabbage with some olive oil and place cut-side down on a baking tray. Cook in the preheated oven for about 15–20 minutes.

3. Meanwhile, in a small dish combine the miso, lemon juice, remaining olive oil and the salt.

4. Remove the cabbage from the oven, turn the halves over and drizzle the dressing over the top. Return to the oven for another 10–15 minutes, until golden brown.

5. Scatter with toasted hazelnuts to serve.

VEGAN | GLUTEN FREE | DAIRY FREE

UNDER 100 CALORIES

PER SERVING | **43cals** | PROTEIN **2g** | CARBS **6g** | FIBRE **2g**

Tomato, Mint and Cucumber Salad

SERVES **2** | PREP **5** mins

Fresh and vibrant, this simple salad or relish goes well with spicy dishes, such as Keema Bowls (see page 116) or as a topping on dahl.

10 cherry tomatoes, diced
2 snack cucumbers, diced
½ small red onion, diced
Juice of ½ small lemon
1 tbsp chopped mint leaves (optional)

1. Mix all the ingredients together in a bowl. Store in the fridge until ready to serve, then bring to room temperature.

VEGAN · GLUTEN FREE · NUT FREE · DAIRY FREE

PER 50G SERVING | **188cals** | PROTEIN **4g** | CARBS **6g** | FIBRE **2g**

UNDER 200 CALORIES

Nut Crumble Topping

MAKES **100g** | PREP **5** mins | COOK **8** mins

100g toasted hazelnuts, finely chopped
1½ tbsp maple syrup

You can buy small packs of toasted hazelnuts, but you can also make your own by dry frying them in a pan – just be careful not to burn them!

1. Preheat the oven to 170°C/Fan 150°C/Gas 3½ and line a baking tray with non-stick baking paper.

2. Tip the nuts on to the lined tray and drizzle with the maple syrup. Use a spatula to turn the nuts to coat them in the syrup.

3. Roast in the preheated oven for 5–8 minutes, turning occasionally.

4. Remove from the oven and set aside to cool on the tray.

5. Store the nut crumble in a sealed jar or airtight container in the fridge.

VEGAN · GLUTEN FREE · DAIRY FREE

UNDER 200 CALORIES

PER SERVING | **104cals** | PROTEIN **1.5g** | CARBS **11.5g** | FIBRE **1.5g**

Smashed Roast Potatoes

SERVES **4** | PREP **10** mins | COOK **40** mins

300g small new potatoes
2 tbsp olive oil
2 long sprigs of rosemary, halved (optional)

No peeling is required here; instead, the potato skins are left on, providing extra fibre. Try to use potatoes of a similar size, so they roast evenly. Potatoes tend to be starchy and can spike blood sugar levels, but small new potatoes are less starchy and a small amount of them, un-peeled, can be a lovely occasional treat.

1. Preheat the oven to 200°C/180°C fan/Gas 6.

2. Cook the potatoes whole in a saucepan of boiling salted water for about 10 minutes, or until just tender but not falling apart. Drain, then leave to dry briefly in the pan.

3. Using a potato masher, gently press the top of each potato to lightly crush it – you don't want it to completely break apart. Season the olive oil with salt and pepper.

4. Lightly oil a large baking tray and top with the rosemary sprigs, if using. Place the smashed potatoes on the tray and brush the tops with the remaining oil. Roast for 12–15 minutes on each side until crisp and golden.

AIR-FRYER TIP

Preheat the air fryer to 190°C. Prepare the potatoes as above. Brush the smashed potatoes with the seasoned oil and air-fry for 10–12 minutes on each side (adding the rosemary halfway through, if using), until crisp and golden.

VEGAN | GLUTEN FREE | NUT FREE | DAIRY FREE

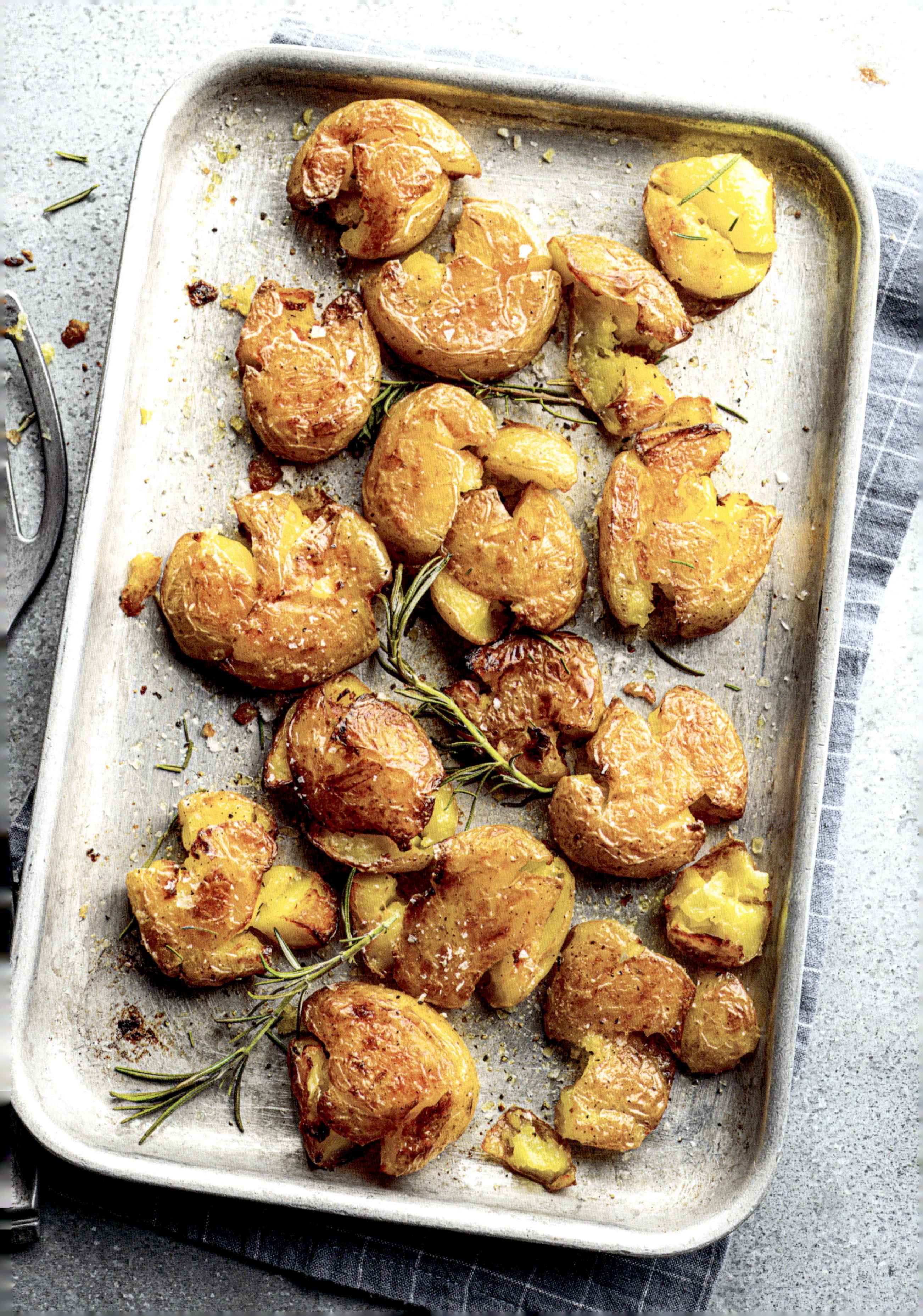

UNDER 200 CALORIES

PER SERVING | 128cals | PROTEIN 1g | CARBS 20g | FIBRE 3g

Sweet Potato Chips

SERVES 3 | PREP 5 mins | COOK 30 mins

300g sweet potatoes, cut into 1cm thick chips (skin left on)
1 tbsp olive oil

Baked rather than fried, these chips make a good side to the baked fish on page 176. The skin is kept on for a fibre boost. Unlike normal potatoes, sweet potatoes have a lower glycaemic index and are rich in antioxidants and nutrients, specifically anthocyanins.

1. Preheat the oven to 220°C/Fan 200°C/Gas 7.

2. Put the sweet potato chips on a baking tray, drizzle over the oil and season with salt and pepper. Toss the chips by hand until coated.

3. Bake in the preheated oven for 20–30 minutes, turning once, until golden and cooked through.

AIR-FRYER TIP

Preheat the air fryer to 190°C if needed. Prepare the sweet potatoes as Step 2 and cook for 15–20 minutes, turning once, until golden and cooked through.

VEGAN · GLUTEN FREE · NUT FREE · DAIRY FREE

DRESSINGS

UNDER 100 CALORIES PER TABLESPOON | **43cals**

Anchovy Vinaigrette

Tangy with a lovely salty umami flavour.

MAKES ABOUT 3 TBSP
PREP TIME 5 MINS
1 garlic clove, peeled and crushed
2 anchovies, diced
1 tbsp balsamic vinegar
1 tbsp extra-virgin olive oil

1. Place all the ingredients in a small bowl. Whisk to combine.

GLUTEN FREE · NUT FREE · DAIRY FREE

PROTEIN **0.5g** | CARBS **1.5g** | FIBRE **0g**

UNDER 100 CALORIES PER TABLESPOON | **37cals**

Yoghurt and Mustard Dressing

A delicious dressing that is both creamy and tangy.

MAKES ABOUT 125ML
PREP TIME 5 MINS
2 tbsp olive oil
100ml full-fat Greek yoghurt
1 tsp lemon juice
½ tsp Dijon mustard

1. Place all the ingredients in a small bowl. Whisk to combine.

VEGGIE · GLUTEN FREE · NUT FREE

PROTEIN **0.5g** | CARBS **0.5g** | FIBRE **0g**

UNDER 100 CALORIES PER TABLESPOON | **73cals**

Cheat's Mayonnaise

An easy and delicious alternative to mayo.

MAKES ABOUT 375ML
PREP TIME 5 MINS
2 eggs
1 tbsp Dijon mustard
250ml extra-virgin olive oil
2 tbsp lemon juice

1. Place all the ingredients in a small bowl. Whisk to combine.

VEGGIE · GLUTEN FREE · NUT FREE · DAIRY FREE

PROTEIN **1g** | CARBS **0g** | FIBRE **0g**

UNDER 100 CALORIES PER TABLESPOON | **66cals**

Green Sauce

Nutritious, flavourful and creamy thanks to the chia seeds, which add protein and fibre too. You can use any herbs you have to hand.

MAKES ABOUT 375ML
PREP TIME 5 MINS
150g baby spinach or parsley leaves
1 tbsp chia seeds
200ml olive oil
1–2 tbsp capers, drained

1. Put all the ingredients in a blender and blend until smooth.

VEGAN · GLUTEN FREE · NUT FREE · DAIRY FREE

PROTEIN **0g** | CARBS **0g** | FIBRE **0g**

UNDER 100 CALORIES

PER TABLESPOON | **67cals**

Herby Tahini Dressing

A creamy, herby sauce that is delicious spooned over salads or as a sauce with fish, chicken and vegetarian dishes.

MAKES ABOUT 6 TBSP
PREP TIME 5 MINS
2 tbsp tahini
2 tbsp extra-virgin olive oil
1 small garlic clove, minced
Juice of 1 lemon
Handful of parsley (about 15g), stalks and leaves

1. Put all the ingredients in a blender and blend until smooth and creamy, adding a splash of water to loosen, if necessary. Season with salt and pepper to taste. The dressing can be stored in the fridge for up to 3 days.

VEGAN | GLUTEN FREE | NUT FREE | DAIRY FREE

PROTEIN **1.5g** | CARBS **0g** | FIBRE **1g**

UNDER 100 CALORIES

PER TABLESPOON | **56cals**

Roasted Garlic Mayo

The perfect accompaniment to roast meat, chicken or fish: roasting mellows and softens the flavour of the garlic. If you have the oven on, simply throw a few whole cloves in to roast alongside. For a garlic mayo with more punch (and if not using the oven), use fresh minced garlic. Reduce the quantity to one clove, then stir it into the remaining ingredients.

MAKES ABOUT 150ML
PREP TIME 5 MINS
COOK TIME 40 MINS
3 large garlic cloves, unpeeled
Splash of olive oil
6 tbsp full-fat plain yoghurt
2 tbsp mayonnaise
1 tbsp lemon juice

1. Preheat the oven to 200°C/Fan 180°C / Gas 6.

2. Put the garlic in a roasting tin with whatever else you are cooking at the time. Roast in the oven for 30–40 minutes, until tender when pressed.

3. Squeeze the softened garlic out of its skin into a bowl and mash with the back of a fork until fairly smooth. Stir in the remaining ingredients and season to taste. The roasted garlic mayo will keep in the fridge for up to 3 days.

VEGGIE | GLUTEN FREE | NUT FREE

PROTEIN **0.7g** | CARBS **0.6g** | FIBRE **0g**

UNDER 100 CALORIES | PER TEASPOON | **7cals**

Creamy Hot Sauce

This creamy dressing is excellent with fish, seafood, chicken and tofu, or spoon it over quinoa, beans or vegetables.

MAKES ABOUT 1½ TBSP
PREP TIME 5 MINS
1 tbsp full-fat Greek yoghurt
¼ tsp hot sauce, or to taste
1 tsp lime juice
Pinch of fajita spice mix (optional)

1. Mix all the ingredients together in a small bowl. Season with salt to serve.

VEGGIE · GLUTEN FREE · NUT FREE

PROTEIN **0g** | CARBS **0g** | FIBRE **0g**

UNDER 100 CALORIES | PER TABLESPOON | **13cals**

Mint Yoghurt Sauce

Excellent with lamb (see page 122) or Indian dishes, this is quick and easy to make and will keep in the fridge for up to 2 days.

MAKES ABOUT 150ML
PREP TIME 5 MINS
6 tbsp full-fat Greek yoghurt
1 small garlic clove, minced
Juice of ½ lemon
2 tbsp chopped mint leaves

1. Mix all the ingredients together in a bowl. Season with salt and pepper to serve.

VEGGIE · GLUTEN FREE · NUT FREE

PROTEIN **0.5g** | CARBS **0.5g** | FIBRE **0g**

UNDER 100 CALORIES

PER TABLESPOON | **55cals**

Soy and Sesame Dressing

This makes an easy dressing for salads, noodles and rice dishes as well as a marinade for chicken, fish and pork.

MAKES ABOUT 2 TBSP
PREP TIME 5 MINS
1 tbsp light soy sauce
1 tbsp sesame oil
1 tsp apple cider vinegar

1. Mix all the ingredients together in a bowl.

VEGGIE | NUT FREE

PROTEIN **0g** | CARBS **1.5g** | FIBRE **0g**

UNDER 200 CALORIES

PER SERVING | **127cals**

Guacamole

Simple and quick to make, this is perfect for adding nutrients and healthy fats to your diet. Serve it as a dip with vegetable sticks, or add a spoonful for a finishing touch to a meal. You can make it creamier by adding a tablespoonful of mayonnaise or yoghurt.

SERVES 2
PREP TIME 5 MINS
1 ripe avocado, halved, destoned and flesh scooped out
½ large lime
1 small garlic clove, minced

1. Mash the avocado in a bowl with the lime juice and garlic until almost smooth. Season and set aside until ready to serve. It can be made about 1 hour ahead of serving and stored in the fridge.

VEGAN | GLUTEN FREE | NUT FREE | DAIRY FREE

PROTEIN **1g** | CARBS **1.5g** | FIBRE **3g**

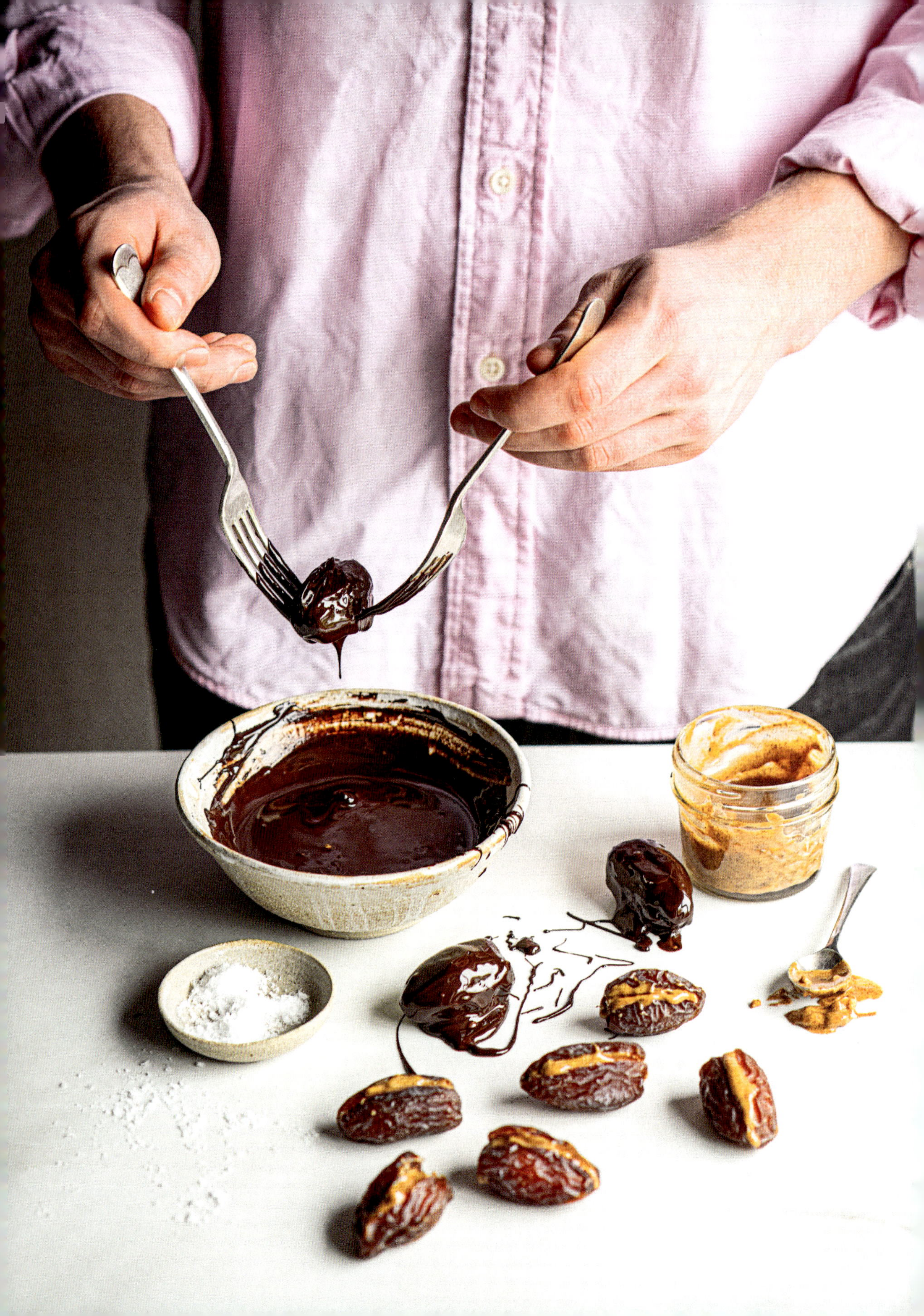

Occasional Treats

UNDER **200** CALORIES

PER SERVING | **138cals** | PROTEIN **3.6g** | CARBS **14.3g** | FIBRE **2.6g**

Bobbly Chocolate Bark

SERVES **10** | PREP **40** mins | COOK **30** mins

1 × 400g tin chickpeas, drained and rinsed
180g dark chocolate (at least 70 per cent cocoa solids), broken into chunks
2 tbsp almond or peanut butter
2 tsp ground cinnamon
Generous pinch of flaked sea salt

So simple and won't send sugars soaring.

1. Preheat the oven to 170°C/Fan 150°C/Gas 3½ and line a 28 × 20cm or 24cm square baking tin with non-stick baking paper.

2. Spread the chickpeas in a single layer in the tin and cook for 25–30 minutes.

3. Meanwhile, combine the chocolate, almond butter and cinnamon in a microwave-safe bowl. Heat in a microwave for 3 minutes until melted.

4. Remove the chickpeas from the oven and pour the chocolate mixture over the top.

5. Scatter with the flaked salt and set aside in fridge to harden.

6. Break into pieces to serve. Store in an airtight container in the fridge or freezer.

AIR-FRYER TIP

You could air fry the chickpeas at 150°C for about 15 minutes, if you prefer, shaking halfway through.

VEGAN | GLUTEN FREE | DAIRY FREE

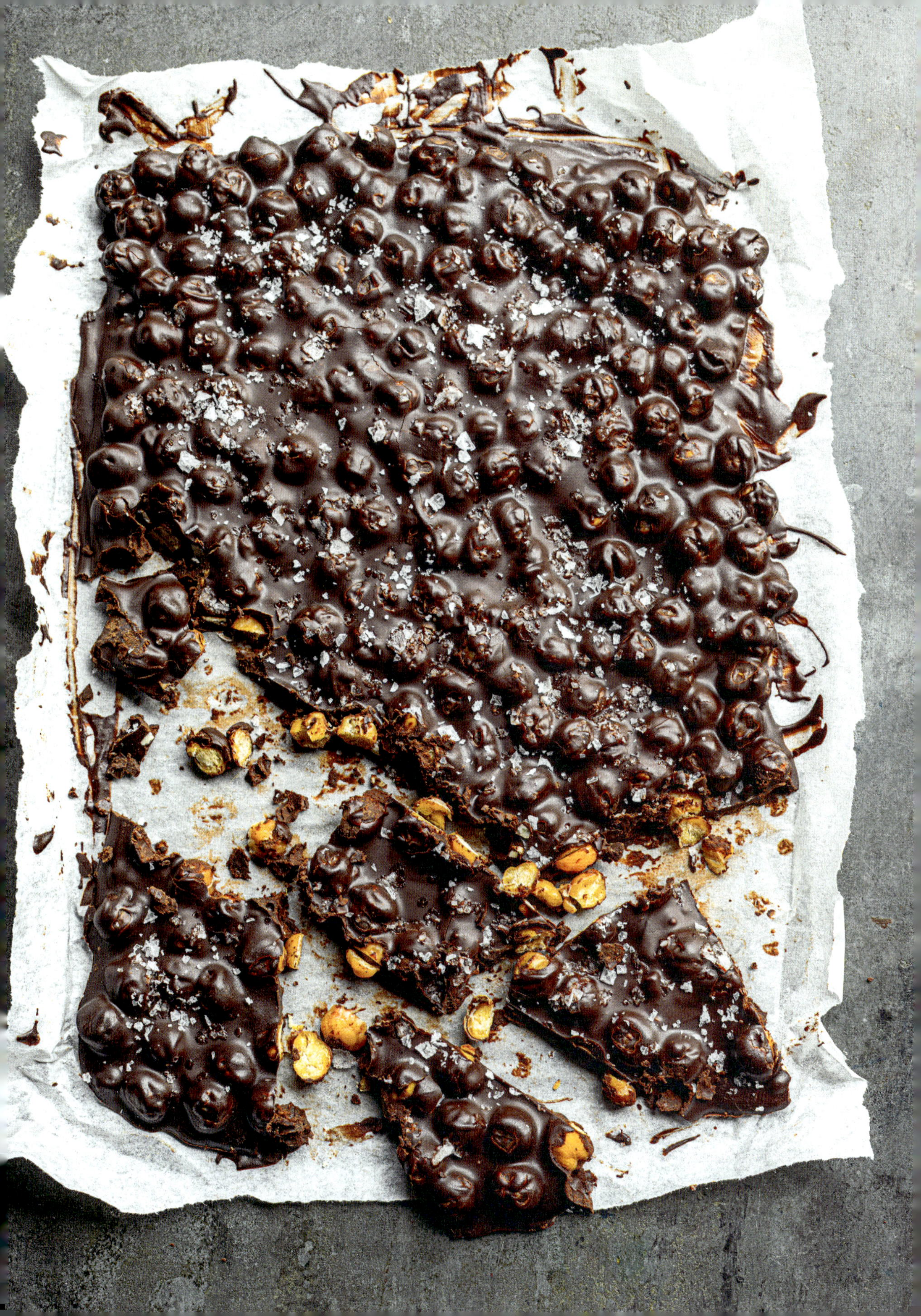

UNDER 200 CALORIES

PER SERVING | **165cals** | PROTEIN **2g** | CARBS **13g** | FIBRE **0.5g**

Minty Grapefruit Ice Cream

SERVES 4 | PREP 3 hours

1 × 540g tin mixed or pink grapefruit segments in syrup, drained (drained weight 290g)
1 × 200g tin coconut cream
2 tbsp full-fat Greek yoghurt
20 mint leaves, plus extra to serve

Tart and bitter-sweet, grapefruit is high in vitamin C. It is also known to reduce cholesterol and improve heart health.

1. Tip the grapefruit into a large jug, setting aside 4 segments to decorate later.

2. Add the coconut cream, yoghurt and a pinch of salt to the jug and blitz with a stick blender for about 40 seconds or until fairly smooth. Add the mint leaves and blitz again for a further 10 seconds.

3. Scrape the mixture into a freezer-proof container and freeze for about 3 hours, until set, stirring occasionally.

4. Allow 5 minutes to soften, if necessary, before serving in bowls with a segment of grapefruit and a few mint leaves placed on top.

VEGGIE · GLUTEN FREE · NUT FREE

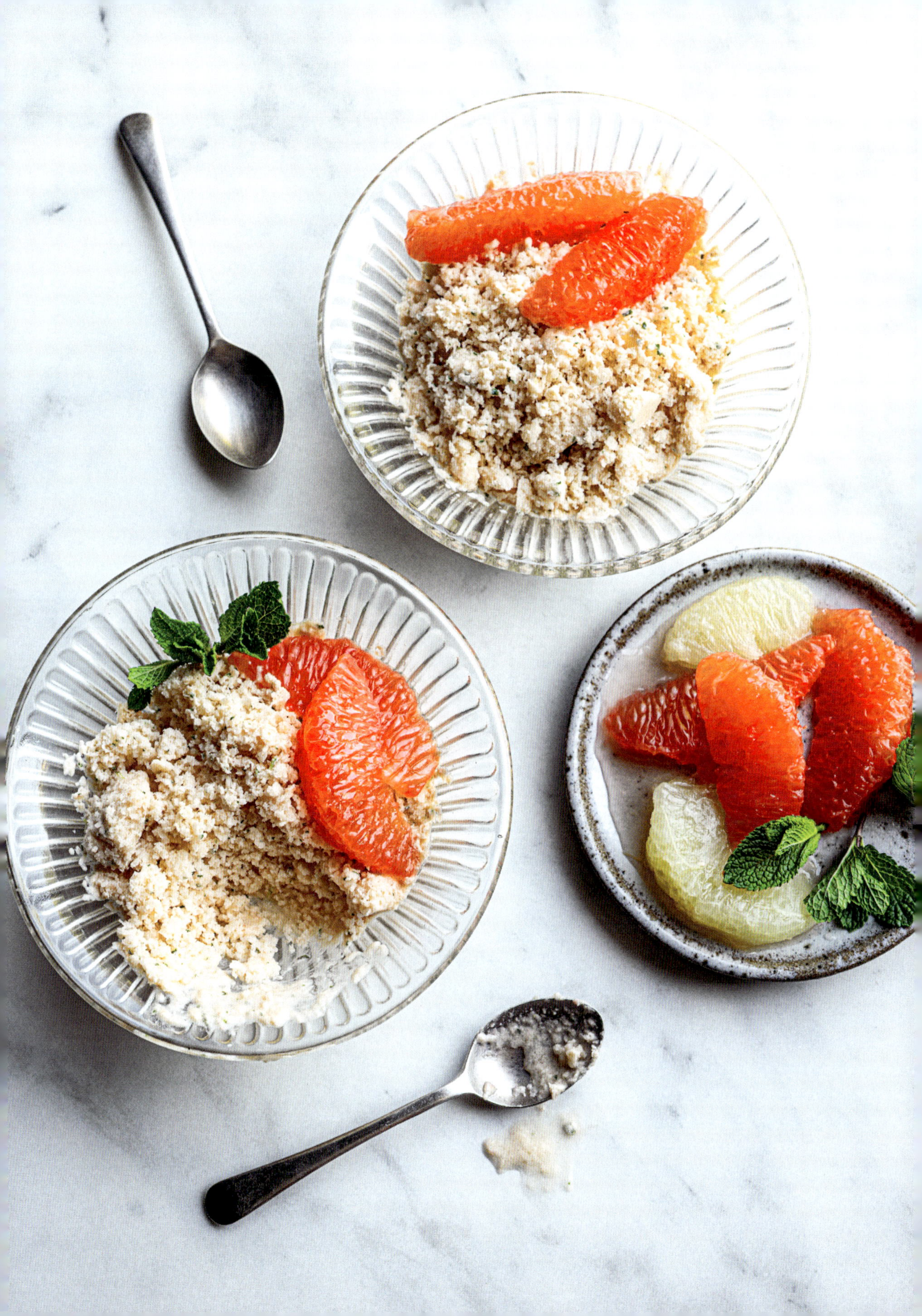

PROTEIN BALLS 3 WAYS

Delicious, portable, nutrient-rich balls for when you are flagging or for muscle recovery. Enjoy the various flavours.

UNDER 200 CALORIES

PER SERVING | **110cals** | PROTEIN **3g** | CARBS **12g** | FIBRE **2g**

Pistachio Bliss Balls

MAKES **12** | PREP **90** mins

80g Medjool dates, pitted
2 tbsp chia seeds
1 tbsp tahini
½ tbsp runny honey
80g rolled oats
80g pistachios
40g dried cranberries

1. Place the dates in just-boiled water for 10 minutes to soften, then drain.

2. Place the dates, chia seeds, tahini and honey in a food processor and blitz until fairly smooth. Scrape down the sides with a spatula.

3. Add the oats, pistachios, cranberries, a pinch of salt and 2 tablespoons of water and blitz again until finely chopped and clumping together. Squeeze the mixture between your fingers – it is ready when it sticks together easily. If it's too dry, add another tablespoon of water.

4. Divide into 12 pieces and roll between your palms.

5. Place them on a plate or tray lined with non-stick baking paper. Put in the fridge or freezer to set for 1 hour. Store the balls in an airtight container in the fridge.

VEGGIE · GLUTEN FREE · DAIRY FREE

PER SERVING | **229cals** | PROTEIN **7g** | CARBS **10g** | FIBRE **3.5g**

UNDER 300 CALORIES

Coconut Protein Balls

MAKES **20** | PREP **2½** hours

12 Medjool dates, pitted
240g ground almonds
85g desiccated coconut
270g nut butter
35g pistachios
1 tsp vanilla extract

1. Place the dates in just-boiled water for 10 minutes to soften, then drain.

2. Tip all the ingredients into a food processor, then blitz until combined.

3. Taking 1 tablespoon of the mixture at a time, roll into 20 golf-ball-sized balls.

4. Place them on a plate or tray lined with non-stick baking paper and set aside for 2 hours before eating. Store the balls in an airtight container in the fridge.

PER SERVING | **90cals** | PROTEIN **2.5g** | CARBS **8g** | FIBRE **1g**

UNDER 100 CALORIES

Ginger Date Energy Balls

MAKES **14** | PREP **70** mins

100g Medjool dates, pitted
125g cashew nuts
2 tsp ground ginger
1 ball stem ginger in syrup, drained and finely chopped
2 tsp ginger syrup
2 tsp cacao or unsweetened cocoa powder
1 tbsp almond butter
1 tbsp chia seeds

1. Place the dates in just-boiled water for 10 minutes to soften, then drain.

2. Place the cashew nuts in a food processor and blitz briefly. Add all the other ingredients and blitz again to a sticky paste.

3. Roll into 14 balls and arrange on a plate or tray lined with non-stick baking paper. Put in the fridge or freezer to set for an hour. They keep well and can be eaten straight from the freezer.

VEGAN | GLUTEN FREE | DAIRY FREE

UNDER 200 CALORIES

PER SERVING | 127cals | PROTEIN 2g | CARBS 19g | FIBRE 1.5g

Easy Nut Butter Bites

MAKES 9 | PREP 20 mins | COOK 1 min

9 Medjool dates, pitted
4½ tsp nut butter
100g dark chocolate (at least 70 per cent cocoa solids), roughly chopped
Pinch of flaked sea salt

Need a treat at short notice and one using ingredients in the store cupboard? These contain only 3 ingredients and, what's more, they are a good source of antioxidants and polyphenols. Nutritious and delicious, these won't send blood sugar levels soaring.

1. Line a small baking tray with non-stick baking paper.

2. Place the dates on the prepared tray, opening them out. Add about ½ teaspoon of nut butter into the body of each date, then gently press them back together.

3. Place the chocolate in a small microwave-safe bowl and heat in the microwave in 10 second bursts until melted.

4. Use 2 forks to lift up each of the dates and dip them in the melted chocolate. Return them to the baking paper, leaving space between each one.

5. Sprinkle the chocolate-covered dates with a small pinch of flaked salt, then place in the fridge or freezer to set.

6. Once the chocolate has hardened, transfer the dates to a freezer-proof bag and store in the fridge or freezer until needed.

VEGAN | GLUTEN FREE

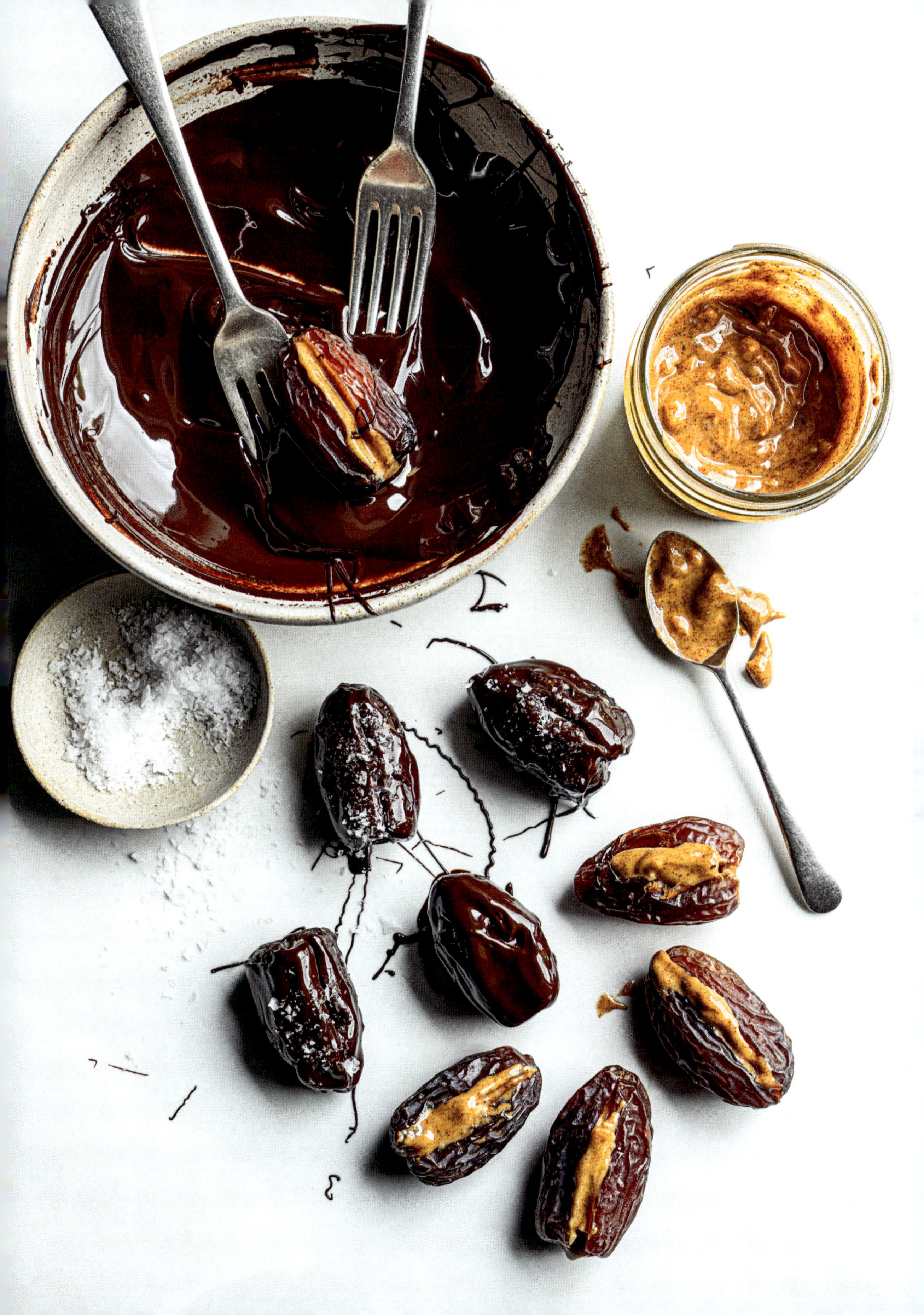

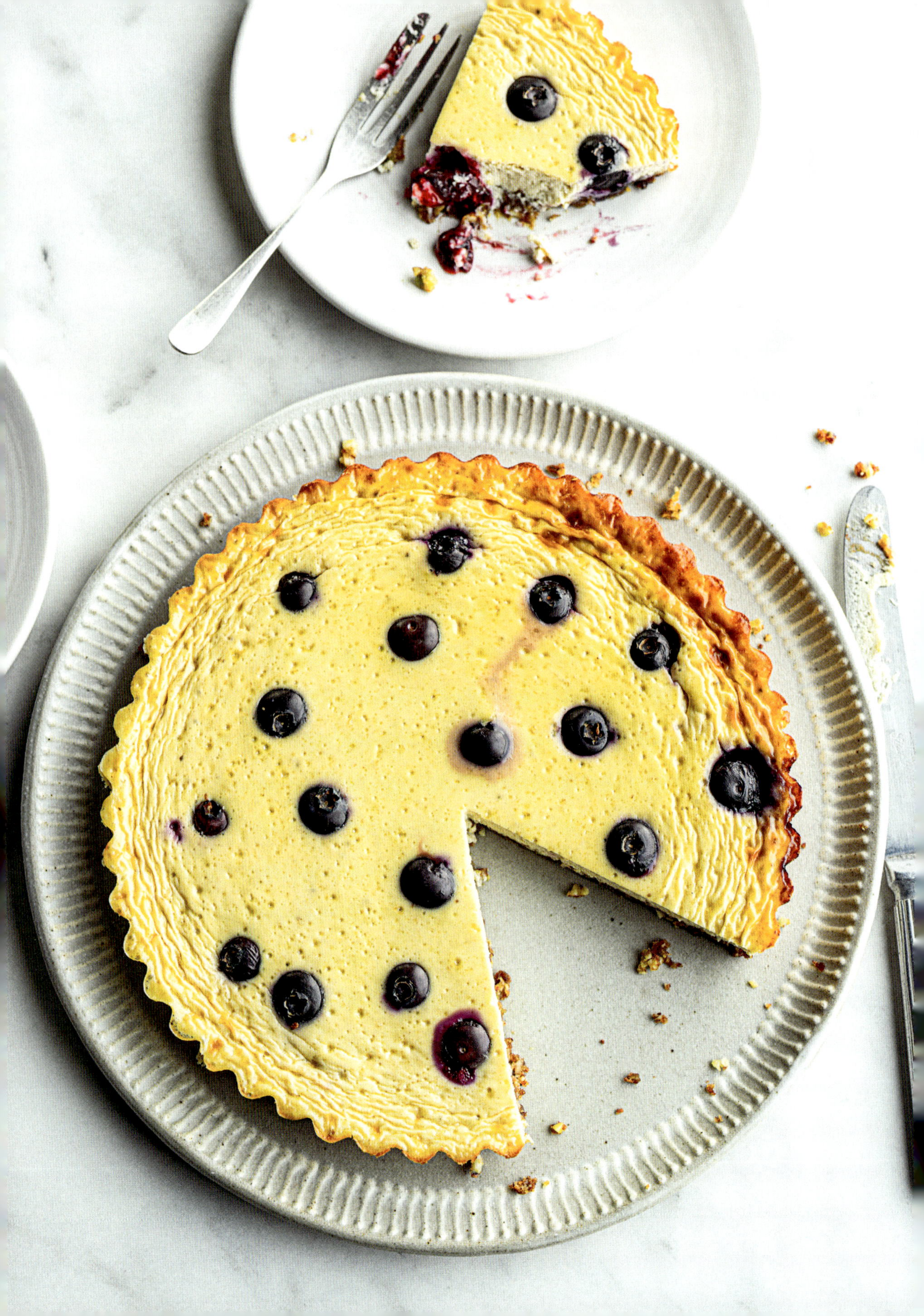

PER SERVING | **219cals** | PROTEIN **12g** | CARBS **15g** | FIBRE **1g**

UNDER **300** CALORIES

Blueberry Cheesecake

SERVES **6** | PREP **10** mins | COOK **30** mins

This gorgeous cheesecake, made with ripe bananas, blueberries and Greek yoghurt, will hardly move the dial when it comes to sugar spikes, thanks to all the protein and fibre.

2 ripe bananas, mashed (about 200g)
240ml full-fat Greek yoghurt (5 or 10 per cent fat)
2 large eggs
1 tbsp blueberries

For the base
100g mixed nuts
50g Medjool dates (or a mix of dates and other dried fruit), pitted and roughly chopped

1. Preheat the oven to 190°C/Fan 170°C/Gas 5 and line the base of a 20cm flan tin or pie dish with non-stick baking paper.

2. Add the mashed bananas, yoghurt and eggs to a bowl and whisk together with an electric whisk to a smooth batter.

3. Blitz the nuts and dates together in a food processor until fine and tacky. Press the date and nut mixture firmly into the prepared dish with the back of a spoon. It should stick together well.

4. Pour the batter on top, then scatter over the blueberries.

5. Bake in the preheated oven for 30 minutes, or until set and just beginning to colour.

6. Leave to cool before serving.

VEGGIE | GLUTEN FREE

UNDER 200 CALORIES

PER SERVING | **177cals** | PROTEIN **5.5g** | CARBS **16g** | FIBRE **1g**

Peaches with Yoghurt and Pistachios

SERVES **2** | PREP **5** mins

4 tbsp full-fat Greek yoghurt
1 × 410g tin peaches in fruit juice, drained
2–3 sprigs of mint, leaves chopped
30g pistachios or walnuts, roughly chopped

Easy comfort food, especially if you have a poor appetite.

1. Divide the yoghurt between two bowls.

2. Divide the peach slices between the bowls, arranging them on top of the yoghurt.

3. Scatter the mint and pistachios over the top of the peaches to serve.

VEGGIE GLUTEN FREE

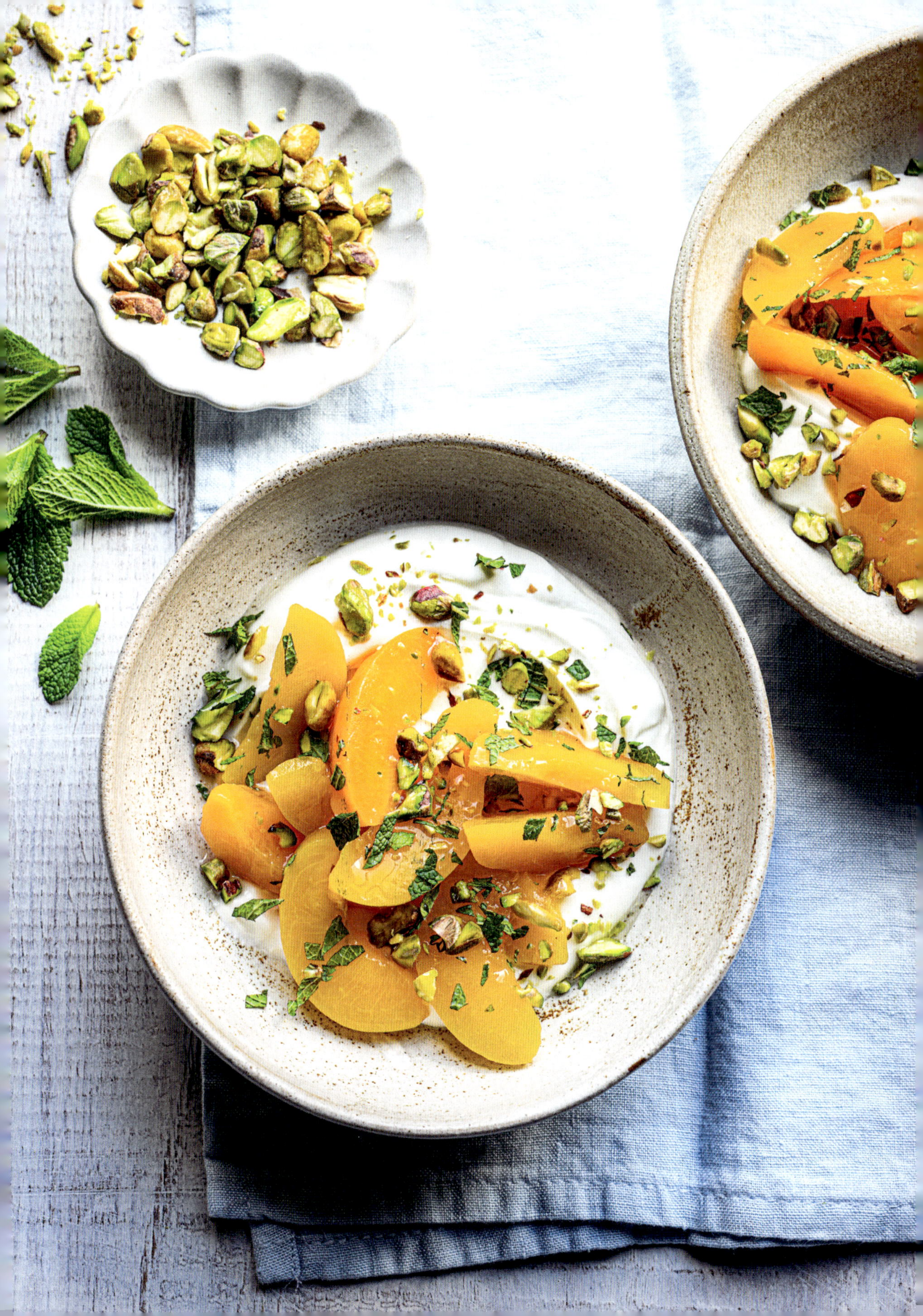

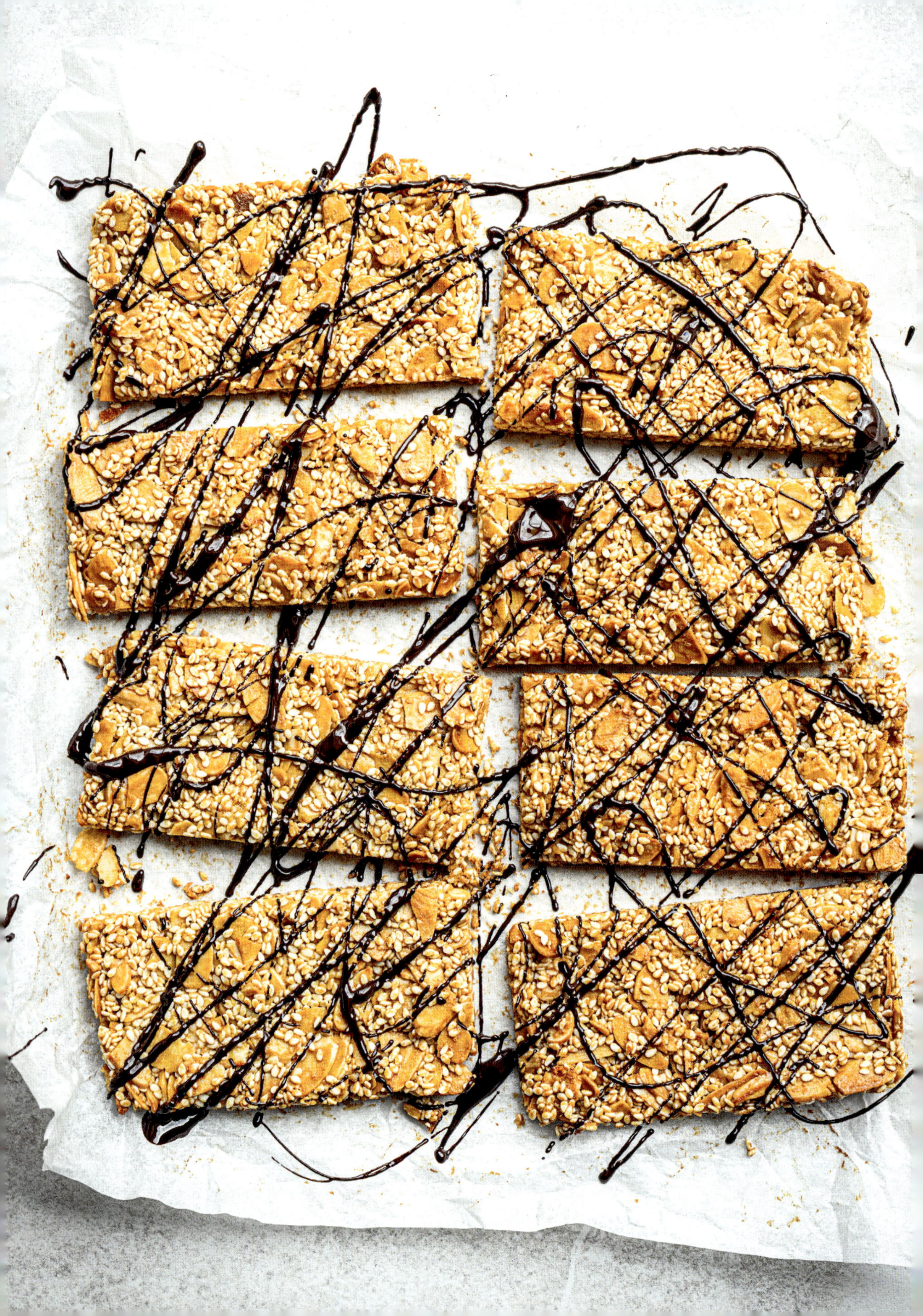

PER SERVING | 260cals | PROTEIN 7g | CARBS 12g | FIBRE 3.5g

UNDER 300 CALORIES

Sesame Crisp

MAKES 8 | PREP 5 mins | COOK 20 mins

100g flaked almonds
100g sesame seeds
2 tbsp tahini
2 tbsp maple syrup or honey
Pinch of sea salt
100g dark chocolate (at least 70 per cent cocoa solids), roughly chopped (optional)

Made with ground sesame seeds, tahini is surprisingly nutritious and ideal as an energy booster. Here we top the nuts and seeds with a drizzle of dark chocolate.

1. Preheat the oven to 170°C/Fan 150°C/Gas 3½ and line a 20cm square baking tin with non-stick baking paper.

2. Combine all the ingredients, except the chocolate, in a medium bowl. Mix to coat everything well.

3. Tip into the prepared tin and spread it out thinly, pressing the mixture firmly into the tin. Mark out 8 biscuits with a knife, then bake in the oven for 15–20 minutes until golden in places. Remove from the oven and leave to cool in the tin.

4. Break into 8 biscuits to serve.

5. If adding a chocolate topping, place the chocolate in a microwave-safe bowl and heat in the microwave in 10 second bursts until melted. Spread the chocolate over the surface of the biscuits and place in the fridge to set.

VEGGIE · GLUTEN FREE

UNDER 200 CALORIES

PER SERVING | **100cals** | PROTEIN **3g** | CARBS **9g** | FIBRE **2.5g**

Black Bean Truffles

SERVES **12** | PREP **75** mins

75g Medjool dates, pitted and chopped
75g dark chocolate (at least 70 per cent cocoa solids), roughly chopped
1 tbsp coconut oil
1 × 400g tin black beans, drained and rinsed (240g drained weight)
2 tbsp unsweetened cocoa powder, plus extra to finish
45g almond butter
1 tsp vanilla extract
Pinch of sea salt

Scrumptious – you would never guess the ingredients. This is an indulgence shared from the Fast 800 programme. We made 12 truffles with one batch of this recipe, but they can be made smaller, if desired.

1. Cover the dates with just-boiled water to soften for 10–15 minutes.

2. Meanwhile, place the chocolate and coconut oil in a microwave-safe bowl and heat in the microwave in 10 second bursts, until melted.

3. Drain the dates, reserving the water. Tip the dates and all the other ingredients into a food processor and blitz until a smooth dough-like batter forms. Add splashes of the date water (or fresh water) to loosen, if needed.

4. Chill the mixture in the fridge for 30–60 minutes to firm up.

5. Divide the mixture into 12 and roll into balls. Place them on a plate or tray lined with non-stick baking paper and chill in the fridge until ready to serve.

6. Dust with a little extra cocoa powder when serving, and enjoy. Store any leftovers in an airtight container in the fridge for up to 5 days.

VEGGIE GLUTEN FREE

PER SERVING | **219cals** | PROTEIN **6g** | CARBS **16.5g** | FIBRE **3.5g**

UNDER 300 CALORIES

Oaty Ginger Biscuits

MAKES **12** | PREP **10** mins | COOK **15** mins

1 large banana, mashed
180g rolled oats
240g ground almonds
3 balls stem ginger in syrup, drained and finely chopped
1 tbsp butter, softened, or coconut oil, melted
Pinch of sea salt

So easy to make and they won't send blood sugar levels soaring.

1. Preheat the oven to 190°C/Fan 170°C/Gas 5 and line a baking tray with non-stick baking paper.

2. Combine all ingredients in a bowl and mix well.

3. Use a dessertspoon to scoop up some of the mixture and place it on the prepared tray. Repeat until all the mixture has been used. You should make 12 biscuits. Bake in the oven for about 15 minutes, until golden.

4. Leave the biscuits to cool on the tray for a few minutes, then transfer to a wire rack to cool completely.

VEGGIE GLUTEN FREE

UNDER 300 CALORIES

PER SERVING | **280cals** | PROTEIN **6g** | CARBS **22.5g** | FIBRE **2g**

Nutty Flapjacks

MAKES **9** | PREP **10** mins | COOK **35** mins

200g rolled oats
150g mixed nuts, chopped
18 Medjool dates, pitted and diced
125g coconut oil or butter
1 tbsp ground cinnamon
Generous pinch of sea salt
1 egg white, whisked
1–2 tbsp maple syrup or honey

Who doesn't love a flapjack? Because the oats in flapjacks are cooked and left to cool, they are converted to resistant starch, which reduces the carb load, does not cause blood sugar spikes and benefits your gut microbiome. Perfect for a lunch box.

1. Preheat the oven to 170°C/Fan 150°C/Gas 3½, and line an 18cm square baking tin with non-stick baking paper.

2. In a bowl, combine the oats and nuts.

3. Place 1 tablespoon of water in a small pan with the dates over a medium heat to soften. Press the dates against the side of the pan with a wooden spoon occasionally to make a paste. Add the coconut oil, cinnamon and salt and bring to a gentle simmer, adding extra water, if needed.

4. Remove the pan from the heat and stir the date mixture into the oats and nuts. Add the egg white and maple syrup, and mix well.

5. Press the oat mixture firmly into the prepared tin and bake in the oven for 30 minutes.

6. Remove from the oven and leave to cool in the tin before slicing into 9 pieces.

VEGGIE | GLUTEN FREE | DAIRY FREE

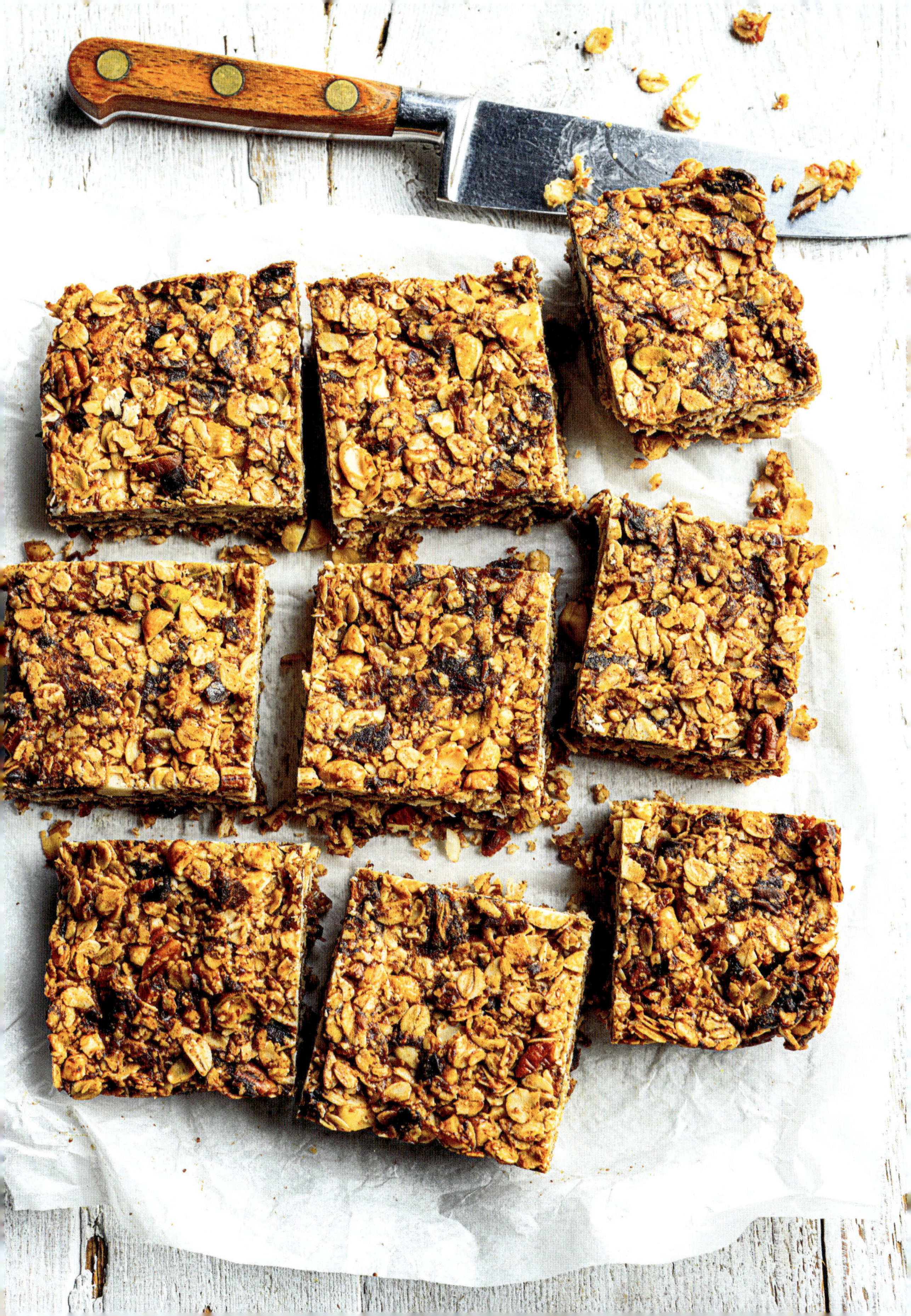

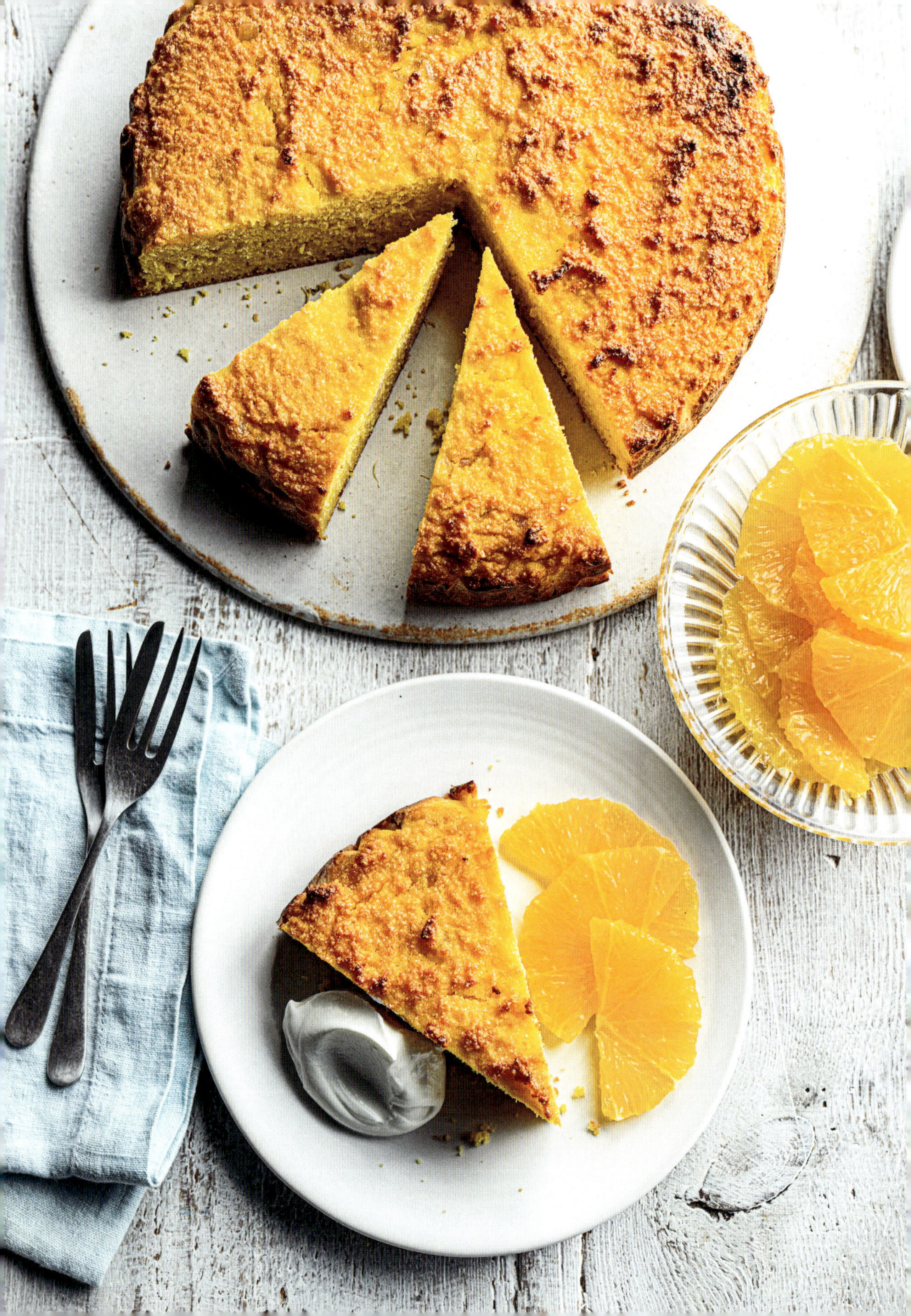

PER SERVING | **290cals** | PROTEIN **10g** | CARBS **20g** | FIBRE **3.5g**

UNDER 300 CALORIES

Orange and Polenta Cake

SERVES **8** | PREP **10** mins | COOK **30** mins

This glorious orange and ginger cake is gluten free with a firm texture and plenty of fibre. It is sweetened with stem ginger balls in syrup.

20g butter, softened
3 eggs
Pinch of sea salt
200g ground almonds
100g polenta
1 tsp baking powder
4 balls stem ginger in syrup, diced
Finely grated zest and juice of 2 oranges
1 orange, peeled and thinly sliced, to serve

1. Preheat the oven to 190°C/Fan 170°C/Gas 5 and line a 20cm cake tin with non-stick baking paper.

2. In a medium bowl, whisk the butter with an electric whisk, then add the eggs one at a time, whisking between each addition.

3. Add the salt, then stir in the ground almonds, polenta, baking powder, ginger and orange zest and juice. Mix well.

4. Pour the cake mixture into the prepared tin and bake in the oven for 25–30 minutes, until golden brown and a knife inserted into the centre comes out clean.

5. Leave to cool for a few minutes, then turn out and finish cooling on a wire rack.

6. Decorate with thin slices of orange to serve.

VEGGIE | GLUTEN FREE

UNDER 200 CALORIES

PER SERVING | **166cals** | PROTEIN **5g** | CARBS **14g** | FIBRE **2g**

Sweet Potato Chocolate Brownie

SERVES **9** | PREP **5** mins | COOK **35** mins

1 medium sweet potato (skin on), diced
3 tbsp coconut oil
100g Medjool dates, pitted and diced
3 tbsp unsweetened cocoa powder
1 tsp vanilla extract
2 tbsp ground flaxseed
3 medium eggs
¼ tsp sea salt
80g dark chocolate chips

There are lots of wonderful nutrients in the skin of the sweet potato, so make sure you use the whole vegetable!

1. Preheat the oven to 200°C/Fan 180°C/Gas 6 and line a 20cm square baking tin with non-stick baking paper.

2. Place the diced sweet potato in a medium microwave-safe bowl with ½ tablespoon of water. Cook on high in the microwave for about 5 minutes, or until soft.

3. Add all the remaining ingredients to the bowl, except the chocolate chips, and mix well, using a stick blender (or use a food processor).

4. Stir in the dark chocolate chips, then tip the mixture into the prepared tin and bake in the preheated oven for 20–30 minutes.

5. Leave to cool slightly in the tin, then turn out onto a wire rack and cool completely before cuttin into 9 squares.

VEGGIE | GLUTEN FREE | NUT FREE

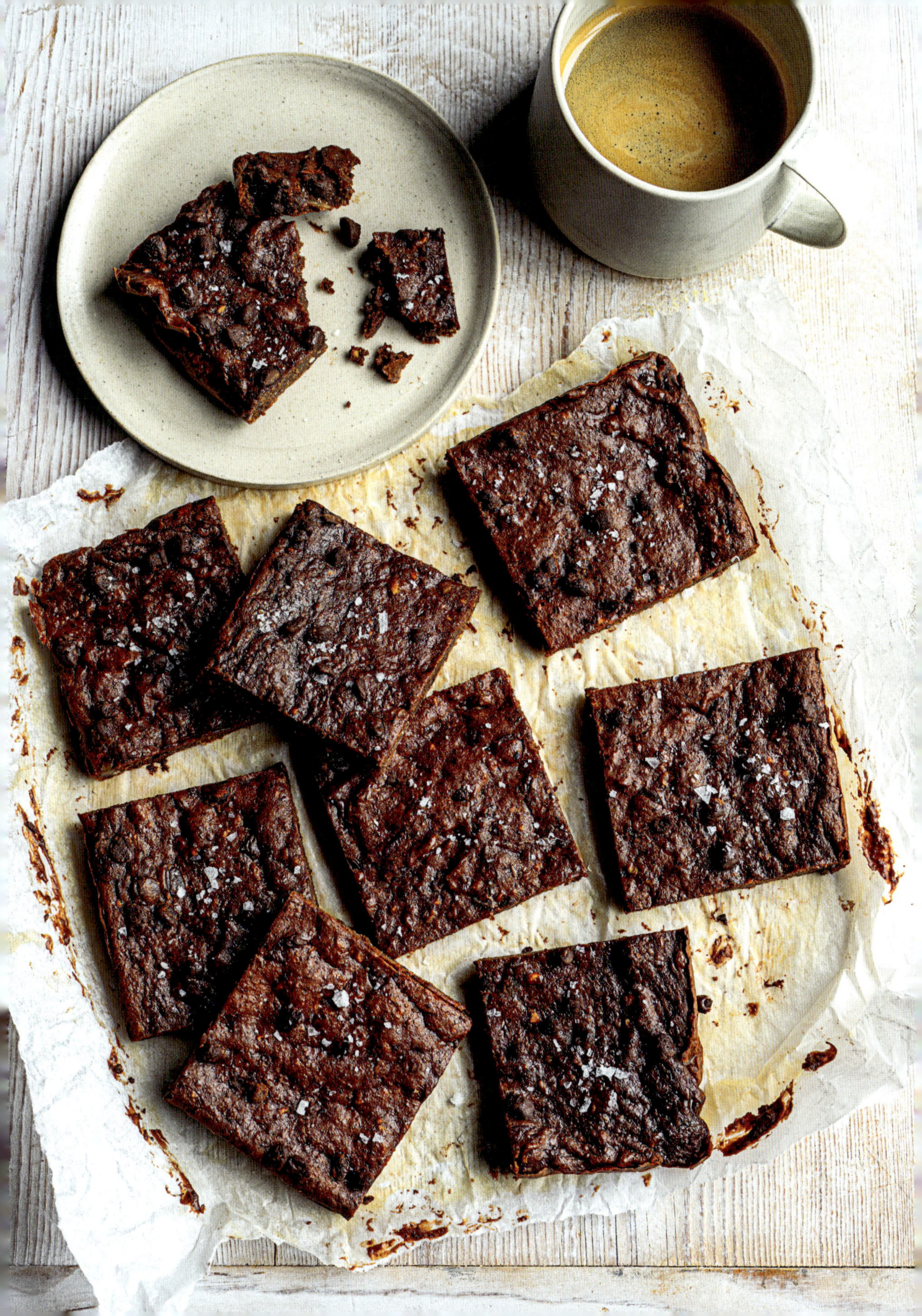

UNDER 300 CALORIES

PER SERVING | **273cals** | PROTEIN **4.7g** | CARBS **30.9g** | FIBRE **5.3g**

Apple Crumble

SERVES **2** | PREP **10** mins | COOK **25** mins

1 apple, cored and cut into 2cm chunks
20g frozen blueberries
10g rolled oats
10g butter, diced and softened
5g almonds, chopped
½ tsp ground cinnamon
30ml full-fat Greek yoghurt

With ground almonds and Greek yoghurt, you can still enjoy a homemade apple crumble. This recipe is much-loved by the Fast 800 programme.

1. Preheat the oven to 180°C/Fan 160°F/Gas 4.

2. Place the apple and blueberries in a saucepan with a splash of water over a medium heat and cook for 10–15 minutes, until soft.

3. Meanwhile, combine the oats, butter, almonds and cinnamon in a bowl. Mix well until it sticks together.

4. Spoon the apple mixture into a small baking dish and top with the oats. Bake in the oven for 5–10 minutes or until golden brown.

5. Serve with a scoop of Greek yoghurt.

VEGGIE GLUTEN FREE

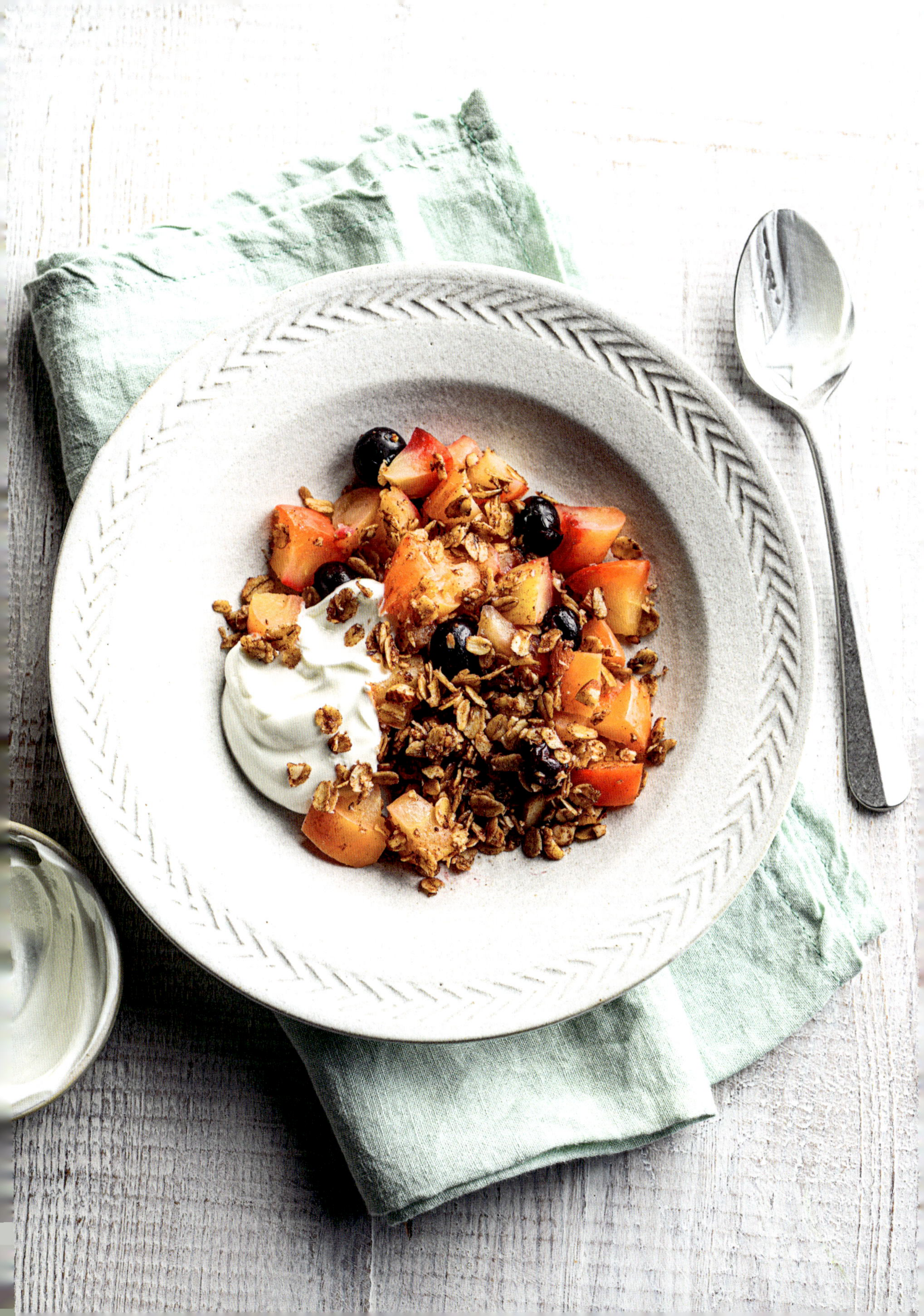

UNDER 300 CALORIES

PER SERVING | **209cals** | PROTEIN **9.5g** | CARBS **3g** | FIBRE **3.5g**

Instant Healthy Seeded Bread

SERVES **2** | PREP **5** mins | COOK **1½** mins

½ tsp butter, softened (or coconut oil), plus extra for greasing
2 tbsp ground flaxseed
1 tbsp mixed seeds
Good pinch of sea salt
2 tbsp ground almonds
½ tsp baking powder
1 egg

Full of fibre and protein, this bun is fun to make in less than 5 minutes in the microwave. Perfect for breakfast, to accompany soup, or to make a sandwich for lunch.

1. Grease a small microwave-safe dish with butter.

2. Combine all the ingredients in a bowl and mix vigorously.

3. Fashion the dough into a bun approximately 2cm thick and place in the buttered dish. Cook in the microwave for about 60 seconds, then for another 20 second burst, if it is not quite cooked through.

4. Set aside to cool, then cut horizontally to make 2 slices.

VEGGIE | GLUTEN FREE

Your Fast 800 toolkit

Traffic lights quick food check

A guide to help you see at a glance which foods are to be encouraged, which eaten in moderation and which to avoid. This is a rough guide only, as people respond differently to different foods.

green

Foods you can eat freely – calories still to be counted on fasting days on all but the non-starchy veg

- Non-starchy vegetables, including salad, leafy greens, broccoli, courgettes, onions and mushrooms
- Fish
- Nuts and seeds
- Tofu
- White meat
- Extra-virgin olive oil and rapeseed oil
- Herbs and spices
- Tomatoes, peppers, peas and aubergines
- Full-fat fermented dairy, including cheese, yoghurt and fromage frais (these are borderline orange – enjoy in moderation)
- Lowish-sugar fruit, including berries and hard fruits (e.g. apples and pears) and citrus fruits – preferably at the end of a meal
- Eggs

orange

Foods you can eat in moderation or occasionally

- Full-fat dairy, such as milk and butter
- Coconut oil or coconut milk
- Diced bacon or chorizo for garnish or flavour
- Beans, lentil and quinoa (NB these are in the green category if you are vegetarian)
- Whole grains
- Wholegrain seeded or sourdough bread
- Wholemeal/seeded pitta or flatbread
- Wholemeal pasta
- Wholemeal/ stoneground flour
- Unprocessed, unsweetened cereals
- Red meat (up to two times a week)
- Moderately starchy root veg, such as swede, parsnip and sweetcorn
- Butternut squash and pumpkin
- Sweet tropical fruits (e.g. mango and pineapple)

red

Foods to avoid if possible

- Most pastries, cakes, snacks and biscuits
- White pasta/bread/rice
- White flour
- Highly processed foods
- Low-fat dairy products
- Highly processed oils, especially anything with trans fats
- Pre-prepared convenience food with lots of unrecognisable ingredients!
- Sugars and sweets

Easy ways to add protein

Research points to the importance of eating adequate amounts of protein – ideally at least 60g or more a day. It's harder for vegetarians to achieve their daily protein requirement on 800–1000 calories, so they may need to increase their intake slightly to ensure they get their nutrients, and that's OK. Using protein supplement shakes can also help you maintain protein (see thefast800.com for more info on meal replacement shakes). These simple, calorie-counted solutions are particularly useful if you haven't got time to cook a full recipe or you just want to beef up a plate of non-starchy veg.

Meat

75g cooked chicken breast (115cals, 22.5g protein)
2 slices roast turkey breast, around 50g (76cals, 17g protein)
1 tbsp diced chorizo, around 10g (40cals, 2.5g protein)
1 tbsp chopped fried back bacon, around 7g (24cals, 1.5g protein)
2 thin slices ham, around 40g (43cals, 7g protein)
2 slices roast beef, around 80g (140cals, 26g protein)
4 slices salami or cured chorizo, around 20g (88cals, 4g protein)
1 rasher cooked back bacon, around 20g (61cals, 5g protein)

Fish

75g frozen cooked prawns, defrosted (52cals, 11.5g protein)
45g tuna, canned in oil (72cals, 11.5g protein)
3 drained anchovies in oil (17cals, 2g protein)
1 smoked mackerel fillet, around 70g (211cals, 15g protein)
2 slices smoked salmon, around 50g in total (92cals, 11.5g protein)
100g roasted or poached salmon (239cals, 24.5g protein)

Dairy and egg

1 medium boiled egg (78cals, 7g protein)
1 tbsp grated cheese, around 10g (41cals, 2.5g protein)
1 tbsp cottage cheese (14kcals, 2g protein)
30g mature Cheddar (124cals, 7.5g protein)
30g halloumi, sliced, lightly fried in 1 tsp olive oil for 4–5 mins (130cals, 6g protein)
40g Greek-style yoghurt (53cals, 2g protein)
50g feta (124cals, 7.5g protein)
20g Parmesan (82cals, 7g protein)
50g soft blue cheese, such as Roquefort, (187cals, 10g protein)
50g soft cheese, such as Brie (171cals, 10g protein)

Vegetarian

Handful of nuts, around 10g total weight, e.g. walnuts, pecans, hazelnuts (71cals, 2g protein)
15g almonds (95cals, 4g protein)
2 tsp sesame seeds, around 10g (63cals, 2g protein)
2 tbsp mixed seeds, around 20g (122cals, 5.4g protein)
100g tofu (123cals, 12.5g protein)
80g cooked edamame beans (110cals, 9g protein)
100g cooked puy lentils (143cals, 11g protein)
40g mushrooms fried in 1 tsp olive oil (33cals, 1g protein)
2 tbsp hummus, around 50g (160cals, 3.5g protein)
100g tinned beans (109cals, 7g protein)
100g cooked lentils (143cals, 11g protein)
100g cooked quinoa (185cals, 6g protein)

Easy ways to add fibre

We used to think that fibre was irrelevant, but the research is clear and it is actually a crucial part of our diet.

Fibre supports good gut health and a thriving gut microbiome, which in turn helps regulate digestion, as well as helping you feel full for longer and stabilising blood sugars. Beyond that, fibre produces substances that help to regulate immunity, reduce inflammation in the body and can even improve mood. And don't forget the importance of fibre in keeping us regular too – a particular issue with GLPs.

We will show you practical and delicious ways to incorporate fibre into most meals. Start slowly – if you are not used to eating enough fibre, give your gut time to adapt to avoid wind! You are doing really well if you are generally hitting 25g fibre a day.

Food / Amount of fibre per 100cals

Psyllium husks (40g)	Kiwi fruit (5g)
Blackberries (12.5g)	Red lentils (5g)
Raspberries (12.5g)	Apples (4.5g)
Artichokes (10g)	Blueberries (4.5g)
Broccoli (9.5g)	Chickpeas (4.5g)
Spinach (9.5g)	Flaxseed (4.5g)
Asparagus (9g)	Oranges (4.5g)
Pak choi (8g)	Wholegrain bread (4.5g)
Cauliflower (8g)	Almonds (4g)
Black beans (7.5g)	Avocados (4g)
Chia seeds (7g)	Popcorn (3.5g)
Red kidney beans (7g)	Sweet potatoes (3.5g)
Carrots (6.5g)	Bananas (3g)
Strawberries (6.5g)	Oats (3g)
Beetroot (5.5g)	Prunes (3g)
Pears (5.5g)	Potatoes (2.5g)
Butter beans (5g)	Quinoa (2g)

Enjoy healthy complex carbs

Healthy wholegrains, beans and lentils

As these foods often take longer to cook, you can save yourself time by cooking larger quantities and freezing them in portions. Try crumbling in half a stock cube during cooking for added flavour. Beans and pulses are a particularly good source of protein for vegetarians and, like wholegrains, they are good for gut bacteria, too. We have included some wholegrains in small quantities in some of our recipes. But if you have calories to spare you might add 1 or 2 tablespoons to a dish. On a non-fasting day, you can add 2–3 heaped tablespoons to your meal without counting. Here are a few options:

- 1 tbsp cooked brown rice (21cals)
- 1 tbsp cooked quinoa (18cals)
- 1 tbsp cooked bulgur wheat (13cals)
- 1 tbsp cooked Puy lentils (18cals)
- 1 tbsp cooked pearl barley (19cals)

- **Cauliflower** makes an excellent swap as it's very low in calories and high in nutrients.
- **Cauli-rice** Make cauli-rice by grating or blitzing half a cauliflower, or buy it ready-made from the supermarket freezer cabinet.
- **Courgetti spaghetti** Follow the recipe on page 191 or buy courgettes already spiralised in some supermarkets.
- **Smashed Minty Peas** (see page 232)
- **Charred Miso Cabbage** (see page 233)
- **Kimchi** (see page 225)
- **Roasted vegetable wedges** Choose non-starchy veg, such as cabbage, courgette, aubergine, asparagus, beetroot, Brussels sprouts and peppers.
- **Cabbage linguine** Use ½ Savoy cabbage for 2 people. Remove the core, finely slice the cabbage then steam for about 5 minutes.
- **Konjak 'Zero' noodles or spaghetti** (Shiritaki) Originally from Japan, these contain remarkably few calories and plenty of fibre.

How to make your greens even tastier

Green and non-starchy vegetables are so healthy and such an important part of the Fast 800 that we encourage you to eat these freely, filling half your plate at each meal. Steam, boil or microwave them, and then try some of the following ideas to make them taste even better. We list both 'no-calorie counting' options, for when you are at your 800cals limit, and low-calorie options for when you've got some calories going spare.

Examples of non-starchy greens and veg:

Cabbage
Spring greens
Chard
Kale
Pak choi
Cavolo nero
Spinach
Fine green beans
Mangetout
Courgette
Broccoli
Salad leaves of all colours – the more colourful, the better the nutritional value (and they look so enticing too)

Ways to add flavour with insignificant calories:

Flaked sea salt and a generous amount of black pepper
A pinch of dried chilli flakes
A pinch of crushed garlic
1 tbsp soy sauce
A squeeze of lemon or lime, e.g. on cabbage, broccoli or cauliflower
1 tbsp apple cider vinegar or balsamic vinegar, e.g. on spinach or cavolo nero
A pinch of herbs
I like to scatter little black nigella seeds on steamed veg, salads and slaws

Low-calorie ways to add flavour:

1 tsp butter – good on any veg (25cals)
1 tsp extra-virgin olive oil – good on any veg (27cals)
1 tsp hoisin sauce, e.g. on wilted spinach or cabbage (12cals)
1 tsp sesame or nigella seeds, e.g. on fine green beans or cabbage (32cals)
1 tsp grated Parmesan scattered on top, e.g. steamed broccoli (8cals)
Jazz up greens by frying the veg in ½ tablespoon olive oil with ½ garlic clove (you could add 1 teaspoon light soy sauce, if you like), e.g. cabbage, mangetout, broccoli or chard (52cals)
Drizzle dressing on a large green or mixed salad

The Fast 800 stores

Fresh meat and fruit and veg may be nice to have, but I'm also a big fan of cooking from stores. Frozen veg, such as peas, spinach or cauliflower florets, are already conveniently prepared and chopped; they provide high-quality nutrients and, because they last for many weeks in the freezer, you know they're always available. Likewise, tins of chickpeas, tomatoes, tuna or jars of red peppers are brilliant staples, sitting there, ready to be pulled out of the cupboard and thrown together for a quick meal. Remember, if you have the right foods to hand, you are much less likely to get sidetracked or tempted by unhealthy ones. This list is intended as a guide. Please don't feel you have to go out and buy every item on it! Be selective and start with the foods you think you are most likely to eat.

Oils and vinegars
Extra-virgin olive oil, or the least refined oil you can afford
Cold-pressed rapeseed oil (for high temperature frying)
Coconut oil
Apple cider vinegar
Balsamic vinegar

Tinned
Tomatoes
Chickpeas
Coconut milk
Beans: kidney, mixed beans, haricot, butter beans, black beans
Puy lentils
Fish: tuna, sardines, salmon, mackerel, anchovies

Dried
Stock cubes
Wholemeal flour
Baking powder
Wholegrains
Oats
Brown/red/black or wild rice
Pearl barley
Quinoa
Puy lentils, red lentils

Jars and bottles
Red peppers
Piquant peppadew peppers
Capers
Jalapeños
Stem ginger in syrup

Herbs and spices
Oregano or mixed herbs
Thyme
Medium curry powder
Cumin seeds
Turmeric powder
Smoked paprika
Black pepper
Chilli flakes
Sea salt

Nuts and seeds
Mixed unsalted nuts
Ground almonds
Flaked almonds
Cashews
Walnuts
Pecans
Mixed seeds

Flavourings, sauces and pastes
Harissa paste
Pesto
Thai red or green curry paste
Medium curry paste
Dark soy sauce
Tomato purée
Plum sauce
Light soy or tamari sauce
Hoisin sauce
Miso paste

Frozen
Chicken breasts
Prawns
Spinach
Peas
Edamame
Mixed veg
Raspberries, mixed berries
Broccoli, cauliflower

Fridge
Eggs
Full-fat live Greek yoghurt
Cheese – mature Cheddar, goat's cheese, feta, Parmesan, halloumi
Leafy greens and salad
Fresh garlic
Fresh ginger
Parsley
Coriander
Cooked chicken
Chorizo
Bacon
Smoked mackerel
Lemons and limes
Full-fat mayo
Mustard
Sauerkraut

Sweet things
Medjool dates
Maple syrup
Vanilla extract
Dark chocolate (ideally 70 per cent cocoa solids or higher)

Making meals work for the whole family

Because the Fast 800 programme is based on a healthy, lowish-carb Mediterranean-style diet, it is extremely flexible – whether you want to bump up a low-calorie recipe to eat on a non-fasting day or to feed other members of your household. While Michael was doing some 800–1000 calorie days during lockdown, we all ate together – the children and I eating freely, while Michael skipped any starchy carbs, like bread or potatoes, and occasionally ate a couple of tablespoons of brown rice, quinoa or Puy lentils. The simple message is that you can expand the portion sizes of our recipes and add in extras where and how you wish.

When you are making a meal such as a stew, curry or a substantial salad, simply double up portions and/or add a veg side dish (see pages 222–38) and/or extra protein (see page 272). Breakfast may be doubled up, too, or become a brunch or lunch. Soups are wonderfully adaptable – add toasted seeds, bacon, chorizo or grated cheese (see page 272 for more tasty and high-protein toppings) and/or a slice of wholemeal seeded bread.

Increase your complex carbs, such as beans, lentils and wholegrains, by adding an extra 2–3 heaped tablespoons of these foods on a non-fasting day, and encourage the rest of the family to eat these, too. When it comes to bread, it's about choosing carefully, as white bread and a slice of seeded wholemeal sourdough are two entirely different species, and this is also true for your non-dieting family. Encourage them to choose wholegrain, seeded or sourdough wherever possible.

Equally, urge all the family to choose fruit which is moderately low in sugar, like berries, apples and pears, and to enjoy these with full-fat live Greek yoghurt.

7-day meal plans

These meal plans are intended to give you a taste of how the different options might work. There are plans for when you want to eat 2 meals a day and for when you want to eat 3 meals. We have included meal plans for meat and fish eaters, as well as for vegetarians.

Do feel free to use up your leftovers and swap in different recipes you like the look of and to repeat days, so you don't have to cook two days in a row – whatever best suits you. Just keep an eye on the nutritional information on the recipe pages to make sure you are keeping protein high (more than 60g daily, if you can) and starchy carbs and sugar lowish (try not to go over 75g carbs on most days).

Remember, the 800–1000cals a day is just a ballpark figure. Calories, although useful, are not an accurate science and there is considerable variation between calorie counters. The meat-free meal plans, for example, come in slightly over the 1000cals a day, in order to get the recommended amount of protein. Going over by 50cals here and there is not going to make a significant difference to your rate of weight loss. Just remind yourself that any reduction below 1000cals a day is going to have a substantial impact. And beyond that, it's the quality of the food that really matters. Eating 800cals of pastries is going to be far worse for you than 1000cals on a Mediterranean-style diet!

If you are vegetarian, you may also wish to swap in a suitable high-protein shake to top up your protein (see thefast800.com for options); and if you are vegan, adding in high-protein shakes may be the only way to do this diet.

On days when you have calories to spare, you might want to add a dressing to your salad or try some of the other ideas on page 274 to jazz up your non-starchy vegetables. You can also include a portion of hard fruit, such as an apple or pear, or a handful of berries, to take you just over the 800cals – eat this either with breakfast or straight after a meal. The important thing, if you want to encourage fat-burning, is to stick to a lowish carb diet, avoid snacking between meals, and ideally add in some Time Restricted Eating (see page 19 for more on this).

2 Meals a Day, with Meat

Day 1	**Cals / Prot / Carb**	**Total Cals**	**Total Prot**
Lunchbox Puttanesca	376 / 19 / 33		
Chicken Poke Bowl	541 / 54 / 29	**917**	**73**
sprinkle with chia seeds to boost fibre/protein			
Day 2			
Brunch Wrap (Chicken Avo)	392 / 39 / 32		
Meatballs with Tomato and White Beans	414 / 27 / 16	806	66
serve with steamed broccoli to boost fibre			
Day 3			
Warm Lentils with Halloumi	433 / 21 / 20.5		
Moroccan-spiced Chicken Stew	414 / 44 / 31	**847**	**65**
serve with steamed spinach to boost fibre			
Day 4			
Quick Tuna Stir-fry	480 / 36 / 13		
Hoisin Pork Lettuce Wrap	335 / 36 / 17	**815**	**72**
sprinkle with flaxseeds to boost fibre/protein			
Day 5			
Brunch Wrap (Smoked Salmon)	341 / 20 / 32		
Turkey Goujons with Red Pepper Dip	590 / 54 / 7.5	**931**	**74**
serve with steamed cauliflower to boost fibre			
Day 6			
Pepper Pots	502 / 24 / 21		
Spanish Pork and Chorizo Srew	367 / 41 / 16	**869**	**65**
serve with small slice of wholegrain bread and steamed spinach to boost fibre			
Day 7			
Scrambled Eggs with Parmesan and Greens	356 / 24.5 / 19		
Mediterranean One-pan Chicken with Roasted Garlic	318 / 33 / 18		
serve with steamed broccoli to boost fibre			
and Sweet Potato Chips	192 / 2 / 30.5		
Treat: Blueberry Cheesecake	219 / 12 / 15	**1,085**	**71.5**

3 Meals a Day, with Meat

Day 1	Cals / Prot / Carb	Total Cals	Total Prot
Satisfying Raspberry Overnight Oats	319 / 12.5 / 26		
Crushed Pea and Edamame Toast with Avocado	406 / 18.5 / 25.5		
sprinkle with chia/flaxseeds to boost fibre/protein			
Ginger and Spring Onion Poached Chicken	241 / 43 / 4	**966**	**74**
serve with green vegetables			
Day 2			
Harissa scrambled eggs	290 / 17.5 / 3		
Chorizo, White Bean and Avocado Salad	307 / 10 / 10		
Chicken and Black Bean Traybake	352 / 36 / 23	**958**	**63.5**
serve with steamed broccoli for fibre boost			
Day 3			
Berry and Cinnamon Smoothie	221 / 9 / 24.5		
Simple Minestrone	262 / 16 / 27		
Poached Ginger Salmon with Broccoli	491 / 41 / 18	**949**	**66**
Day 4			
Easy Breakfast Eggy Muffins	118 / 9 / 0.5		
No-cook Prawn Burrito Bowl	391 / 23 / 24		
sprinkle with flaxseeds to boost fibre/protein			
Keema Bowls	375 / 31 / 15	**884**	**63**
serve with steamed spinach to boost fibre			
Day 5			
Apricot Protein Pot	202 / 10 / 21.5		
Mackerel with Horseradish and Beetroot Dip	251 / 15.5 / 7		
Chargrilled Chicken with Pineapple Salsa	240 / 42 / 6		
serve with Sweet Potato Chips	192 / 2 / 30.5	**885**	**69.5**
and rocket salad/ flaxseeds to boost fibre/protein			
Day 6			
Mexican-style Scrambled Tofu	432 / 24 / 18		
Bruschetta with Prosciutto and Tomato	194 / 9.5 / 17		
serve with rocket leaves to boost fibre			
Caribbean Fish Traybake	310 / 32 / 24	**936**	**65.5**
serve with steamed asparagus to boost fibre			
Day 7			
Scambled Egg with Parmesan and Greens	356 / 24.5 / 19		
Pear, Blue Cheese and Walnut Blinis x 2	118 / 4 / 6		
Beany Beefy Bourguignon	505 / 36 / 19		
serve with steamed spinach to boost fibre			
Treat: Ginger Date Energy Balls	90 / 2.5 / 8	**1,069**	**67**

2 Meals a Day, Vegetarian

Day 1	Cals / Prot / Carb	Total Cals	Total Prot
Warm Lentils and Halloumi	433 / 21 / 20.5		
sprinkle with chia/flaxseeds for fibre/protein boost			
10-minute Smoked Tofu and Quinoa Bowl	447 / 33 / 25		
with Miso Fibre Cracker	82 / 3 / 7		
and Pistachio Bliss Ball	110 / 3 / 12	**1,072**	**60**
Day 2			
Almost-instant High-Protein Pizza	297 / 22.5 / 3		
serve with Berry and Cinnamon Smoothie	221 / 9 / 24.5		
Fridge-raid Supper	412 / 22 / 14		
sprinkle with Smoky Seeds	39 / 1.5 / 2		
and scatter over 50g feta	124 / 7.5 / 1	**1,093**	**62.5**
Day 3			
Pizza Omelette	470 / 27.5 / 2.5		
sprinkle with flaxseeds to boost fibre/protein			
Broccoli and Almond Pesto Pasta	453 / 29 / 34		
add 100g canned beans to sauce	109 / 7 / 12		
serve with rocket leaves to boost fibre		**1,032**	**63.5**
Day 4			
Scrambled Eggs with Parmesan and Greens	356 / 24.5 / 19		
serve with Galia Melon and Almond Smoothie	200 / 6 / 22		
Roasted Cauliflower, Chickpea and Halloumi Salad	452 / 24.5 / 28		
serve with High-fibre Protein Cracker	92 / 4.5 / 2	**1,100**	**60.5**
Day 5			
Simple Minestrone	262 / 16 / 27		
serve with Coconut Bliss Ball	229 / 7 / 10		
One-pot Kimchi Tofu	353 / 23 / 28		
serve with Charred Miso Cabbage	320 / 10.5 / 14	**1,164**	**60**
Day 6			
Baked Eggs with Spinach, Feta and Toasted Seeds	370 / 26.5 / 3.5		
serve with Easy Cheesy Crispy Biscuit	64 / 3.5 / 0.5		
Crispy Katsu Tofu Steaks	538 / 29 / 13.5	**972**	**60.5**
serve with Steamed Broccoli to boost fibre			
Day 7			
Garlicky Cauliflower Cheese	534 / 31 / 20		
serve with steamed spinach to boost fibre			
Meat-free Ragu	284 / 18 / 20		
serve with Steamed Broccoli to boost fibre			
Treat: Blueberry Cheesecake	219 / 12 / 15	**1,037**	**61**

3 Meals a Day, Vegetarian

Day 1	Cals / Prot / Carb	Total Cals	Total Prot
Satisfying Raspberry Overnight Oats	319 / 12.5 / 26		
Almost-instant High-protein Pizza	297 / 22.5 / 3		
serve with rocket leaves to boost fibre			
Fridge-raid Supper	412 / 22 / 14		
and scatter over 50g feta	124 / 7.5 / 1	**1,152**	**64.5**
Day 2			
Apricot Protein Pot	202 / 10 / 21.5		
Lentil and Tomato Soup	250 / 14 / 25		
serve with Easy Cheesy Crispy Biscuit	128 / 7 / 1		
Broccoli and Almond Pasta	453 / 29 / 34	**1,033**	**60**
Day 3			
Mexican-style Scrambled Tofu	432 / 24 / 18		
Baked Eggs with Spinach, Feta and Toasted Seeds	370 / 26.5 / 3.5		
Beetroot Salad with Puy Lentils, Goats' Cheese and Toasted Walnuts	393 / 14 / 11.5	**1,195**	**64.5**
Day 4			
Easy Breakfast Eggy Muffins	118 / 9 / 0.5		
10-minute Smoked Tofu and Quninoa Bowl	447 / 33 / 25		
Falafel Burgers with Pitta Pockets	414 / 16 / 32		
serve with 2 tbsp grated cheese	82 / 5 / 1	**1,061**	**63**
and watercress to boost fibre			
Day 5			
Chocolate Protein Pot	185 / 10 / 19		
Omelette Spring Roll	364 / 20 / 17		
One-pot Kimchi Tofu	353 / 23 / 28		
serve with 80g cooked edamame beans	110 / 9 / 6	**1,012**	**62**
Day 6			
Boiled Egg with Seedy Sprinkles	117 / 9 / 0		
and Soy Seedy Sprinkles	37 / 1.5 / 2		
Garlicky Cauliflower Cheese	534 / 31 / 20		
serve with Smashed Minty Peas	100 / 5.5 / 8		
Meat-free Ragu	284 / 18 / 20	**1,072**	**65**
serve with green vegetables to boost fibre			
Day 7			
High-protein pancakes (sweet)	318 / 14.5 / 19		
Simple Minestrone	262 / 16 / 27		
Crispy Katsu Tofu Steaks	538 / 29 / 13.5		
serve with steamed broccoli to boost fibre	100 / 3 / 9	**1,218**	**62.5**

Index of recipes by calories

Index

DR JACK MOSLEY is the son of Dr Clare Bailey Mosley and the late Dr Michael Mosley, pioneer of the hugely popular 5:2 diet and the Fast 800 books and programme: The Fast 800. Jack studied medicine at Newcastle University and received a Distinction in his Masters of Research in diabetes with Professor Roy Taylor, whose remarkable work proved the transformative effect of weight loss and diet on type 2 diabetes, leading many hundreds of thousand putting their diabetes into remission. Jack worked as a doctor in emergency medicine in the UK and Australia and now works as a GP registrar. His first book, *Food Noise*, was published in 2025 and was a *Sunday Times* number 1 bestseller.

DR CLARE BAILEY MOSLEY is a GP who has supported hundreds of patients to lose weight, reduce their blood sugar levels and put their diabetes in remission at her surgery in Buckinghamshire. She is the author of the bestselling *8-Week Blood Sugar Diet Recipe Book, The Clever Guts Diet Recipe Book, The Fast 800 Recipe Book, The Fast 800 Easy, The Fast 800 Treats Recipe Book* and *Eating Together: A Recipe for Healthier, Happier Families.*

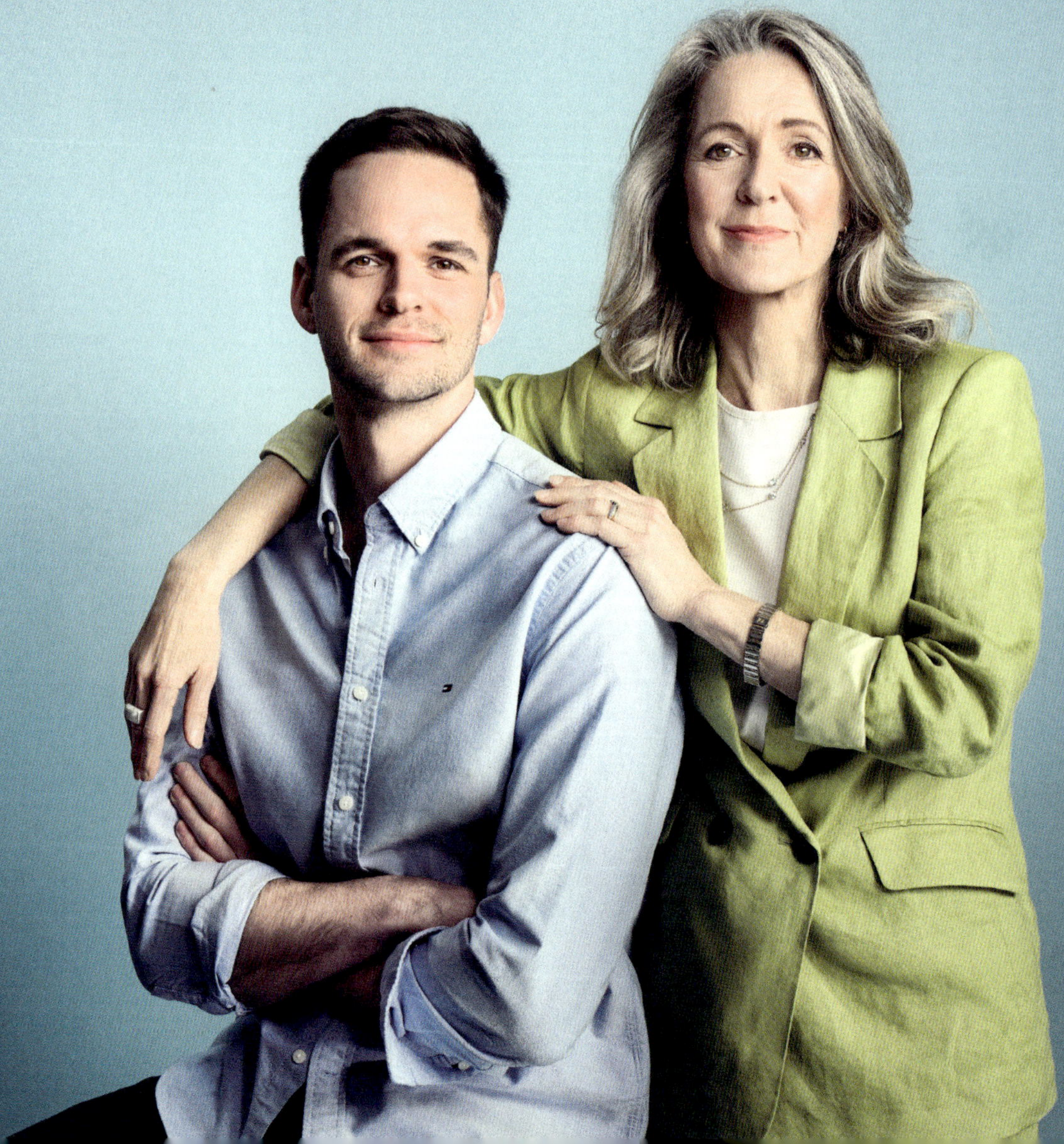